Springer Series on Epidemiology and Public Health

Series editors

Wolfgang Ahrens, Leibniz Institute for Prevention Research and Epidemiology—BIPS, Bremen, Germany

Iris Pigeot, Leibniz Institute for Prevention Research and Epidemiology—BIPS, Bremen, Germany

The series has two main aims. First, it publishes textbooks and monographs addressing recent advances in specific research areas. Second, it provides comprehensive overviews of the methods and results of key epidemiological studies marking cornerstones of epidemiological practice, which are otherwise scattered across numerous narrow-focused publications. Thus the series offers in-depth knowledge on a variety of topics, in particular, on epidemiological concepts and methods, statistical tools, applications, epidemiological practice and public health. It also covers innovative areas such as molecular and genetic epidemiology, statistical principles in epidemiology, modern study designs, data management, quality assurance and other recent methodological developments. Written by the key experts and leaders in corresponding fields, the books in the series offer both broad overviews and insights into specific areas and topics. The series serves as an in-depth reference source that can be used complementarily to the "The Handbook of Epidemiology," which provides a starting point of orientation for interested readers (2nd edition published in 2014 http://www.springer.com/public+health/book/978-0-387-09835-7). The series is intended for researchers and professionals involved in health research, health reporting, health promotion, health system administration and related aspects. It is also of interest for public health specialists and researchers, epidemiologists, physicians, biostatisticians, health educators, and students worldwide.

More information about this series at http://www.springer.com/series/7251

Karin Bammann · Lauren Lissner
Iris Pigeot · Wolfgang Ahrens
Editors

Instruments for Health Surveys in Children and Adolescents

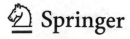 Springer

Editors
Karin Bammann
Working Group Epidemiology of
 Demographic Change, Institute for Public
 Health and Nursing Research (IPP)
University of Bremen
Bremen, Germany

Lauren Lissner
Department of Public Health and
 Community Medicine, Sahlgrenska
 Academy
University of Gothenburg
Gothenburg, Sweden

Iris Pigeot
Leibniz Institute for Prevention Research
 and Epidemiology—BIPS
Bremen, Germany

and

Faculty of Mathematics
 and Computer Science
University of Bremen
Bremen, Germany

Wolfgang Ahrens
Leibniz Institute for Prevention
 Research and Epidemiology—BIPS
Bremen, Germany

and

Faculty of Mathematics
 and Computer Science
University of Bremen
Bremen, Germany

ISSN 1869-7933   ISSN 1869-7941   (electronic)
Springer Series on Epidemiology and Public Health
ISBN 978-3-030-07541-5   ISBN 978-3-319-98857-3   (eBook)
https://doi.org/10.1007/978-3-319-98857-3

This Springer imprint is published by the registered company Springer Nature Switzerland AG
The registered company address is: Gewerbestrasse 11, 6330 Cham, Switzerland

Preface

Epidemiology is one of the basic sciences of public health. It helps shaping practices and policies for pursuing the universal goals to prevent disease and promote health through the life course. A key tool of epidemiology is the population-based field study where primary data are gathered to investigate defined research questions. The European projects IDEFICS and I.Family, funded within the 6th and 7th European Framework Programme, respectively, are studies on prevalence, aetiology and prevention of lifestyle-related diseases focusing on overweight and obesity in children and their families. Over a decade, the IDEFICS and I.Family studies undertook a major research endeavour of collecting standardised data from children, families, neighbourhoods, kindergartens, preschools and schools in eight European countries. This resulted in a rich picture of the daily lives and living contexts of children and their families, who were followed over several years. This book presents the design, methods and instruments for data collection used in the IDEFICS and I.Family studies, which we would like to share with other researchers in the field.

For this purpose, we invited the key experts to explain the development and background of the instruments applied for the surveys and to summarise current knowledge. We had the opportunity to work together with these experts within the framework of the IDEFICS and I.Family studies. Therefore, we would like to acknowledge the outstanding expertise of all contributors and their efforts in providing the best available knowledge on the instruments and methods presented in the chapters that follow. We are grateful for their valuable contributions and their enthusiastic support in producing this book.

During our fieldwork, we faced some major challenges. As enchanting as they are, children are complicated study subjects. Because young children are still in their development, they are intellectually not able to follow abstract directions, which hampers their participation in experiments and test settings. Moreover, when quantitative questionnaires are impossible for them to complete, questionnaire data have to be obtained from proxy respondents, usually the parents. But information on children's behaviours that is not under parental observation as well as on undesirable parenting practices cannot be assessed by this route. Also, for legal and ethical reasons, both the children and their parents have to consent to each survey procedure. This is straightforward, but it multiplies the effort and time going into the consenting process, including age-appropriate explanations for each procedure, and complicates scheduling and other survey logistics.

Another difficulty is that the IDEFICS and I.Family projects were multi-centre studies conducted in eight European countries stretching from Sweden to Cyprus and from Spain to Estonia. While it is quite feasible to overcome challenges of a multi-centre study with strict standardisation and quality control, conducting pan-European fieldwork is not an easy task. Europe, although homogenous in many ways, has considerable between-country heterogeneity in lifestyle and culture. This may require country-specific research solutions, e.g. dietary questionnaires adapted to local food cultures. Other challenges arise from differences in data protection regulation, ethical standards and varying attitudes towards respecting privacy during physical measurements.

Finally, diet- and lifestyle-related diseases constitute an infinitely wide topic due to their multi-factorial aetiologies. Thus, we had to walk a fine line between excessive burden on subjects, survey teams, budgets and general logistics on one hand, and collecting too little data to answer a wide range of scientific research questions, on the other. This point is especially challenging as there is never an ideal set of variables. Rather, this remains a point of constant discussion and sometimes, modification. This is compounded with the longitudinal design of our study which requires comparability of questions asked to individuals over time, wherever possible.

The book is organised as follows: Chapter 1 gives an overview of the design of the IDEFICS and I.Family studies and briefly introduces the methods described in detail in subsequent chapters of this book. Chapter 2 additionally introduces a modular control and documentation system to guide and track the recruitment of study participants in epidemiological studies. The remaining twelve chapters focus on certain instruments used in the overall examination and survey programme. Each chapter gives the rationale for choosing the respective instrument and closes with practical experiences gained during fieldwork. All instruments and the General Survey Manuals of both studies that comprise all standard operating procedures are provided on the following website: www.leibniz-bips.de/ifhs upon registration. Each third partner who wants to use a specific instrument or standard operating procedure is kindly requested to cite the chapter where the instrument or standard operating procedure is described. Instructions on the reference style are given towards the end of each respective chapter.

This book not only introduces the instruments used for our surveys but also describes survey experiences in which practice does not always follow theory. Reactions of respondents can be unexpected and unpredictable, but meeting these challenges can also enrich epidemiological surveys and result in methodological refinements. We wish you the best of luck for your own research adventures. We sincerely hope that the book and the online material will be of value to other research teams.

Bremen, Germany   Karin Bammann
May 2018   Lauren Lissner
                                                                      Iris Pigeot
                                                                  Wolfgang Ahrens

Acknowledgements

The development of instruments, the baseline data collection and the first follow-up work as part of the IDEFICS study (www.idefics.eu) were financially supported by the European Commission within the Sixth RTD Framework Programme Contract No. 016181 (FOOD). The most recent follow-up including the development of new instruments and the adaptation of previously used instruments was conducted in the framework of the I.Family study (www.ifamilystudy.eu) which was funded by the European Commission within the Seventh RTD Framework Programme Contract No. 266044 (KBBE 2010–14).

We thank all families for participating in the pretests and extensive examinations of the IDEFICS and I.Family studies. We are also grateful for the support from school boards, headmasters and communities. Finally, we would like to thank Regine Albrecht, Ina Alvarez and Frauke Günther for their continuous and outstanding engagement. Without their efforts, this volume would not have been possible. They have devoted many hours to this book over and above their other responsibilities. Last but not least we are grateful to Eva Hiripi of Springer Publishers for her support and confidence in us.

Contents

Contributors

Wolfgang Ahrens Leibniz Institute for Prevention Research and Epidemiology—BIPS, Bremen, Germany; Faculty of Mathematics and Computer Science, University of Bremen, Bremen, Germany

Karin Bammann Leibniz Institute for Prevention Research and Epidemiology – BIPS, Bremen, Germany; Working Group Epidemiology of Demographic Change, Institute for Public Health and Nursing Research (IPP), University of Bremen, Bremen, Germany

Leonie-Helen Bogl Leibniz Institute for Prevention Research and Epidemiology—BIPS, Bremen, Germany; Institute for Molecular Medicine (FIMM), University of Helsinki, Helsinki, Finland

Mirko Brandes Leibniz Institute for Prevention Research and Epidemiology—BIPS, Bremen, Germany

Claudia Brünings-Kuppe Leibniz Institute for Prevention Research and Epidemiology—BIPS, Bremen, Germany

Kirsten Buchecker Department of Food Science, Technologie-Transfer-Zentrum (TTZ Bremerhaven), Bremerhaven, Germany; University of Applied Sciences Bremerhaven, Bremerhaven, Germany

Charis Chadjigeorgiou Research and Education Institute of Child Health, Strovolos, Cyprus

Swati Chopra Leeds Institute of Rheumatic and Musculoskeletal Medicine, University of Leeds, Leeds, UK

Ilse De Bourdeaudhuij Ghent University, Ghent, Belgium

Stefaan De Henauw Ghent University, Ghent, Belgium

Gabriele Eiben University of Gothenburg, Gothenburg, Sweden

Annarita Formisano Unit of Epidemiology and Population Genetics, Institute of Food Sciences, National Research Council, Avellino, Italy

Natalia Lascorz Frauca University of Zaragoza, Zaragoza, Spain

Katharina Gallois Leibniz Institute for Prevention Research and Epidemiology— BIPS, Bremen, Germany

Andrea Gottlieb Unit 12 "Research Services", Academic Affairs, University of Bremen, Bremen, Germany

Wencke Gwozdz Department of Management, Society and Communication, Copenhagen Business School, Frederiksberg, Denmark; Justus-Liebig-University Giessen, Giessen, Germany

Kathrin Günther Leibniz Institute for Prevention Research and Epidemiology— BIPS, Bremen, Germany

Holger Hassel Hochschule für Angewandte Wissenschaften Coburg, Coburg, Germany

Antje Hebestreit Leibniz Institute for Prevention Research and Epidemiology— BIPS, Bremen, Germany

Hannah Jilani Leibniz Institute for Prevention Research and Epidemiology— BIPS, Bremen, Germany

Jaakko Kaprio Institute for Molecular Medicine (FIMM), University of Helsinki, Helsinki, Finland

Kenn Konstabel National Institute for Health Development, Tallinn, Estonia; Institute of Psychology, University of Tartu, Tartu, Estonia; School of Natural Sciences and Health, Tallinn University, Tallinn, Estonia

Éva Kovács University of Pécs, Pécs, Hungary

Fabio Lauria Unit of Epidemiology and Population Genetics, Institute of Food Sciences, National Research Council, Avellino, Italy

Lauren Lissner Section for Epidemiology and Social Medicine (EPSO), Department of Public Health and Community Medicine, Sahlgrenska Academy, University of Gothenburg, Gothenburg, Sweden

Annette Lübke Zentrum Für Netze (ZfN), University of Bremen, Bremen, Germany

Lea Maes Ghent University, Ghent, Belgium

Dénes Molnár Department of Pediatrics, University of Pécs, Pécs, Hungary

Luis A. Moreno Facultad de Ciencias de la Salud, Growth, Exercise, NUtrition and Development (GENUD) Research Group, Universidad de Zaragoza, Zaragoza, Spain

Borja Muñiz-Pardos GENUD Research Group, University of Zaragoza, Zaragoza, Spain

Staffan Mårild Department of Paediatrics, Institute for Clinical Sciences, The Queen Silvia Children's Hospital, The Sahlgrenska Academy at University of Gothenburg, Gothenburg, Sweden

Annunziata Nappo National Research Council, Avellino, Italy

Robert Ojiambo Department of Medical Physiology, Moi University, Eldoret, Kenya

Valeria Pala Fondazione IRCCS Istituto Nazionale dei Tumori, Milan, Italy

Jenny Peplies Working Group Epidemiology of Demographic Change, Institute for Public Health and Nursing Research (IPP), University of Bremen, Bremen, Germany; Leibniz Institute for Prevention Research and Epidemiology—BIPS, Bremen, Germany

Iris Pigeot Leibniz Institute for Prevention Research and Epidemiology—BIPS, Bremen, Germany; Faculty of Mathematics and Computer Science, University of Bremen, Bremen, Germany

Yannis Pitsiladis Department of Movement, Human and Health Sciences, University of Rome "Foro Italico", Rome, Italy; Collaborating Centre of Sports Medicine, University of Brighton, Eastbourne, UK

Hermann Pohlabeln Leibniz Institute for Prevention Research and Epidemiology—BIPS, Bremen, Germany

Stefan Rach Leibniz Institute for Prevention Research and Epidemiology—BIPS, Bremen, Germany

Achim Reineke Leibniz Institute for Prevention Research and Epidemiology—BIPS, Bremen, Germany

Lucia A. Reisch Department of Management, Society and Communication, Copenhagen Business School, Frederiksberg, Denmark

Alfonso Siani Epidemiology and Population Genetics, Institute of Food Science, National Research Council, Avellino, Italy

Marc Suling Leibniz Institute for Prevention Research and Epidemiology—BIPS, Bremen, Germany

Michalis Tornaritis Research and Education Institute of Child Health, Strovolos, Cyprus

Toomas Veidebaum National Institute for Health Development, Tallinn, Estonia

Vera Verbestel Ghent University, Ghent, Belgium

Germán Vicente-Rodríguez GENUD (Growth, Exercise, Nutrition and Development) Research Group, University of Zaragoza, Zaragoza, Spain; Department of Public Health, Ghent University, Ghent, Belgium

Garrath Williams Department of Politics, Philosophy and Religion, Lancaster University, Lancaster, UK

Maike Wolters Leibniz Institute for Prevention Research and Epidemiology—BIPS, Bremen, Germany

Chapter 1
The IDEFICS/I.Family Studies: Design and Methods of a Large European Child Cohort

Wolfgang Ahrens, Karin Bammann and Iris Pigeot

Abstract Many unfavourable health outcomes such as excess body weight and resulting cardiovascular and metabolic sequelae have developmental origins and track into adulthood. The IDEFICS and I.Family studies investigated the impact of dietary, behavioural and socioeconomic factors on non-communicable chronic diseases in a large diverse sample of European children. The baseline examination of 16,229 children aged 2–9.9 years (mean age: 6.0 years; standard deviation: 1.8) from Belgium, Cyprus, Estonia, Germany, Hungary, Italy, Spain and Sweden took place between September 2007 and June 2008. Two years later, 11,041 (68%) of these children and 2555 newly recruited children participated in the second round of examinations (mean age: 7.9 years; standard deviation: 1.9) where the same examination protocols were utilised as at baseline. In the interval between the two surveys, the children participated in a controlled trial of a community-oriented primary prevention programme to reduce overweight and obesity. A third round of examinations was conducted in 2013/2014 (mean age: 10.9 years; standard deviation: 2.9) to investigate the influence of familial characteristics on the children's development with focus on diet and health outcomes. For this, we also invited siblings and at least one parent of the index child. Parents reported sociodemographic, behavioural, medical, nutritional and other lifestyle data for their younger children, themselves and their families while adolescents reported for themselves. Physical examinations of the offspring included anthropometry, blood pressure, heel ultrasonography, physical fitness, accelerometry as well as the collection of

On behalf of the IDEFICS and I.Family consortia

W. Ahrens (✉) · I. Pigeot
Leibniz Institute for Prevention Research and Epidemiology—BIPS, Bremen, Germany
e-mail: ahrens@leibniz-bips.de

W. Ahrens · I. Pigeot
Faculty of Mathematics and Computer Science, University of Bremen, Bremen, Germany

K. Bammann
Working Group Epidemiology of Demographic Change, Institute for Public Health and Nursing Research (IPP), University of Bremen, Bremen, Germany

© Springer Nature Switzerland AG 2019
K. Bammann et al. (eds.), *Instruments for Health Surveys in Children and Adolescents*, Springer Series on Epidemiology and Public Health,
https://doi.org/10.1007/978-3-319-98857-3_1

1

DNA from saliva and physiological markers in blood and urine. The built environment, sensory taste perception, neuropsychological traits and other characteristics presumably influencing children's food choice (e.g. fMRI) as well as consumer behaviour were studied in subgroups. By covering the time from early childhood until adolescence, the studies allow the investigation of sensitive developmental periods using a life-course approach. The data set is enriched by further information from the pre-, peri- and postnatal phase gathered from registries and by self-report. The inclusion of parents and siblings and the assessment of peer groups enable the I.Family study to investigate the children as members of families and other social networks.

1.1 Introduction

The European IDEFICS cohort was established in 2007/2008 with one follow-up examination 2 years later and a second follow-up as part of its successor called I. Family in 2013/2014. In addition about 1 year after the completion of the second follow-up in-depth examinations of so-called contrasting groups, i.e. subgroups of children with divergent weight trajectories, were conducted.

The IDEFICS study (Identification and prevention of dietary- and lifestyle-induced health effects in children and infants) started in 2006 and pursued two main aims. First, it assessed the health status of European children with respect to dietary- and lifestyle-induced diseases and disorders with special focus on overweight, obesity and co-morbid disorders. Using a common protocol, children's health status and potential risk factors were measured in a standardised way in eight participating European countries (Ahrens et al. 2011). Second, the IDEFICS study exploited the existing knowledge on modifiable risk factors of overweight and obesity in children to develop, implement and evaluate a controlled intervention programme for primary prevention of obesity (De Henauw et al. 2011).

The I.Family study focussed on the familial, social and physical environment to assess the determinants of eating behaviour and food choice and its impact on health outcomes (Ahrens et al. 2017). Therefore, siblings and parents were invited to the third physical examination together with all so-called index children, i.e. children who previously participated in the IDEFICS study. The study protocol was based on the IDEFICS survey manual with adaptations to account for the older age groups (adolescents and parents) and to address the new research focus. In this way, the IDEFICS/I.Family cohort provides repeated measurements of social and behavioural factors, individual characteristics and medical parameters over the early life course and allows the investigation of developmental trajectories covering the transition from childhood to adolescence.

This chapter gives an overview of the designs of both studies and also refers to the instruments that are introduced in subsequent chapters of this book.

1.2   Overall Design of the IDEFICS Study

The IDEFICS study is a prospective multi-centre cohort study that took place in eight European countries, namely Belgium, Cyprus, Estonia, Germany, Hungary, Italy, Spain and Sweden. Additional centres providing expertise on fatty acid analyses, genetics, physical activity, ethics, consumer research as well as knowledge transfer and public relations were located in France, Italy, Great Britain, Germany, Belgium and Denmark. A detailed description of the initial study design and its survey instruments is given in Ahrens et al. (2006) and Bammann et al. (2006), respectively. A description of the updated study design and of the study population at baseline can be found in Ahrens et al. (2011) which also serves as major reference for the first part of this chapter.

The study design incorporated several components, each of which may be considered as a study of its own. Figure 1.1 (left part) shows the overall timeline and the three major components of the IDEFICS study: (1) at baseline, all children were examined according to a detailed protocol. These children were invited to participate in a second examination at follow-up 2 years later. By this, a child cohort was created allowing for longitudinal investigations. (2) Between the two surveys, about half of the children participated in a community-oriented setting-based intervention that was implemented in one region of each country where the other community served as control region. (3) Further, three nested case–control studies were performed to investigate the aetiology of (a) obesity and

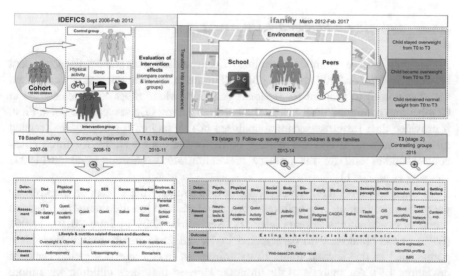

Fig. 1.1 Design and major components of the IDEFICS and the I.Family studies *Source* Ahrens et al. (2017)

overweight (Bammann et al. 2014), (b) bone health (Herrmann et al. 2015) and (c) insulin resistance. (4) Additional studies in selected countries were initiated such as a study of the influence of the food environment on children's dietary behaviour in one German survey centre (Buck et al. 2013) and of the built environment on their physical activity (Buck et al. 2011, 2015) in three countries (Germany, Italy, Sweden).

In total, 16,229 children aged 2–9.9 years were recruited in the population-based baseline survey in the eight European survey countries listed above which corresponds to 51% of all children who have been invited to participate in the IDEFICS study. Potential selection effects at baseline were investigated in the Swedish sample. Here, families with single parenthood, foreign background, low education and low income were underrepresented. However, body mass index (BMI) had no selection effect (Regber et al. 2013).

The children were approached via kindergarten and school settings which facilitated their enrolment and the implementation of intervention activities. Parents of the children were approached by letter and invited to participate. The informed consent, which was signed by parents, offered the option to participate in the full examination programme or only in parts of it. As requested by the ethics review consensus report of the European Commission, each child was informed orally by a study nurse immediately before examination about the modules using a simplified preformulated text. This was done to ensure that each participating child gave verbal assent before participating in a given module.

1.2.1   Baseline and Follow-Up Surveys

All children were examined at baseline (T_0) according to a standardised protocol between September 2007 and June 2008. Timing of recruitment was synchronised across countries to account for seasonal variation, where most countries started in October and continued until April. The baseline survey (T_0) served two aims. First, it provided data for cross-sectional analyses of risk factors for obesity and related disorders. Second, it was the starting point for the cohort study, for three case–control studies and for the primary prevention study (Ahrens et al. 2011; De Henauw et al. 2011).

In order to assess their development and to evaluate the effects of the primary prevention programme, the children were then followed longitudinally by a second round of examinations 2 years later (T_1, September 2009 to June 2010). 11,041 (68%) of the children who participated in T_0 and 2555 newly recruited children participated in this second round of examinations (mean age: 7.9 years; standard deviation: 1.9). An analysis of the dropouts showed that these children were more likely to be overweight, to report low well-being scores and to come from low-educated or single-parent families. Moreover, attrition was positively associated with a high degree of item non-response at baseline (Hense et al. 2013). In the

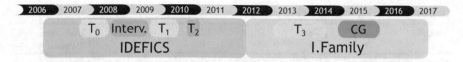

Fig. 1.2 Timeline of the follow-up examinations of the IDEFICS cohort and its extension by the I.Family study *Source* Ahrens et al. (2017) (T_0 = baseline survey; T_1 = first follow-up examination; T_2 = mailed survey; T_3 = second follow-up examination; CG = contrasting groups; extended examination in subgroups of the cohort)

German sample, an extended recruitment effort at baseline was not associated with a higher chance of attrition at follow-up (Langeheine et al. 2017).

The same instruments and examination protocols were used at T_0 and at T_1. To assess sustainability of the implemented intervention activities, a mail survey was conducted at T_2 (September 2010–December 2010); see Fig. 1.2.

1.2.2   Examination Modules

The IDEFICS study involved researchers from different disciplines with a variety of research topics. Hence, it was clear that the final set of survey instruments was a compromise between scientific ambition and feasibility. Since the overall project duration was limited to 5 years, the planned schedule for the surveys was tight. Within 6 months, each survey centre had to examine 2000 children, amounting to about 80–90 children per week. Preferably, all examinations of a child took place on the same day. However, in some cases this was not feasible, as for instance when a physician or nurse was not available for drawing blood. Usually, the survey teams established mobile examination sites that moved between participating schools and preschools. Alternative examination sites were established at the premises of the research centre, in a public building or in a hospital.

It had to be considered that a part of the examinations such as measurement of weight, waist circumference, bioelectrical impedance (BIA) and blood drawing required a fasting status of the child, and other parts required the parents, respectively, guardians to be present in some of the participating countries. The pretest showed that the order of survey modules (see Table 1.1) needed to be adapted to local conditions although there were minimum requirements for all survey centres (e.g. modules requiring fasting status had to be applied first) (Suling et al. 2011). The examination protocol was composed of compulsory modules and optional extensions (see below). The average duration of a child's examination was estimated to last about 1.5 h for the core protocol plus approximately 50 min for the full set of optional modules of the extended protocol. Parents were asked to fill in the questionnaires (see below) prior to or in parallel to their child's examination.

Table 1.1 Modules of the IDEFICS surveys

Module	Tasks	Estimated duration (min)
Reception and farewell	Welcome, handing over study documents, open questions, check completeness of interview, labels and documents, appointments, farewell	15
Physical examinations with fasting status	Application of anaesthetic patch and drawing of blood, anthropometry I (weight and leg-to-leg BIA, waist circumference)	8
Physical examinations (no fasting status required)	Medical interview, blood pressure and pulse rate, anthropometry II (height, skinfolds, other circumferences), heel ultrasound	25
Biological samples	Handing out urine cup and explanation of procedure to parents and acceptance of urine sample, saliva collection	10
24HDR	24 h dietary recall incl. assessment of school meal data for same day; second recall in 20% subsample	25
Accelerometers	Handing over and explanation of accelerometer	10
Data from official records	Centre-specific	Centre-specific
Parental questionnaires	Parental questionnaire I and II (self-administered)	0
Food tasting	Sensory perception tests (20% subsample; ages 6 +)	25
Physical fitness	Physical fitness tests (ages 6+)	25

Only instruments suitable for large-scale population-based surveys were eligible, where preference was given to established and validated methods. Moreover, each instrument and measurement had to be suitable and ethically acceptable for use in small children, time-efficient and robust against observer effects. Interviews, for examples, had generally to be conducted as proxy interviews, since children at such a young age are not able to give reliable information.

The examination modules used at baseline survey were selected in order to cover the assessment of body composition (e.g. overweight/obesity) and other health indicators (e.g. bone health) as outcome variables and putative key risk factors (e.g. diet). Moreover, innovative components, e.g. sensory tests and alternative measurements, e.g. a 24-hour dietary recall (24HDR), to assess diet were integrated into the set of measurements. In order to obtain objective growth data from the infancy period and the period preceding T_0, we also collected maternity cards and records of routine child visits.

The core protocol included all modules that were offered to all children in each country. Children were asked to provide venous blood, saliva and urine. In addition, stool samples were collected in a subgroup. The extended protocol covered modules that were optional or were only applied in subsamples of children, either (1) because they were not feasible in small children (e.g. physical fitness tests, tests on sensory taste perception), or (2) because they were too time-consuming (e.g.

questionnaires/experiments to assess to role of commercials in food choice; see Chap. 10 of this book) or (3) because they were too expensive (e.g. bone stiffness, analysis of vitamin D). Where age was the only limiting factor, it was intended to apply the extended protocol to all primary school children, while in all other cases a 20% random sample of children was selected. Accelerometry was only performed in about half of the children because of a limited number of devices. The final set of survey instruments consists of various questionnaires, physiological measurements, the collection of biological samples and the performance of several tests (see Table 1.2) which are briefly summarised here and described in more detail in the respective chapters of this book.

Reception and farewell: This module comprises reception and farewell that had to be repeated if the survey schedule of a child was distributed over several appointments. Each appointment involved a procedure for check of documents and samples, a check to ensure that identification (ID) labels were attached to each document or sample container and a check whether interviews were complete.

Physical examinations with fasting status: The physical examinations in the IDEFICS survey were organised into two modules, one comprising all examinations requiring the participating children to be in a fasting status for at least eight hours and one comprising all examinations where this was not necessarily required. This division allowed the survey centres to plan more freely their daily schedule according to their local conditions.

The fasting module comprises measuring of leg-to-leg bioelectrical impedance (BIA), body weight and waist circumference, and blood drawing. Fasting venous blood was collected from each consenting child. If venous blood could not be obtained, capillary blood was taken when possible. After finishing the fasting module, a beverage and a healthy snack were offered to the children.

Physical examinations (no fasting status required): This module comprises a face-to-face interview of the parents on the medical history of the child, the inspection of drug packages and a series of measurements. These include body height, blood pressure, hip and mid-upper arm circumferences and skinfold thicknesses. To lower the burden of survey centres and of study subjects and since some of the survey centres had less experience with skinfold measurements, only two sites (biceps, subscapular) were mandatory, whereas two additional sites (triceps, supra-illiac) were optional. For assessing bone stiffness, the heel ultrasound Lunar Achilles Insight was used. For more details on the two modules, we refer to Chap. 3 of this book.

The medical history of a child was obtained in a face-to-face interview with one parent. In order to keep the interview as short as possible, basic information on the pregnancy that was considered to be more easily recalled was assessed through self-administered questions in the parental questionnaire. In addition, all medications the child had taken within the week preceding the interview were recorded.

Biological samples: This module comprises urine and saliva collection. For blood collection see above. Morning urine was collected by the parents using a urine collection kit that was handed out on a prior occasion to the parents together with an instruction sheet. Saliva was collected for deoxyribonucleic acid

Table 1.2 Variables and age-specific instruments applied in the baseline survey of the IDEFICS study (cf. Bammann et al. 2006)

Module/instrument	Assessment methods	Variables
Physical examination —fasting status mandatory	Measurements	Weight with leg-to-leg BIA (TANITA BC 420 SMA with adapter) Waist circumference (SECA 200)
Physical examination —fasting status not required	Measurements	Blood pressure and pulse rate (automated sphygmomanometer Welch Allyn 4200B-E2 with cuffs) Standing height (SECA 225) Skinfold thicknesses (Holtain Caliper) Circumferences: mid-upper arm, hip, neck (SECA 200) Heel ultrasound (optional; Lunar Achilles Insight)
Medical history	Face-to-face interview	Ten pages containing the following sections: Health and diseases of the family Pregnancy information for the child Health information of the child Drug use of the child
Parental questionnaire —core questions	Self-administered questionnaire (parents)	26 pages containing the following sections: General information Day care, preschool and school Pregnancy and early childhood Family lifestyle Health and well-being Leisure time activities and consumer behaviour Children's spending Sociodemographic information
Parental questionnaire —diet	Self-administered questionnaire (parents)	Ten pages including questions on attitudes and eating habits and a detailed FFQ
24-hour dietary recall (24HDR)	Computer-assisted personal interview (parents)	Computer-aided 24HDR (proxy interview); complemented by recording of school meals
Questionnaire for preschools and schools	Mix of methods	Eight pages containing the following sections: Advertising and sponsorship Availability of food
Teachers and caretakers questionnaire	Self-administered questionnaire (teacher)	Seven pages including questions on attitudes, opinions, own eating behaviour, own physical activity.
Physical fitness tests (≥ 6 years)		Flamingo balance test Backsaver sit and reach Handgrip strength Standing broad jump 40-m sprint Shuttle run test

(continued)

Table 1.2 (continued)

Module/instrument	Assessment methods	Variables
Biological samples	Saliva	Selected SNPs in candidate genes
	Morning urine	Cortisol, glucose, albumin, creatinine, sodium, calcium, phosphate, magnesium, potassium
	Fasting blood	On-site: glucose, total cholesterol, HDL cholesterol, triglycerides Fatty acid test strips: fatty acid profile (subsample of children) Central lab: core markers: insulin (in serum), CRP (in serum), HbA1c (in EDTA whole blood); additional markers of bone metabolism: calcium, NTX-peptide, vitamin D (in serum, in subsample); additional hormones of energy/fat metabolism: leptin, adiponectin (in serum, in subsample)
Accelerometers	Measurement	Physical activity [ActiGraph GT1 M (in preschool children), ActiTrainer (in school children)]
Food tasting (≥ 6 years; subsample)	Forced choice tests	Threshold of taste for sweet, salty, bitter and umami Preferences of taste for sweet, salt, fat, umami and artificial flavour

FFQ Food frequency questionnaire; *SNP* Single-nucleotide polymorphisms; *HDL* High-density lipoprotein; *CRP* C-reactive protein; *EDTA* Ethylenediaminetetraacetic acid

(DNA) extraction with different collection procedures depending on age. Central laboratories were used for the majority of biological parameters. A biosample logistics database was used to record information on collection, processing, storage and shipping of all biological materials. Each centre used an individual copy of this database which provides an overview of the material collected locally. These individual copies were merged into the central database. For more details, we refer to Chap. 4 of this book.

24-hour dietary recall: A single 24-hour dietary recall (24HDR) was assessed in the full sample of IDEFICS children, and a second one was administered in a 20% subsample. The computer questionnaire containing the 24HDR was offered as a self-administered instrument at the survey centre to be filled in by the parents (proxy report). For each of the 24HDRs, school meal consumption was recorded for each child for the same day through observation by field staff at the school premises. For more details, we refer to see Chap. 5 of this book.

Accelerometers: Physical activity was measured by a 3-day accelerometer recording (two weekdays, one weekend day) partly complemented by heart rate recordings. Two different devices were used: the ActiGraph GT1 M for accelerometer measurements and the ActiTrainer (consisting of an ActiGraph and a Polar heart rate monitor) for the measurements combining acceleration and heart rate. Due to the limited number of devices, heart rate measurements were restricted to children 6 years and older for whom data on physical fitness were collected (see below). For more details, we refer to Chap. 7 of this book.

Data from official records: Survey centres were asked to assess additional data from official records, e.g. medical records, where possible, to complete the information on the individual child. For more details, we refer to Chap. 8 of this book.

Parental questionnaires: Two questionnaires were completed by the parents. The first one (IDEFICS parental questionnaire; see Chap. 9 of this book) contains questions, e.g. on sex and date of birth of the child, use of day-care services, school and preschool, pregnancy and early childhood, family lifestyle, health and well-being, and on sociodemographic factors; the second one assesses dietary behaviour and frequency of food intake (see Chap. 6 of this book). Parents were instructed to bring the completed questionnaires to the survey centre, where completeness was checked and help was offered for omitted questions. Alternatively, it was possible to complete the parental questionnaires in a face-to-face interview, in a telephone interview or in a group session. However, any alternative mode of completion had to be documented in the electronic appointment system (see Chap. 2 of this book).

Food tasting (for children ≥ 6 years): Taste thresholds for basic tastes and food preferences of the children were assessed in an experimental setting. For this, standardised methods according to International Organization for Standardization ISO 3972 commonly used in the food industry were adapted for the IDEFICS surveys. This module was performed in a subsample of 20% of the children. Moreover, since the pretest showed that younger children need considerably more time and responses were lacking precision, we restricted the module to children 6 years and over. For details, we refer to Chap. 12 of this book.

Physical fitness (for children ≥ 6 years): This module consists of a battery of physical fitness tests in order to assess motor skills and aerobic fitness in the children. Since a maximum test was part of the test battery (shuttle run test), a person capable of giving emergency first aid to children had to be present during these tests. This module was only performed in children 6 years and older since it became apparent in the preparatory phase that it was not possible to perform the tests with younger children in a reasonable time. The module was carried out in group sessions, e.g. during physical education classes. For more details, we refer to Chap. 13 of this book.

1.2.3 Case–Control Studies

The IDEFICS study aimed to investigate the aetiology of major disorders, namely (1) obesity and overweight (Bammann et al. 2014), (2) bone health (Herrmann et al. 2015) and (3) insulin resistance, all of which may be regarded as important lifestyle and nutrition-related health outcomes in children. Each of these three conditions was analysed in a case–control study to assess the interplay of various risk factors including biological markers that could only be analysed in subsamples of the cohort. In all three case–control studies, additional variables such as bone metabolic markers, peripheral hormones involved in energy intake regulation like insulin and leptin and specific genetic markers were assessed to allow for in-depth analyses in relation to environmental and behavioural factors.

1.2.4   Intervention Study

The intervention study was designed as a community-oriented and setting-based primary prevention trial, based on the five-step intervention mapping protocol (Verbestel et al. 2011; Bartholomew et al. 2006). The IDEFICS prevention programme was developed under participation of all relevant actors, e.g. through focus groups (Haerens et al. 2009, 2010). Local policy actors were involved to target the obesogenic environment. Based on a literature review, several intervention targets for the IDEFICS intervention programme were selected for which previous interventions had shown at least promising evidence of positive effects. The programme was standardised to enable a comparison between countries although certain aspects were culturally adapted during a preparatory phase (Pigeot et al. 2015a).

The evaluation of the overall programme addressed (1) its development, i.e. costs, expenditure of time, practical problems and solutions, (2) the process, i.e. participation, feasibility, acceptance and sustainability (see Chap. 11 of this book) and (3) the effect on various endpoints. The results of the intervention are published in a supplement volume of Obesity Reviews (Pigeot et al. 2015b).

1.2.5   Training and Quality Management

All measurements followed detailed standard operation procedures (SOPs) that were documented in the IDEFICS General Survey Manual (for access see Sect. 1.6) and finalised after the pretest of all survey modules (Suling et al. 2011). Field personnel from each survey centre participated in central training and organised local training sessions thereafter to ensure the implementation of methods and procedures according to the General Survey Manual. To be more specific, the field work training was organised as a two-step procedure. Training sessions held in English took place centrally and were followed by local training sessions in each survey centre in the local language since the local field staff in the different European countries was not necessarily capable to understand training lessons in English. The central training for the baseline survey was held in Bremen, Germany, as a 4-day meeting in July 2007. Participants from each survey centre were present where for all but one survey centre the desirable minimum number of two participants was reached. Training material was distributed to the survey centres electronically. An additional, 2-day central training session on anthropometry with a particular focus on skinfold measurements was held in Glasgow, Scotland, in August 2007.

The coordinating centre conducted site visits of each survey location during both field surveys to check adherence of field staff to the SOPs. During the IDEFICS baseline survey (T_0) from September 2007 until May 2008, each of the survey centres was visited by the central quality control at least once. The site visits are a means for external quality control of the examinations performed in the surveys and are part of the IDEFICS quality plan. Ideally, they were complemented by internal quality control means. The internal checks were implemented by all survey centres on a non-formal basis. Questionnaires were developed in English and translated to local languages. The quality of translations was checked by back translation. All survey centres used the same technical equipment. Measurement devices and supplies for biological sampling were purchased centrally to maximise comparability of data.

Despite national differences in recruiting study subjects, a common set of variables was collected to document the participation proportion and the reasons for non-participation. For those centres that contacted parents directly with a mailed letter, a documentation software, called MODYS, was provided to record and monitor all contact attempts and by this to guide the recruitment process (see Chap. 2 of this book).

Databases and computer-assisted questionnaires included automated plausibility checks. A barcode sticker with the subject identification number (ID) was attached to each recording sheet, each questionnaire module and each vial of biological material. Where possible a bar code reader was used to enter the data. In all other cases, the ID had to be entered twice before the document could be entered in the respective database. All numerical variables were entered twice independently, and deviating entries were corrected (Ahrens et al. 2011). Inconsistencies identified by additional plausibility checks were rectified by the survey centres. All corrections were documented centrally such that the changes in the analysis data set can be traced back to the raw data set which was archived under lock and key.

To further check the quality of data, subsamples of study subjects were examined twice to calculate the inter- and intra-observer reliability of anthropometric measurements (Stomfai et al. 2011). The reliability of tests on taste perception was assessed in a group of German children (Knof et al. 2011). In addition, the reliability of questionnaires was checked by re-administering the Children's Eating Habits Questionnaire (CEHQ) and selected questions of the parental questionnaire to a convenience sample of study participants (Lanfer et al. 2011; Herrmann et al. 2011). Food consumption assessed by the CEHQ was validated against selected nutrients measured in blood and urine (Huybrechts et al. 2011). The new method to analyse the fatty acid profile in a dried drop of blood was compared to the standard analysis of serum and erythrocytes from venous blood. A validation study was carried out to compare uni-axial and tri-axial accelerometers in children and to validate them using doubly labelled water as the gold standard (Bammann et al. 2011; Ojambo et al. 2012) and to also validate body composition measures using a three-compartment model (Bammann et al. 2013). Ultrasonometry was compared to DEXA to assess the correlation between bone mineral density and bone stiffness in a sample of children from Sweden and Belgium (Sioen et al. 2011). Annually, a quality report was written and discussed with the project review board of the European Commission.

1.3   Overall Design of the I.Family Study

I.Family pursued two strategic objectives, i.e. (1) to understand the interplay between barriers and drivers towards a healthy food choice, physical activity and lifestyle factors, and their associations with related health outcomes and (2) to develop and disseminate strategies to induce changes promoting a healthy dietary behaviour in European consumers, especially children, adolescents and their parents.

I.Family is the successor of the IDEFICS study involving the same eight cohort centres to re-examine the index children and to extend the examinations to family members. Other centres from the Netherlands, Great Britain, Finland and Denmark with expertise in functional magnetic resonance imaging, physical activity, ethics, public relations, genetics, and consumer research supported the study. A detailed description on how the I.Family study extends the IDEFICS study can be found in a recent publication by Ahrens et al. (2017) which serves as the basis for the second part of this chapter.

The parents of the index children were informed about this new examination by personal letters with a brief description of the aims and components of the study as well as a consent form with further details asking for their willingness to participate in I.Family. These letters were either sent directly to the families or delivered by the teacher of an index child. Additional phone calls by the study personnel helped to explain the aims and examinations of the study in more detail. Ethical approval was again obtained from the local ethics committees where similar procedures were followed as in the IDEFICS study with the main difference that children from 12 years onwards were asked for their written consent in addition to their parents.

1.3.1   Follow-Up Survey

The I.Family study started with the second follow-up examination (T_3) (Fig. 1.1, right part) in 2013/2014, when the age range of index children was between 7 and 17 years. The mean age (standard deviation) of participating children was 6.0 (1.8) years at T_0, 7.9 (1.9) years at T_1 and 10.9 (2.9) years at T_3 with a similar proportion of boys and girls. The role of familial characteristics, family structure and family life in relation to the children's development was a major focus of I.Family. We therefore invited, in addition to the index children, all siblings in the age range from 2 to 18 years. In addition, we strived for at least one parent of each index child to participate and to provide information on their household. In this way, we examined

9617 children at T_3, of whom 7105 participated in one of the previous examinations. In total, 6167 families with on average two children and 4.1 members (including parents) per family participated.

The IDEFICS and the I.Family studies allowed us to establish the largest pan-European children's cohort to date, to perform longitudinal analyses of biological markers and lifestyle behaviours in combination with social, cultural and environmental factors and to investigate the impact of these factors on children's health and development over the early life course. Some major results are summarised in Ahrens et al. (2017), but we expect much more exciting insights into children's health trajectories to come.

1.3.2 Contrasting Groups

Three subgroups of children with divergent weight trajectories, so-called contrasting groups, were further examined about 1 year after completion of T_3 (stage 1) as illustrated in Fig. 1.1, right part (T_3, stage 2) according to an extended protocol. The contrasting groups were defined at T_3 based on weight status at baseline and average change in BMI z-scores per year as follows: (1) children with normal weight at baseline and follow-up and no change of ±0.1 in BMI z-score per year; (2) children who retained overweight or obesity at baseline and follow-up and no change of ±0.1 in BMI z-score per year; and (3) children with excessive weight gain were those who started with a BMI z-score above −0.1 at baseline and who gained more than +0.1 in BMI z-score per year during the follow-up period. These contrasting groups are particularly informative to understand the major determinants and prognostic factors that help explain the differences in weight development.

1.3.3 Examination Modules

Follow-up examinations (T_3, stage 1): The examination programme at T_3 covered the majority of the modules employed at baseline and at first follow-up. Questionnaire modules that were originally designed for proxy interviews, i.e. for parents responding for their children, were adapted for completion by adolescents and parents, respectively (see Table 1.3), and addressed the following topics (see Chap. 9 of this book):

- *Parents for themselves and their family*: general information about the respondent/the family; family life and rules; meal habits of the family; parenting style; attitudes towards TV advertisements; sociodemographic characteristics; smoking and alcohol consumption; body image; physical activity; sleeping habits; dietary behaviour, dieting and food frequency.

Table 1.3 Overview of examination modules and their mode of application at T_3 (stage 1) in children, adolescents and their parents

Instrument	Target group	Estimated duration (min)	Completed by/measured in		
			Children	Adolescents	Parents
In the examination centre					
Reception and informed consent, farewell					
Welcome, handing over study documents, informed consent discussion	All subjects	5	x	x	x
Check completeness of received questionnaires, interviews and documents	All subjects	5	x	x	x
Farewell	All subjects	5	x	x	x
Self-administered paper questionnaire					
Food and beverage preference questionnaire	All subjects ≥ 6 years	7	x	x	x
Peer network questionnaire	Adolescents ≥ 12 years	4		x	
Maturation stages (pictorial representation)	All children ≥ 8 years	2	x	x	
Tablet (self-administered tablet questionnaire)					
Teen questionnaire	Adolescents ≥ 12 years	40		x	
Computer-assisted personal interviews (CAPIs)					
Interview on kinship and household	All children	5			x legal guardian
Medical interview (health and diseases of the family and of the child, drug use of the child)	All children	12			x biological parent/ grandparent
Interview on pregnancy and early childhood (different modules for index children and siblings)	All children	7			x biological mother

(continued)

Table 1.3 (continued)

Instrument	Target group	Estimated duration (min)	Completed by/measured in		
			Children	Adolescents	Parents
Physical examinations (anthropometry)					
... in a fasting state					
Weight and BIA (TANITA 418/420)	All subjects	2	x	x	x
Height (SECA 225/213)	All subjects	1	x	x	x
Waist circumference (SECA 201)	All subjects	2	x	x	x
... in a non-fasting state					
Blood pressure and pulse rate	All children	8	x	x	Optional
Skinfold thickness (triceps, biceps, subscapular)	Index children	4	Optional	Optional	
Bone stiffness (Achilles)	All subjects	9	Optional, strongly adviced	Optional, strongly adviced	Optional, strongly adviced
Handgrip strength (physical fitness)	All children	3	x	x	Optional
Collection of biosamples					
Timed urine (handing out urine cup and explanation of procedure)	All children	1	x	x	
Venous blood (application of anaesthetic patch and drawing of blood)	All subjects	5	x	x	Optional
Saliva (DNA from mouth mucosal cells; Oragene DNA self-collection kits)	Siblings, biol. parents and index children with no/insufficient amount of DNA	5	x	x	x

(continued)

Table 1.3 (continued)

Instrument	Target group	Estimated duration (min)	Completed by/measured in		
			Children	Adolescents	Parents
SACANA 24 h dietary recall					
Completion of first SACANA in the examination centre, second and third at home	All subjects ≥ 8 years	25	x	x	x
Computerised self-administered tests (CSATs)—neuropsychological tests					
The "hungry donkey" task (HDT)—in children Bechara gambling task (BGT)—in adults	All subjects ≥ 8 years	6	x (HDT)	x (HDT)	Optional (BGT)
Stop signal task	All subjects ≥ 8 years	7	x	x	Optional
Berg's card sorting test	All subjects ≥ 8 years	10	x	x	Optional
Accelerometry (7 days cycle)					
Handing out, explanation of procedure, handing out accelerometer diary (physical activity, sleep duration, sleep quality)	All children	3	x	x	Optional
Health records					
Maternity cards and records of routine child visits (where available)	Children	Depending on data source	x	x	x
At home					
Self-administered paper questionnaires					
Children's questionnaire (proxy report, completed by a parent together with the child, no more than two proxies per family)	Children 2–11 years	38	x (proxy report)		
Parent's questionnaire (from one parent, second parent optional)	Parents	31			x

(continued)

Table 1.3 (continued)

Instrument	Target group	Estimated duration (min)	Completed by/measured in		
			Children	Adolescents	Parents
Family questionnaire (one questionnaire per family)	Parents	47			x
Accelerometer diary (parental proxy report for children 2–11 years; self-report for children 12–15 years and self-report for parents available)	All subjects wearing an accelerometer	5	x (proxy report)	x	Optional

Adapted from supplementary Table 1, Ahrens et al. (2017)

- *Parents for their children (below the age of 12 years)*: general information about the child; physical activity; sleeping habits; dietary behaviour, dieting and food frequency; media consumption; well-being; children's spending.
- *Adolescents (≥ 12 years) for themselves*: general information about the teen; well-being; teen's spending; media consumption; physical activity; sleeping habits; dietary behaviour, dieting and food frequency; family life and rules; body image; impulsiveness; smoking and alcohol consumption; school grades.

The focus on families required the development of a kinship questionnaire assessing the biological and social ties of each index child within his/her family (see Chap. 14 of this book). Additional measurement tools were developed to assess neuropsychological traits using tests on decision making, set shifting capacity and inhibitory capacity. Maturation stages according to Tanner were assessed with pictograms. The medical history was reported by parents for both their children and for themselves.

At T_3, the questionnaire on dietary habits and food consumption frequency was combined with the general questionnaire and offered to teens and their parents for self-completion on a tablet PC (see Chap. 6 of this book). The computer-assisted 24-hour dietary recall (24-HDR) used in the IDEFICS study was amended and delivered as a Web-based version, called SACANA (see Chap. 5 of this book), which was offered to all participants from 8 years onwards. It was recommended to complete the first 24-HDR at the examination centre and another two 24-HDRs on non-consecutive days including one weekend day during the next 2 weeks. Parents were asked to assist smaller children (<11 years) in completing their 24-HDR.

All other questionnaires were completed by parents about themselves or their children if they were younger than 12 years and by adolescents themselves if they were at least 12 years old.

In addition to completing questionnaires and interviews, participants went through an extensive set of examinations and tests. Children or parents could refuse their participation in any examination module at any time. An overview of all modules, the target groups (children, adolescents or parents) and the estimated time needed to complete the respective modules are given in Table 1.3.

Extended examination protocol for contrasting groups (T$_3$, stage 2): An enhanced protocol including expression of genes related to food choice and measurement of brain activation, sensory taste perception, objective measurements of sleep quality and duration, sedentary time, screen time, physical activity and impact of the built environment was performed in the contrasting groups. Preference tests performed at T_0 and T_1 were repeated in contrasting groups and combined with taste intensity tests in both children and their parents. In a subsample of a few hundred children, stool samples were collected at T_1, at T_3 and in contrasting groups to analyse changes in the gut microbiome longitudinally.

The measurement of physical activity using accelerometers was combined with GPS sensors in Germany, Italy and Spain. The influence of the built environment on physical activity and health outcomes was investigated by combining accelerometry data with information on the physical environment obtained from geographic information systems (GIS). Functional magnetic resonance imaging of the brain (fMRI) assessed brain activation by visual food cues in a small subgroup of parent–child pairs.

1.3.4 Quality Management

As in all previous examinations of the IDEFICS study, quality management was enforced by central trainings of field staff, detailed standard operating procedures documented in the I.Family General Survey Manual (for access see Sect. 1.6), site visits during the field phase, central data management, central processing of biological samples and calibration studies to ensure comparability of measurements over time and across survey centres. A panel of statisticians supported the state-of-the-art data analysis.

1.4 Publication Policy, Data Management and Access to the Data

The data set was made available for analysis on a protected central data server for remote online analyses. Access to the data is restricted to authorised members of the study consortium. Researchers with access to the analysis data are prohibited from accessing person identifying data that were separated from any measurement data and stored under lock and key. A central statistical platform was established by the coordinating centre to provide appropriate statistical software tools and validated programmes, to carry out central statistical analyses and to consult and support all partners with their data analyses. Due to the prospective nature of this ongoing cohort study, the full anonymisation of study data is ruled out and use of data requires a mutual agreement between the IDEFICS/I.Family consortium and interested third parties on a case-by-case basis. Corresponding requests should be directed to the study coordinator.

1.5 Conclusions

The inclusion of different European populations is vital to capture the influence of various cultural and genetic backgrounds, social environments and dietary habits. However, the multi-centre study design and the varying environments required extra efforts to achieve a maximum degree of harmonisation of measurements, instruments, procedures for data collection and laboratory work, data management and statistical analyses: thus, the central purchase of all necessary equipment and material and the provision of SOPs to apply uniform criteria on a European level for a gender-sensitive assessment of physical constitution, metabolic status and the standardised measurement of obesity was crucial. In combination with regular quality control and intensive training of field staff, the implementation of the same methodological standards across many different European countries was feasible. But the roll-out of the detailed examination protocol was demanding and labour intensive. Our study also demonstrated the feasibility of combining observational, experimental and interventional components in one multi-level study.

The involvement of children posed specific challenges beyond the ones usually faced in studies of adults due to the need to develop instruments suitable for different age groups and to combine proxy information with respondents' self-reports. Of particular concern were the more stringent ethical constraints, especially since the measurements taken were obtained from healthy children, as e.g. the blood draw and the need to obtain informed consent from both parents and the child him-/herself. Since our study addressed very young children, parents often had to be actively involved beyond their consent. This was a real challenge which added to the burden of the field staff that already faced a lot of logistical challenges, e.g. by having to organise measurements for 80 to 100 small children per week in fasting status. In addition, caution had to be taken that the intervention did not induce adverse health effects in the children and that children being overweight or obese were not stigmatised.

The overall study programme had to be restricted in order to limit the burden for study participants. Especially children may become impatient very fast or may become detracted if the programme takes too much time. Moreover, measurements in children take usually longer than in adults. In addition, several devices had to be adapted for children as, e.g. the TANITA scale used for measuring BIA which could not be used in 2-year-old children due to too small feet, and the belts for accelerometers which had to be shortened.

But despite these restrictions, we were able to overcome most of the challenges. Thus, we were able to collect venous blood from healthy young children and to obtain ethical approval for blood and genetic analyses. Based on the collected blood samples, we were, for instance, able to derive age- and sex-specific reference values for biomarkers in pre-adolescent children which have been published in a supplement volume of the International Journal of Obesity (Ahrens et al. 2014). Furthermore, these samples gave us the unique opportunity to establish a biobank for future research allowing in-depth research on health outcomes and prognostic markers and a precious resource for the prospective investigation of long-term health effects in children.

1.6   Provision of Instruments and Standard Operating Procedures to Third Parties

The General Survey Manuals that provide among others all standard operating procedures can be accessed on the following website: www.leibniz-bips.de/ifhs after registration.

Each third partner referring to the General Survey Manuals is kindly requested to cite this chapter as follows: Ahrens W, Bammann K, Pigeot I, on behalf of the IDEFICS and I.Family consortia The IDEFICS/I.Family studies: design and methods of a large European child cohort. In: Bammann K, Lissner L, Pigeot I, Ahrens W, editors. Instruments for health surveys in children and adolescents. Cham: Springer Nature Switzerland; 2019. p. 1–24.

Acknowledgements The development of instruments, the baseline data collection and the first follow-up work as part of the IDEFICS study (www.idefics.eu) were financially supported by the European Commission within the Sixth RTD Framework Programme Contract No. 016181 (FOOD). The most recent follow-up including the development of new instruments and the adaptation of previously used instruments was conducted in the framework of the I.Family study (www.ifamilystudy.eu) which was funded by the European Commission within the Seventh RTD Framework Programme Contract No. 266044 (KBBE 2010–14).

We thank all families for participating in the extensive examinations of the IDEFICS and I. Family studies. We are also grateful for the support from school boards, headmasters and communities.

Statement of Ethics

Approval by the appropriate Ethics Committees was obtained by each of the eight centres doing the field work. Study children did not undergo any procedure before both they and their parents had given consent for examinations, collection of samples, subsequent analysis and storage of personal data and collected samples. Study subjects and their parents could consent to single components of the study while abstaining from others. A common data protection protocol ensuring confidentiality of all collected data was approved by all survey centres. Access to study data is only granted to persons who have committed themselves to our confidentiality rules in writing.

References

Ahrens W, Bammann K, De Henauw S, Halford J, Palou A, Pigeot I, et al. IDEFICS consortium. Understanding and preventing childhood obesity and related disorders—IDEFICS: a European multilevel epidemiological approach. Nutr Metab Cardiovasc Dis. 2006;16(4):302–8.

Ahrens W, Bammann K, Siani A, Buchecker K, De Henauw S, Iacoviello L, et al. IDEFICS consortium. The IDEFICS cohort: design, characteristics and participation in the baseline survey. Int J Obes (Lond). 2011;35(Suppl 1):S3–15.

Ahrens W, Moreno LA, Pigeot I, editors. Obesity determinants and reference standards for health parameters in pre-adolescent European children: results from the IDEFICS study. Int J Obes (Lond). 2014;38 Suppl 2.

Ahrens W, Siani A, Adan R, De Henauw S, Eiben G, Gwozdz W, I.Family consortium, et al.. Cohort profile: The transition from childhood to adolescence in European children—how I. Family extends the IDEFICS cohort. Int J Epidemiol. 2017;46(5):1394–5j.

Bammann K, Peplies J, Sjöström M, Lissner L, De Henauw S, Galli C, IDEFICS consortium, et al. Assessment of diet, physical activity biological, social and environmental factors in a multi-centre European project on diet- and lifestyle-related disorders in children (IDEFICS). J Public Health. 2006;14(5):279–89.

Bammann K, Sioen I, Huybrechts I, Casajús JA, Vicente-Rodríguez G, Cuthill R, IDEFICS consortium, et al. The IDEFICS validation study on field methods for assessing physical activity and body composition in children: design and data collection. Int J Obes (Lond). 2011;35(Suppl 1):S79–87.

Bammann K, Huybrechts I, Vicente-Rodriguez G, Easton C, De Vriendt T, Marild S, IDEFICS consortium, et al. Validation of anthropometry and foot-to-foot bioelectrical resistance against a three-component model to assess total body fat in children: the IDEFICS study. Int J Obes (Lond). 2013;37(4):520–6.

Bammann K, Peplies J, De Henauw S, Hunsberger M, Molnar D, Moreno LA, IDEFICS consortium, et al. Early life course risk factors for childhood obesity: the IDEFICS case-control study. PLoS ONE. 2014;9(2):e86914.

Bartholomew LK, Parcel GS, Kok G, Gottlieb NH. Planning health promotion programs: an Intervention Mapping Approach. 1st ed. San Francisco: Jossey-Bass; 2006.

Buck C, Pohlabeln H, Huybrechts I, De Bourdeaudhuij I, Pitsiladis Y, Reisch L, et al. Development and application of a moveability index to quantify possibilities for physical activity in the built environment of children. Health Place. 2011;17(6):1191–201.

Buck C, Börnhorst C, Pohlabeln H, Huybrechts I, Pala V, Reisch L, IDEFICS/I Family consortia, et al. Clustering of unhealthy food around German schools and its influence on dietary behavior in school children: a pilot study. Int J Behav Nutr Phys Act. 2013;10:65.

Buck C, Tkaczick T, Pitsiladis Y, De Bourdehaudhuij I, Reisch L, Ahrens W, et al. Objective measures of the built environment and physical activity in children: from walkability to moveability. J Urban Health. 2015;92(1):24–38.

De Henauw S, Verbestel V, Marild S, Barba G, Bammann K, Eiben G, IDEFICS consortium, et al. The IDEFICS community oriented intervention program. A new model for childhood obesity prevention in Europe? Int J Obes (Lond). 2011;35(Suppl 1):S16–23.

Haerens L, De Bourdeaudhuij I, Barba G, Eiben G, Fernandez J, Hebestreit A, IDEFICS consortium, et al. Developing the IDEFICS community-based intervention program to enhance eating behaviors in 2- to 8-year-old children: findings from focus groups with children and parents. Health Educ Res. 2009;24(3):381–93.

Haerens L, De Bourdeaudhuij I, Eiben G, Lauria F, Bel S, Keimer K, IDEFICS consortium, ct al. Formative research to develop the IDEFICS physical activity intervention component: findings from focus groups with children and parents. J Phys Act Health. 2010;7(2):246–56.

Herrmann D, Suling M, Reisch L, Siani A, De Bourdeaudhuij I, Maes L, IDEFICS consortium, et al. Repeatability of parental report on prenatal, perinatal and early postnatal factors: findings from the IDEFICS parental questionnaire. Int J Obes (Lond). 2011;35(Suppl 1):S52–60.

Herrmann D, Pohlabeln H, Gianfagna F, Konstabel K, Lissner L, Mårild S, IDEFICS consortium, et al. Association between bone stiffness and nutritional biomarkers combined with weight-bearing exercise, physical activity, and sedentary time in preadolescent children. A case-control study. Bone. 2015;78:142–9.

Hense S, Pohlabeln H, Michels N, Mårild S, Lissner L, Kovacs E, et al. Determinants of attrition to follow-up in a multicentre cohort study in children—results from the IDEFICS study. Epidemiol Res Int. 2013;2013:936365.

Huybrechts I, Börnhorst C, Pala V, Moreno LA, Barba G, Lissner L, the IDEFICS consortium, et al. Evaluation of the children's eating habits questionnaire used in the IDEFICS study by relating urinary calcium and potassium to milk consumption frequencies among European children. Int J Obes (Lond). 2011;35 Suppl 1:S69–78.

Knof K, Lanfer A, Bildstein MO, Buchecker K, Hilz H, IDEFICS consortium. Development of a method to measure sensory perception in children at the European level. Int J Obes (Lond). 2011;35(Suppl 1):S131–6.

Lanfer A, Hebestreit A, Ahrens W, Krogh V, Sieri S, Lissner L, IDEFICS consortium, et al. Reproducibility of food consumption frequencies derived from the Children's Eating Habits Questionnaire used in the IDEFICS study. Int J Obes (Lond). 2011;35(Suppl 1):S61–8.

Langeheine M, Pohlabeln H, Ahrens W, Rach S, IDEFICS consortium. Consequences of an extended recruitment on participation in the follow-up of a child study: results from the German IDEFICS cohort. Paediatr Perinat Epidemiol. 2017;31(1):76–86.

Ojiambo R, Konstabel K, Veidebaum T, Reilly J, Verbestel V, Huybrechts I, IDEFICS consortium, et al. Validity of hip-mounted uniaxial accelerometry with heart-rate monitoring vs. triaxial accelerometry in the assessment of free-living energy expenditure in young children: the IDEFICS validation study. J Appl Physiol. 2012;113(10):1530–6.

Pigeot I, De Baranowski T, Henauw S, IDEFICS Intervention Study Group. The IDEFICS intervention trial to prevent childhood obesity: design and study methods. Obes Rev. 2015a;16 (Suppl 2):S4–15.

Pigeot I, De Henauw S, Baranowski T. The IDEFICS (Identification and prevention of Dietary- and lifestyle-induced health EFfects In Children and infantS) trial outcomes and process evaluations. Obes Rev. 2015b;16(Suppl 2):S2–3.

Regber S, Novak M, Eiben G, Lissner L, Hense S, Sandström TZ, et al. Assessment of selection bias in a health survey of children and families—the IDEFICS Sweden-study. BMC Public Health. 2013;13:418.

Sioen I, Goemare S, Ahrens W, De Henauw S, De Vriendt T, Kaufman JM, IDEFICS consortium, et al. The relationship between paediatric calcaneal quantitative ultrasound measurements and dual energy X-ray absorptiometry (DXA) and DXA with laser (DXL) as well as body composition. Int J Obes (Lond). 2011;35(Suppl 1):S125–30.

Stomfai S, Ahrens W, Bammann K, Kovács E, Mårild S, Michels N, IDEFICS consortium, et al. Intra- and inter-observer reliability in anthropometric measurements in children. Int J Obes (Lond). 2011;35(Suppl 1):S45–51.

Suling M, Hebestreit A, Peplies J, Bammann K, Nappo A, Eiben G, IDEFICS consortium, et al. Design and results of the pre-test of the IDEFICS study. Int J Obes (Lond). 2011;35(Suppl 1): S30–44.

Verbestel V, De Henauw S, Maes L, Haerens L, Mårild S, Eiben G, et al. Using the intervention mapping protocol to develop a community-based intervention for the prevention of childhood obesity in a multi-centre European project: the IDEFICS intervention. Int J Behav Nutr Phys Act. 2011;8:82.

Chapter 2
MODYS—A Modular Control and Documentation System for Epidemiological Studies

Achim Reineke, Iris Pigeot, Wolfgang Ahrens and Stefan Rach

Abstract The quality of data collected in epidemiological observational research critically depends on the appropriate procedures for recruitment of study subjects. In this chapter, we describe the requirements and standard procedures for contacting, recruiting and documenting in field studies. We present a software tool, MODYS (**mo**dular control and **d**ocumentation **system**), that was specifically designed to control and document all recruitment steps in population based studies. The general design of MODYS is outlined, and its implementation for the IDEFICS study is presented in detail. Furthermore, the analysis of paradata recorded by MODYS is demonstrated with examples from the IDEFICS study.

2.1 Introduction

Collecting primary data on study subjects is an integral part of most epidemiological field studies. A high quality of the collected data is crucial, since errors introduced at this early step of a study can hardly be corrected thereafter. Thus, the statistical data analysis and, ultimately, the validity of the conclusions drawn are profoundly dependent on the quality of the data collected. In epidemiology, overall quality depends not only on the study design and the validity and reliability of the instruments or measurements (see related chapters in this book) but also on the procedures used to recruit study participants. Subjects recruited for a given study

On behalf of the IDEFICS and I.Family consortia.

A. Reineke (✉) · I. Pigeot · W. Ahrens · S. Rach
Leibniz Institute for Prevention Research and Epidemiology—BIPS, Bremen, Germany
e-mail: areineke@leibniz-bips.de

I. Pigeot · W. Ahrens
Faculty of Mathematics and Computer Science, University of Bremen, Bremen, Germany

© Springer Nature Switzerland AG 2019
K. Bammann et al. (eds.), *Instruments for Health Surveys in Children and Adolescents*, Springer Series on Epidemiology and Public Health,
https://doi.org/10.1007/978-3-319-98857-3_2

should represent the targeted study population as closely as possible. To ensure that every eligible member of the underlying population has equal chances to be enrolled into the study, highly standardised recruitment procedures have to be defined and applied. The implementation of such standardised procedures demands a high degree of training and control. A detailed documentation is necessary to allow for a proper monitoring of the recruitment process and the evaluation of its outcomes (Lacey and Savage 2016; Vandenbroucke et al. 2007). Such documentation should provide detailed information about critical steps in the recruitment procedure that are amenable to improvements. It should also enable researchers to identify subgroups that are under-represented and to investigate possible determinants of non-response (Stang 2003), i.e. to perform a non-responder analysis or to over-sample in order to eventually optimise the recruitment.

In this chapter, central processes that are necessary for the recruitment of study participants will be introduced before principles of the documentation are presented. We will focus on MODYS, a modular software system for epidemiological studies developed by the Unit IT, Data Management and Medical Documentation in close collaboration with the Unit Field Work of the Leibniz Institute for Prevention Research and Epidemiology—BIPS, Bremen, Germany. MODYS was specifically designed to control and document all recruitment steps while collecting primary data in a field-based study. This comprises all contact attempts and recruitment steps beginning with recording contact details of potential study participants through the final outcome: participation or non-participation.

The software will be described in detail in Sect. 2.3, and its implementation will be illustrated by examples from the IDEFICS/I.Family cohort (Ahrens et al. 2011, 2017). The chapter concludes with a discussion of possible extensions of this tool and its use in multi-centre studies.

2.2   General Requirements for Recruitment Monitoring, Documentation and Response Calculation

The recruitment procedure of a population-based study involves all steps from the identification and selection of eligible study subjects over the various approaches to contact potential participants up to their final decision whether to take part in the study or not. The pathways and means to approach potential study participants have to be adapted to the field setting. An example is given in Fig. 2.1. Usually, it is recommended to send a first contact letter, explaining the purpose of the study and providing general information about it. Subsequently, several approaches are typically needed to get in contact with subjects to obtain consent or refusal for participation or to identify and update invalid contact details (Dillman et al. 2009; Stang et al. 1999). Subjects who refuse may be asked to complete a short

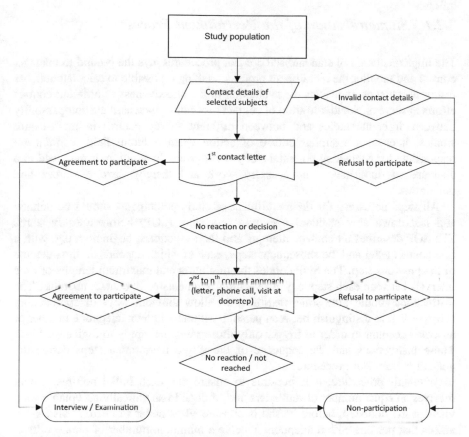

Fig. 2.1 Flow chart of a typical recruitment procedure

non-responder questionnaire to collect information allowing the assessment of possible selection effects. Visits at the doorstep enable the identification of invalid addresses but may also lower the threshold for participation of persons who are yet undecided.

In the context of a general trend towards decreased participation in surveys, specific problems typically include invalid or outdated contact details, missing phone numbers, non-adherence to appointments and non-response to contact attempts. To face these and other challenges, a more complex recruitment procedure is often required, as shown in Fig. 2.1.

Ultimately, the recruitment process needs to be recorded for each individual to provide all data necessary for a detailed response calculation, to monitor the recruitment process and to control the compliance with the defined procedures.

2.2.1 Standardisation of the Recruitment Process

The implementation of standardised contact procedures lays the ground to manage, control and monitor the recruitment process, making it possible to calculate reliable response statistics. It enables the evaluation of the effectiveness of different contact efforts in surveys. Standardisation of contact procedures increases the comparability between different studies and between different survey centres in multi-centre studies. It ensures a similar course of action when different field workers are responsible for contacting potential study participants. In addition, it may lead to a decrease in duplicate or unnecessary work and thereby save resources and manpower.

All steps necessary for the recruitment of study participants should be defined and laid down as a standard operating procedure (SOP) before a study starts. The SOP describes all contact attempts and their outcomes, beginning, e.g. with a first contact letter and the subsequent steps, each of which depends on the outcome of the previous step. The SOP defines the minimum and maximum lengths of time intervals between each step, e.g. for sending reminders or re-contact attempts. The instructions should give some flexibility to allow different ways of approaching subjects, e.g. to distinguish between persons without a known telephone number or an email account in order to trigger only those steps that apply to a given subject. These instructions and the sequence of the single recruitment steps define the general recruitment procedure.

With this procedure, it is possible to ensure that each initial non-respondent receives an equal number of reminders and, if done in an ethically acceptable way, visits at the doorstep, before he/she is considered as never reached. It also guarantees that persons with a telephone receive a minimum number of phone calls at pre-defined points in time during the day before the next step in the procedure is taken.

Besides the standardised contact procedures, different codes and coding instructions are necessary. As mentioned above, all attempts must be documented. A free textual description or notice entails the risk of varying descriptions of the same result. Thus, pre-defined descriptions with codes listed in a thesaurus ensure a standardised documentation. Based on this, the next steps in the recruitment procedure can be triggered. The same requirements apply to the documentation of the reasons for non-participation.

In addition to the definition of a standardised recruitment procedure, tools (preferably electronic) should be used to support and guide the field workers in their daily work. These include convenient databases or automatic reminder systems that support adherence of the field workers to the SOP and may thus contribute to the quality assurance of the recruitment.

2.2.2 Documentation and Monitoring of Recruitment

A reliable and seamless documentation of the field work to monitor the progress of a study must also have clear and comprehensible instructions. Such documentation entails each task in the recruitment procedure, each completed step on a case-by-case basis. The individual recruitment history of a person is made up of the sequence of these steps. The analysis of such recruitment histories helps to identify difficulties in scheduling interviews and reasons for non-participation (Cotter et al. 2002). The documentation can be used to assess the effectiveness of specific recruitment steps (e.g. how many contact attempts result in which increment of the response proportion) or to check if the projected number of interviews can be completed within the study period. These recruitment histories may thus be used to identify effective recruitment strategies while considering individual characteristics of potential participants. Such information allows a more reliable planning of the further course of the recruitment, the resources needed, the schedule and the budget. Altogether, the documentation has to be structured in a way that all elements of a recruitment history are neatly summarised for a given person although they may be generated by different field workers.

The documentation of each activity should at least include the following information (Cotter et al. 2002; Stoop et al. 2010):

- identification number (ID) of potential study participant
- contacted person (e.g. study participant, next of kin)
- date and time of the activity
- ID of field worker
- type of activity/mode of contact
- result of the activity.

To minimise the workload in documenting all steps of the recruitment history and to improve acceptance by field workers, the procedures should become an integral and mandatory component of the recruitment process.

Besides guidance and monitoring of the recruitment process, the collected information provides more detailed response statistics and allows analyses of reasons for non-participation. The documentation system may, for instance, routinely return the proportion of subjects who refused, have never been reached, were too ill, have moved away or were unable to speak the language.

2.2.3 Calculation of Response Proportions
in Population-Based Studies

Although epidemiologists are aware of the fact that selection bias may weaken descriptive studies and limit the external validity of analytical (association) studies (Jöckel and Stang 2013; Nohr et al. 2006; Rothman et al. 2013; Stang and Jöckel

2004), many publications lack a thorough reporting of the response proportion and the way it is calculated. In 1997, Asch and co-authors summarised a review of 321 mail surveys published in 1991 in medical journals and found that in 30% of them neither the response proportion nor the information necessary to calculate it were reported (Asch et al. 1997). In 2006, Morton and co-authors screened 355 peer-reviewed research articles published in the ten highest-impact general epidemiology and public health journals in the first four months of 2003 and found that 56% of case-control, 68% of cohort and 41% of cross-sectional studies failed to report any information on participation proportions (Morton et al. 2006).

But even if a response proportion is reported, its meaning may differ from study to study, mostly because the denominator is defined in different ways. The proportion of interest may be the proportion of non-respondents, the proportion of those never contacted or the overall proportion of participants. The subgroups entered in the nominator and the denominator of the ratio will differ correspondingly which will in turn affect the proportion reported. The problem already starts with the definition of who is eligible for a study and thus eligible to be counted in whatever ratio the researcher is interested in. A meta-analysis by Schnell (1997), for example, showed that the general definition of non-eligible respondents differed systematically between institutions.

Already in 1980, the commission of the "Council of American Survey Research Organizations" (CASRO) suggested a standardised definition of the response proportion. In 1998, the American Association for Public Opinion Research published a report (last update in 2016; AAPOR 2016) on standard definitions for surveys conducted by telephone, for in-person interviews in a sample of household surveys and for mail or for Internet surveys of specifically named persons.

The different versions of the response proportion that are reported in publications are mainly due to the fact that there is no consensus about the meaning of the word "response". For instance, although the numerator for the calculation of a response proportion may in most cases be obvious, i.e. the number of subjects actually participating in a study. Sometimes, all subjects giving consent are counted in the numerator although not all of them eventually take part in the study. In studies consisting of more than one module (e.g. examination, interview, self-completion questionnaire, biological sampling or repeated measurements), the proportion may be related to subjects participating in just one or all study modules. In one mailed survey, the return of a questionnaire may be counted as a response while in another survey only returned questionnaires that were completed may be counted. Lynn et al. (2002) gave a recommendation on how to calculate standardised response proportions, emphasising that response proportions are "very important quality and performance indicators" in surveys.

Besides the various possible definitions of the numerator in calculating the response proportion, the definition of the denominator is even more diverse. While some researchers may report the proportion of subjects participating relative to all persons eligible, others relate this proportion to only those who were successfully contacted. It is common practice to remove all (potentially eligible) subjects from the denominator, who are considered as "neutral" dropouts with regard to any selection effects. For example, subjects who had died or moved out of the study region at the date of sampling may be considered as such neutral "dropouts" as they did not belong to the study population. Often persons who suffer from severe illness are excluded although they may not be considered as neutral. However, exclusion from the denominator of subjects who were never reached may introduce bias as these subjects may systematically differ in many regards from those who were successfully contacted. Since a low response may lead to the rejection of an article submitted to a scientific journal, researchers may be tempted to exclude as many subjects as possible form the denominator in order to raise the reported response proportion. Thus, reporting of a mere response proportion is not informative. Instead, it should be stipulated that each study report has to include a response calculation that includes a detailed breakdown, both of study subjects considered and of subjects excluded as non-eligible for the study (Morton et al. 2006; Lacey and Savage 2016; Schulz et al. 2010; Vandenbroucke et al. 2007).

To report a reproducible response proportion, detailed information about the recruitment has to be recorded for each participant. It is, for instance, necessary to record the specific reason for non-participation to decide whether a non-participant could be counted as a "neutral" dropout (e.g. an illness rendering participation impossible or having left the study population at the time of sampling). For subjects never reached, the number and type of contact attempts have to be recorded. In the ideal case, the individual recruitment history is available for each potential study participant (preferably in electronic form). For this reason, field workers need convenient tools to support and standardise documentation. The documentation effort can be minimised by automated procedures as they will be presented below.

2.2.4 Maintenance of Personal Identifiers and Pseudonyms

Personal identifiers (PID) like names, addresses, telephone numbers, email addresses or social security numbers are needed to get in contact with the potential study participants or to retrieve secondary data on them. These data (and other contact details) have to be recorded for each person, regardless of his/her participation in the study. Even PIDs of non-responders will be stored until the end of the recruitment period as to avoid repeated contact approaches of individuals who already refused to participate. Maintenance of PIDs is mandatory in order to keep them up to date, i.e. to correct invalid addresses and to record changes of contact details, e.g. if a person has moved after being selected for the study. Sometimes, PIDs are outdated or incomplete. In this case, a later completion is necessary, e.g. by adding telephone numbers or email addresses of persons for whom initially only names and/or only postal addresses were available.

PIDs have to be protected from unauthorised access, and therefore, the corresponding database has to be stored in a protected environment where access requires specific authorisation. In general, it is a good practice to store and process PIDs separately from other study data. Separation of study data and personal identifiers needs to be reflected in the organisational structure, where field staff may only have access to PIDs while scientists may only have access to pseudonymised study data.

Often, it is necessary to preserve the link between PID and study data, e.g. in longitudinal studies, in case that a participant withdraws his/her consent after recruitment or in case that implausible data need to be verified. For this purpose, a link variable, a pseudonym, has to be assigned to each study participant that is stored together with the PID as well as the study data. Collected data that allow re-identifying a participant without access to the PID, e.g. deoxyribonucleic acid (DNA), require special pseudonyms. Several pseudonyms may be assigned to each study participant.

The management of these pseudonyms has to be done very carefully, because mistakes can lead to disastrous, often irreversible consequences for the dataset. To use a simple paper sheet to write down the assigned pseudonyms is possible but not preferable. Software tools or databases with functions to assign, store, revoke and retrieve pseudonyms reduce the probability of errors significantly.

All tasks and duties described in this section may be supported by an electronic recruitment system. Key functions of such a tool for the standardised management, monitoring and documentation of the recruitment process are outlined in the following section using the modular control and documentation system (MODYS) for illustrative purposes as an example.

2.3   MODYS: An Electronic Recruitment System

Based on long-standing experience in population-based studies and the development of tools for field work, an electronic recruitment system called MODYS (**mo**dular control and **d**ocumentation **sy**stem) was developed at the Leibniz Institute for Prevention Research and Epidemiology—BIPS (for access see Sect. 2.6). MODYS is designed as a management and documentation tool to support the field staff while recruiting study participants. It has evolved over several years and was successfully used in various field studies.

In the previous sections, we discussed requirements which have to be fulfilled by a well-designed electronic recruitment system. Besides its ability to standardise recruitment procedures and to produce response calculations, MODYS was constructed to optimise the workflow. Thus, MODYS serves as a steering tool guiding the field staff through all steps of the pre-defined study procedures on a case-by-case basis while enabling researchers to monitor adherence to the recruitment protocol.

Our system provides all functionalities that field workers need for their daily work, typically as semi-automated tasks. It also provides an easy-to-use user interface as well as all information needed to keep an overview of the current status and pending tasks; for example, who has to be called by phone in the evening and who has to receive a reminder letter. Keeping all contact information and history in such an organised system allows the project staff to efficiently deal with vast amounts of information (Cotter et al. 2002). The project staff is able to easily review a participant's history of contact attempts, appointments made as well as individual needs of respondents. To use this system, neither advanced user knowledge (e.g. serial letter creation) nor any programming skills are necessary. This is ensured by menus and drop-down lists guiding the user through everyday routines.

By mirroring all steps that have to be followed according to the recruitment pathway, MODYS guides the field workers through the whole procedure. MODYS triggers each step depending on the outcome of the previous one and provides reminders after pre-defined time intervals. By supporting the use of mail merge for letters and/or emails, MODYS substantially enhances recruitment efficiency. An automatic reminder system supports the adherence of the field workers to the pre-defined procedures and thus forms a central constituent of the quality assurance of a field study.

MODYS offers sufficient flexibility to manage a variety of situations encountered during the recruitment process. If, for example, a study subject is reluctant to participate at a given point in time, it may be imperative to suspend the pre-defined procedure for this subject and to re-contact him/her at a later point in time that is more convenient for this individual. Thus, MODYS allows field workers to consider the individual needs of potential participants in order not to put their willingness to participate in the study at risk.

There is no common recruitment procedure that fits all types of study designs. Therefore, the basic architecture of MODYS can be adapted to the specific requirements of all major study designs and to different workflows without the need to re-program its core components.

2.3.1 Architecture

The recruitment procedure is made up by a sequence of single steps, each having a predecessor and a successor, often with bifurcations as illustrated in Fig. 2.2. Each step is represented by a node. Successors of a step are connected by edges. The procedure starts at the top of the tree and progresses from node to node depending on the outcome of the predecessor until one of the end nodes is reached.

In MODYS, the nodes in the tree are represented by the so-called stations. Each station fulfils a specific task or action (e.g. generating a letter or generating a report). By allowing up to two successors, stations can be arranged in a tree-like structure. For each potential study participant, a data record is generated including the personal identifiers and a position marker (PM). The PM flags the progress of the given person in the recruitment procedure. Once a station is completed (e.g. a letter was mailed and documented), the PM is moved to the subsequent station. Each PM (and so each potential study participant) moves through the tree depending on the decisions taken in previous stations.

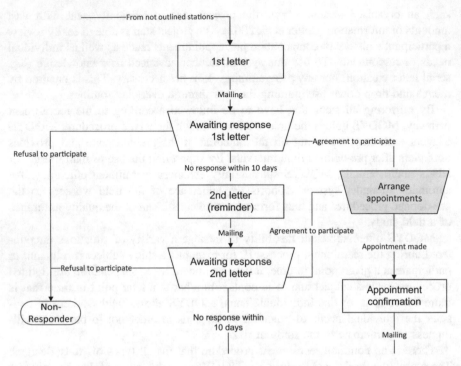

Fig. 2.2 Excerpt of the workflow managed by MODYS in the IDEFICS study. Not shown are the procedures used to contact registries (e.g. for checking address information), to contact groups of participants and to provide feedback information to participants

Figure 2.2 illustrates an excerpt of the workflow managed by MODYS as implemented in the IDEFICS study. The procedure starts with an initial letter asking for participation. To initiate this step, the PM of the potential study participant is assigned to the station "1st letter" (station type "letter") that generates and prints the initial contact letter. After the letter has been printed, the corresponding PM is shifted to the next station called "Awaiting response 1st letter" (station type "work list"). In the example, three different outcomes are possible: no reaction, agreement or refusal. If there is no reaction by the potential study participant within ten days, the corresponding PM will be shifted to the subsequent station "2nd letter (reminder)" to trigger a reminding letter. This will be done by the system without user interaction. "2nd letter (reminder)" is also a station of the type "letter". After the second letter has been printed, the PM is shifted to station "Awaiting response 2nd letter" and the process continues. The second possible outcome could be a refusal. In this case, the reason for the refusal to participate will be asked for and recorded by the field worker (not shown in the figure). The corresponding PM is then shifted to the final station "Non-responder" where the process ends. In case of an agreement to participate, the third possible outcome, the PM is shifted to the station "Arrange appointments". This is a station of the type "work list". The field worker selects a subject out of the list, contacts him/her and makes an appointment for the physical examination. Afterwards, the PM is shifted to the station "Appointment confirmation" and a confirmation is mailed to the respondent.

In each station, all information needed is displayed depending on the station type and the planned task. For example, in a station of type letter, the names of all subjects are shown for whom the previous step was completed. The field worker can now choose a single subject, a defined number or all out of the list. Subsequently, the station generates the corresponding letters and shifts the PMs.

To enhance its flexibility and maintenance friendliness, MODYS has a modular architecture. All stations related to similar procedures are of the same type and trigger similar forms and system routines. Each of these types implements a special action and consists of an on-screen form and the related program code. Different types of stations are implemented in MODYS. Some generate letters, while others manage telephone contacts and still others support appointments. If necessary, additional stations types can be added to the system. The sequence of stations can be configured freely and can be changed simply by changing the definition of the successors.

2.3.2   Standardisation of Contact Procedures

Standardisation of the workflow is a main advantage of an electronic recruitment system like MODYS. All contact attempts are carried out in a well-defined sequence with unambiguous branching points. The system ensures that all steps of the contact procedure take place in a defined order. No study participant can get lost or can be forgotten. The system provides capabilities to store, manage and use all data and information needed to get in contact with each potential respondent and to carry out the necessary recruitment steps (see Fig. 2.3).

The main contact form (see Fig. 2.3) displays all information needed by a field worker to communicate with a potential participant. It includes name, address, date of birth, telephone numbers, the current station, all appointments and other basic data. In addition, the event log containing all tasks and performed contact approaches is included. This ensures that all field workers involved in the study are fully informed of the current recruitment status for a given subject with individual needs of participants recorded during previous contact attempts.

The number and sequence of all recruitment steps are defined by the configured stations, as described in Sect. 2.3.1. In addition, all contact descriptions (options), possible results of contact attempts and all possible non-responder codes are defined and listed for a given study.

The contact descriptions document the kind of contact, e.g. a phone call, email or letter. Such descriptions should be short and clear, e.g. "phone call conducted", "invitation letter sent" or "examination finished". The contact results describe the outcome of the contact attempt, for example, the willingness to participate or the successful arrangement of an appointment for examination or interview. Undefined

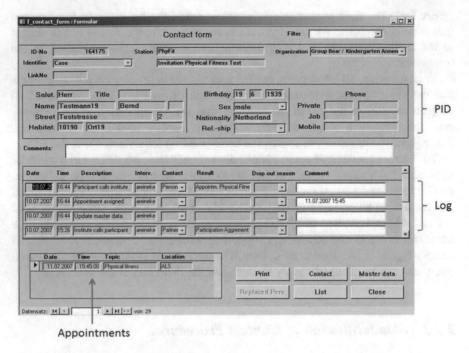

Fig. 2.3 Main contact form in MODYS

or open results are also specified, e.g. to document an unsuccessful phone call if the person was not reached. The items on the list of non-responder codes classify the reasons for non-participation. They consist of a short descriptive text and a unique code. The codes are categorised by type of non-response to allow classification, e.g. as "neutral" or "non-neutral". Rules implemented in the system define permitted combinations of contact descriptions, contact results and non-responder codes.

MODYS offers pre-defined descriptions and codes that can be chosen from drop-down menus for each contact attempt and each performed task. The resulting actions are performed automatically by the system, as, e.g. the progression to the appropriate subsequent recruitment step.

2.3.3 Documentation

MODYS provides an integrated documentation component. The system records all events like contact outcomes or the progression from one step to the next including actions performed automatically by the system. This creates an individual recruitment history for each participant that is automatically saved by the system. All events can be traced by different field workers to allow a shared management of the recruitment.

ID	Date	Time	Description	Operator	Contacted person	Result	Non-Resp. code	Note
0815	07.09.2007	08:24	Initial letter	SJ		Printed		
0815	10.09.2007	10:59	Call from centre	SJ		No contact		
0815	11.09.2007	14:21	Call from centre	AR	Husband	Open-ended		At home after 3 PM
0815	14.09.2007	17:12	Call from centre	HH	Participant	Appointm. fixed		Appointm: 02.10.2007
0815	14.09.2007	17:30	Appointm. confirmation	HH		Printed		
0815	02.10.2007	10:03	Examination result	IG		Finished		
0815	07.10.2007	12:07	Feedback	SJ		Printed		

Fig. 2.4 Example of an event log generated by MODYS

Each event is recorded with a date and time stamp, a description of the event (pre-defined list of contact descriptions), the name of the field worker eliciting the action, the contacted person, the outcome of the action (pre-defined list of contact results), a code for non-participation (pre-defined list of non-responder codes) and optional free text notes (see Fig. 2.4). These records constitute the paradata of the survey (Kreuter et al. 2010) that are used to monitor and manage the recruitment process and to calculate response statistics.

Contact attempts and performed tasks in MODYS are documented in a standardised way which allows pooling of paradata of different studies for research purposes. Furthermore, it supports standardisation of field work procedures across different studies.

2.3.4 Management of Personal Identifiers and Data Protection

MODYS provides several functionalities to manage and use personal identifiers (PID). Names, addresses, telephone numbers or email addresses are stored in the system, are accessible in contact forms and can be printed on letters. Invalid or incomplete data can be corrected or updated by using integrated forms and functions. Each update is documented in an audit trail including the date and time of the update, the name of the field worker and the changed item.

Each contact history supports future individualised contact attempts. The PID and the collected information allow each field worker to keep track of wrong or outdated phone numbers, address changes, as well as any notes that may be pertinent to a particular contact.

Pseudonym management is an integral part of MODYS. The system is capable to store different pseudonyms for each subject. These can easily be assigned, retrieved and used to generate letters or lists. Built-in routines preserve the integrity of the assignments between PID and pseudonym.

The PIDs are protected from unauthorised access by using a database that is kept separated from any other study data. The database is password protected and access is granted solely to persons who are responsible for recruitment. A dedicated server in a protected environment may further enhance data security, e.g. by an additional firewall or a closed network.

2.4   Implementation

The IDEFICS and I.Family studies involved eight European countries with at least two survey locations each. To enrol children into the study, parents were usually approached via schools and kindergartens. Here, we describe the implementation of MODYS as used in the German survey centre to manage a direct contact approach.

2.4.1   MODYS in the German Survey Centres

Implementing MODYS required the definition of the necessary recruitment steps, contact descriptions, contact results and non-responder codes. As usual, completion of these definitions was more demanding than the configuration of MODYS itself. During this process, different alternatives were developed and discarded. MODYS had to meet the requirements of the complex study environment with a survey team travelling to different temporary local examination sites that were set up in schools and health centres in the study region and a mobile examination unit on a van.

In addition to managing the recruitment, MODYS had to support feedback letters to study subjects and the follow-up of residential addresses through queries to the municipal registries of residents. A central MODYS installation at the main survey centre managed the recruitment at two survey locations running in parallel. Potential study participants were first contacted by letters and then by phone, if available.

Although the recruitment procedures differed slightly between the baseline and the follow-up surveys, the configuration of MODYS could be adapted without any reprogramming of its basic architecture.

At baseline, the defined recruitment process consisted of 34 stations (an excerpt is shown in Fig. 2.2). Besides several control stations, fifteen stations of the type "letter" were defined, including invitation letters, reminders, feedbacks and letters to registries. The configuration was completed by 26 contact descriptions, 33 contact results and 14 non-responder codes. While conducting the baseline survey, more than 80,000 contact attempts or process steps were documented for 4434 persons. These data are a valuable source for controlling and monitoring. During the recruitment process, 4801 invitation letters, 3013 first reminders and 1769 second reminders were sent, and 9137 phone calls were made.

2.4.2 Controlling and Monitoring a Study with MODYS Paradata

In the following, several examples taken from the German cohort of the IDEFICS study will illustrate the capability of MODYS to control and monitor recruitment efforts in field surveys.

For the correct calculation of response proportions, it is crucial to consider the reasons for non-participation, because, depending on the sampling procedure and the inclusion criteria of the survey, not all persons in the initial sample may be eligible for the study.

A summary of the reasons for non-participation as assessed at baseline is given in Fig. 2.5. Out of 2405 non-participants, 169 were not eligible for inclusion in the study (non-responder codes 100–150, and 610) and were disregarded in calculating

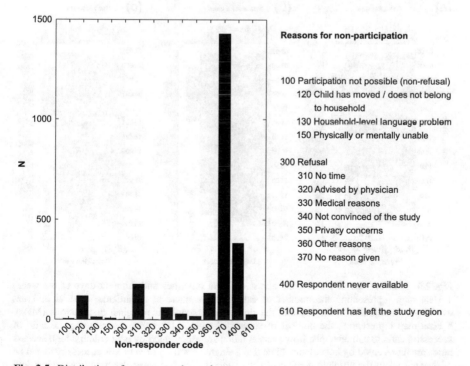

Reasons for non-participation

100 Participation not possible (non-refusal)
    120 Child has moved / does not belong to household
    130 Household-level language problem
    150 Physically or mentally unable

300 Refusal
    310 No time
    320 Advised by physician
    330 Medical reasons
    340 Not convinced of the study
    350 Privacy concerns
    360 Other reasons
    370 No reason given

400 Respondent never available

610 Respondent has left the study region

Fig. 2.5 Distribution of non-responder codes

the response proportion. For 383 potential participants who were never reached (category 400), it cannot be decided whether they belong to the eligible study population or not. To be conservative, eligibility is assumed for such cases. The remaining 1853 non-responders (category 300) gave reasons that do not suggest ineligibility.

Whenever phone numbers are available, calling potential participants increases the probability of participation significantly, as compared to recruitment via land mail (Dillman et al. 2009; Stang et al. 1999). To maximise the chance of reaching a potential participant, it is important to distribute multiple calls to a particular phone number across different daytimes and different days of the week (Slattery et al. 1995). Since all phone call attempts and their results are documented in MODYS, the calls made during a study can be analysed in detail. For instance, the distribution of phone calls made at baseline of the IDEFICS study is depicted by means of heat maps in Fig. 2.6. For each panel, the day of the week and the time are specified on the x- and y-axes, respectively. The cell colouring indicates the absolute number of calls made (Panel A) at a particular time and day of the week, the number of calls which reached the intended respondent (Panel B), or the relative frequency of a call reaching the intended respondent (Panel C). In Panels A and B,

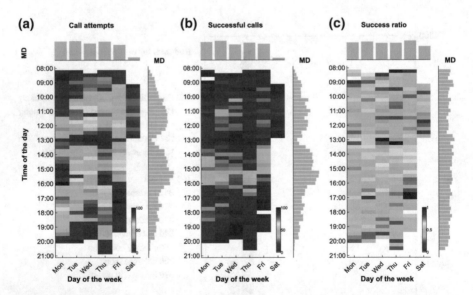

Fig. 2.6 Distributions of phone calls across different daytimes and different days of the week. **a** Heat map representing the number of call attempts made at a particular time at different weekdays. Histograms at the top and the right border represent marginal distributions (MDs). **b** Heat map representing the number of successful calls. **c** Heat map representing the ratio of successful calls to call attempts. Low success ratios are represented by cold colours; high success ratios are represented by hot colours. Note that a single very high or very low success ratio can be misleading when the absolute number of calls attempted at that particular time is not taken into consideration

the bar graphs at the top and at the right border represent the marginal distributions of phone calls. In Panel C, the bar graphs represent the mean ratio of successful calls.

As indicated by the marginal distributions in Panel A, phone calls were roughly equally distributed across the working days, but not across daytimes, as most phone calls were attempted during late morning between 10 a.m. and 12 p.m. as well as early afternoon between 2 p.m. and 4 p.m. As can be seen from Panel B, the increased activity during these timeslots led to an increased absolute number of successful calls within these time windows. The probability of a successful call, however, did not vary substantially by daytime (Panel C).

The paradata documented by MODYS allow for the analysis of the activity of individual study nurses to evaluate performance and, for instance, identify needs for training. In Fig. 2.7, the number of phone calls made (white bar) and successful calls (black bars) is depicted for each study nurse who made more than 100 call attempts. Obviously, the number of call attempts varies considerably between different study nurses, a fact which, however, is likely to be caused by the specific distribution of tasks within the team. Low proportions of successful calls might indicate a need of extra training for the respective study nurse.

In a second step, the results of successful calls could be investigated further. For instance, a comparison between the number of successful calls that led to appointments and the number of calls that eventually resulted in examinations may give valuable insights. For instance, the cancellation of an appointment by a

Fig. 2.7 Number of call attempts and successful calls for different study nurses. Numbers above the bars indicate the proportion of successful calls

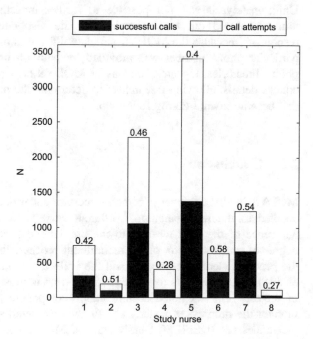

potential participant may suggest that the potential participant may have been talked into making an appointment, although he/she had no real intention to take part in the study.

Recently, Langeheine et al. (2017) analysed paradata of the IDEFICS study recorded with MODYS to investigate the association between recruitment effort and study participation. For cohort studies with adults, it has been shown that participants who were enrolled in a study only after extended recruitment efforts (so-called late responders) are more likely to drop out at a later stage of the study as compared to early responders, that is, participants who enrolled already after few contact attempts (e.g. Cohen et al. 2000; Haring et al. 2009; Nederhof et al. 2012). For children/youth cohorts, however, the recruitment is especially challenging because the consent of both children and parents is required and, therefore, it is not clear, whether the results from adult cohort studies do apply here as well. For instance, it has been reported that parents' failures to provide consent are often not deliberate refusals but rather caused by failures to respond (Fletcher and Hunter 2003). Therefore, extended recruitment strategies are being developed and tested as a countermeasure (e.g. Schilpzand et al. 2015; Wolfenden et al. 2009). Langeheine et al. (2017) demonstrated that, in the German cohort of the IDEFICS study, an extended recruitment effort at baseline was not associated per se with a higher chance to drop out at follow-up. Participants who responded late at baseline, however, were more likely to not be reachable at follow-up, if their contact details contained only a single mobile phone number as compared to participants whose contact details contained landline numbers or more than one phone number. Unfortunately, it was not possible to further investigate why more telephone numbers turned out to be invalid for late responders as compared to early responders, because the MODYS paradata did not allow differentiating whether a particular phone number was provided by participants or collected from public phone directories. Updated versions of MODYS now record all changes made to contact details, allowing researchers to determine the origin of telephone numbers that become invalid during follow-up.

2.5 Conclusion

MODYS is able to cover a complex recruitment procedure, and it can be easily adapted to the requirements of different surveys. Since MODYS supports the adherence of the field workers to the pre-defined procedures, it leads to a high degree of standardisation of the recruitment process. Its functionalities to manage the personal identifiers, the IDs and the collected contact history for each subject enable the field workers to concentrate on what is most important: the recruitment of subjects. The integrated documentation component provides useful paradata to monitor the progress of a study and to generate detailed response statistics.

Besides the IDEFICS/I.Family studies, MODYS is also used in several other studies. One challenging example is the NAKO Health Study (German National

Cohort (GNC) Consortium 2014) where eighteen study centres all over Germany use the system to manage the recruitment of 200,000 study participants.

The architecture of MODYS is open to further implement new functionalities, as, e.g. the integration of a data analysis module. Currently a new version is under development based on up-to-date Web technologies providing a more flexible user interface and data management capabilities to better fulfil the needs of multi-centre studies.

2.6 Provision of MODYS and Standard Operating Procedures to Third Parties

The electronic recruitment system MODYS (test version of Web-based MODYS) including the General Survey Manual that provides among other all standard operating procedures can be accessed on the following website: www.leibniz-bips. de/ifhs after registration. The full program can be provided upon request

Each third partiei using MODYS or the corresponding SOPs, respectively, is kindly requested to cite this chapter as follows:

Reineke A, Pigeot I, Ahrens W, Rach S, on behalf of the IDEFICS and I.Family consortia. MODYS—a modular control and documentation system for epidemiological studies. In: Bammann K, Lissner L, Pigeot I, Ahrens W, editors. Instruments for health surveys in children and adolescents. Cham: Springer Nature Switzerland; 2019. p. 25–45.

Acknowledgements The development of instruments, the baseline data collection and the first follow-up work as part of the IDEFICS study (www.idefics.eu) were financially supported by the European Commission within the Sixth RTD Framework Programme Contract No. 016181 (FOOD). The most recent follow-up including the development of new instruments and the adaptation of previously used instruments was conducted in the framework of the I.Family study (www.ifamilystudy.eu) which was funded by the European Commission within the Seventh RTD Framework Programme Contract No. 266044 (KBBE 2010-14).

We thank all families for participating in the extensive examinations of the IDEFICS and I. Family studies. We are also grateful for the support from school boards, headmasters and communities.

References

Ahrens W, Bammann K, Siani A, Buchecker K, De Henauw S, Iacoviello L, et al. IDEFICS consortium. The IDEFICS cohort: design, characteristics and participation in the baseline survey. Int J Obes (Lond). 2011;35(Suppl 1):S3–15.
Ahrens W, Siani A, Adan R, De Henauw S, Eiben G, Gwozdz W, et al. I.Family consortium. Cohort profile: the transition from childhood to adolescence in European children—how I.Family extends the IDEFICS cohort. Int J Epidemiol. 2017;46(5):1394–1395j.

American Association for Public Opinion Research (AAPOR). Standard definitions: final dispositions of case codes and outcome rates for surveys. Ann Arbor, Michigan: American Association for Public Opinion Research; 2016.

Asch DA, Jedrziewski MK, Christakis NA. Response rates to mail surveys published in medical journals. J Clin Epidemiol. 1997;50(10):1129–36.

Cohen SB, Machlin SR, Branscome JM. Patterns of survey attrition and reluctant response in the 1996 medical expenditure panel survey. Health Serv Outcomes Res Methodol. 2000;1(2): 131–48.

Cotter RB, Burke JD, Loeber R, Navratil JL. Innovative retention methods in longitudinal research: a case study of the developmental trends study. J Child Fam Stud. 2002;11(4): 485–98.

Dillman DA, Phelps G, Tortora R, Swift K, Kohrell J, Berck J, et al. Response rate and measurement differences in mixed-mode surveys using mail, telephone, interactive voice response and internet. Soc Sci Res. 2009;38:1–18.

Fletcher AC, Hunter AG. Strategies for obtaining parental consent to participate in research. Fam Relat. 2003;52(3):216–21.

German National Cohort. (GNC) Consortium. The German National Cohort: aims, study design and organization. Eur J Epidemiol. 2014;29(5):371–82.

Haring R, Alte D, Völzke H, Sauer S, Wallaschofski H, John U, et al. Extended recruitment efforts minimize attrition but not necessarily bias. J Clin Epidemiol. 2009;62(3):252–60.

Jöckel KH, Stang A. Cohort studies with low baseline response may not be generalisable to populations with different exposure distributions. Eur J Epidemiol. 2013;28(3):223–7.

Kreuter F, Couper M, Lyberg L. The use of paradata to monitor and manage survey data collection. In: Proceedings of the joint statistical meetings, American Statistical Association; 2010, p. 282–296.

Lacey JV Jr, Savage KE. 50% response rates: half-empty, or half-full? Cancer Causes Control. 2016;27(6):805–8.

Langeheine M, Pohlabeln H, Ahrens W, Rach S. IDEFICS consortium. Consequences of an extended recruitment on participation in the follow-up of a child study: Results from the German IDEFICS cohort. Paediatr Perinat Epidemiol. 2017;31(1):76–86.

Lynn P, Beerten R, Laiho J, Martin J. Towards standardization of survey outcome categories and response rate calculations. Res Official Stat. 2002;1:61–84.

Morton LM, Cahill J, Hartge P. Reporting participation in epidemiologic studies: a survey of practice. Am J Epidemiol. 2006;163(3):197–203.

Nederhof E, Jörg F, Raven D, Veenstra R, Verhulst FC, Ormel J, et al. Benefits of extensive recruitment effort persist during follow-ups and are consistent across age group and survey method. The TRAILS study. BMC Med Res Methodol. 2012;93:3–15.

Nohr EA, Frydenberg M, Henriksen TB, Olsen J. Does low participation in cohort studies induce bias? Epidemiology. 2006;17(4):413–8.

Rothman KJ, Gallacher JE, Hatch EE. Why representativeness should be avoided. Int J Epidemiol. 2013;42(4):1012–4.

Schilpzand EJ, Sciberras E, Efron D, Anderson V, Nicholson JM. Improving survey response rates from parents in school-based research using a multi-level approach. PLoS ONE. 2015;10(5): e0126950.

Schnell R. Nonresponse in Bevölkerungsumfragen: Ausmaß, Entwicklung und Ursachen. Opladen: Leske und Buderich; 1997.

Schulz KF, Altman DG, Moher D, Group C. CONSORT 2010 Statement: updated guidelines for reporting parallel group randomised trials. J Clin Epidemiol. 2010;63(8):834–40.

Slattery ML, Edwards SL, Caan BJ, Kerber RA, Potter JD. Response rates among control subjects in case-control studies. Ann Epidemiol. 1995;5(3):245–9.

Stang A. Nonresponse research—an underdeveloped field in epidemiology. Eur J Epidemiol. 2003;18(10):929–31.

Stang A, Ahrens W, Jöckel KH. Control response proportions in population-based case-control studies in Germany. Epidemiology. 1999;10(2):181–3.

Stang A, Jöckel KH. Studies with low response proportions may be less biased than studies with high response proportions. Am J Epidemiol. 2004;159(2):204–10.

Stoop I, Billiet J, Koch A, Fitzgerald R. Improving survey response: lessons learned from the European Social Survey. Chichester: Wiley; 2010.

Vandenbroucke JP, von Elm E, Altman DG, Gøtzsche PC, Mulrow CD, Pocock SJ, et al. Strengthening the reporting of observational studies in epidemiology (STROBE): explanation and elaboration. Epidemiology. 2007;18(6):805–35.

Wolfenden L, Kypri K, Freund M, Hodder R. Obtaining active parental consent for school-based research: a guide for researchers. Aust N Z J Public Health. 2009;33(3):270–5.

Chapter 3
Physical Examinations

Karin Bammann, Jenny Peplies, Staffan Mårild, Dénes Molnár,
Marc Suling and Alfonso Siani

Abstract One central element of the IDEFICS and I.Family studies was the physical examination of the child including anthropometric measurements, blood pressure, heel ultrasonography and medical history. These examinations provided measurement data for central outcomes, like nutritional status, and were thus of high importance to the studies. For ease of survey logistics, the examinations were subdivided into two modules that could be performed independently from each other. For each of these measurements, a standard operating procedure was fixed in the General Survey Manuals that had to be followed by the local field staff in each survey centre.

On behalf of the IDEFICS and I.Family consortia

K. Bammann (✉) · J. Peplies
Working Group Epidemiology of Demographic Change,
Institute for Public Health and Nursing Research (IPP),
University of Bremen, Bremen, Germany
e-mail: bammann@uni-bremen.de

K. Bammann · J. Peplies · M. Suling
Leibniz Institute for Prevention Research and Epidemiology—BIPS,
Bremen, Germany

S. Mårild
Department of Paediatrics, Institute for Clinical Sciences,
The Queen Silvia Children's Hospital, the Sahlgrenska Academy
at University of Gothenburg, Gothenburg, Sweden

D. Molnár
Department of Pediatrics, University of Pécs, Pécs, Hungary

A. Siani
Epidemiology and Population Genetics, Institute of Food Science,
National Research Council, Avellino, Italy

© Springer Nature Switzerland AG 2019
K. Bammann et al. (eds.), *Instruments for Health Surveys in Children
and Adolescents*, Springer Series on Epidemiology and Public Health,
https://doi.org/10.1007/978-3-319-98857-3_3

3.1   Introduction

Anthropometric measurements to assess body composition of the child comprise not only body mass index and bioelectrical impedance, but also circumferences and skinfolds to add information on fat distribution. The latter seems to be central for determining the risk of developing some comorbid conditions, e.g. cardiovascular risk factors (Labayen et al. 2006). The range of anthropometric measurements allows calculation of several indicators of weight status and body composition (Gibson 2005; Bammann et al. 2013) and gives valuable insight when comparing different subgroups and between countries.

Resting blood pressure is measured as a central parameter of cardiovascular disease. Hypertension has been shown to be prevalent already in young age (Kavey et al. 2010). Fasting blood is taken to assess laboratory parameters (for details see Chap. 4 of this book).

Heel ultrasonography is used to measure bone stiffness in both feet as an indicator of bone health (Moayyeri et al. 2012).

These measurements are complemented by the parental-reported medical history of the child and the child's family (see Chap. 14 of this book), and by information on past and current drug use.

3.2   Physical Examination Modules

The physical examination modules of the IDEFICS/I.Family baseline and follow-up surveys consist of two different sets of examinations, one for which an 8-h fasting status of the child is mandatory (module physical examination A) and one where this is not the case (module physical examination B). This distinction allows for the adaption of the examination schedule to local needs: in many survey centres, both sets of examinations were carried out in subsequent time slots with the fasting examination before the non-fasting examination. In this case, a healthy snack was organised to take place between these two time slots.

Some survey centres separated the two slots completely. The two modules, which are summarised in Table 3.1, are described in the following.

3.3   Physical Examination A (Fasting Status Mandatory)

The physical examination A module comprises blood drawing, measuring of leg-to-leg bioelectrical impedance, body mass and waist circumference.

The fasting status is assessed by a set of structured questions (see recording sheet for physical examinations A; for access see Sect. 3.7) to be answered by an accompanying parent or other adult. If a child is not accompanied by a parent/

Table 3.1 Examination modules deployed in the IDEFICS/I.Family baseline and follow-up surveys (specific devices used are listed in brackets)

Module	Assessment methods	Variables	References
Physical examination A —fasting status mandatory	Measurements	Weight with leg-to-leg BIA (TANITA BC 420 SMA with adapter) Waist circumference (SECA 200) Blood drawing[a]	Marfell-Jones et al. (2006)
Physical examination B —fasting status not required	Measurements	Blood pressure and pulse rate (automated sphygmomanometer Welch Allyn 4200B-E2 with cuffs) Standing height (SECA 225) Skinfold thicknesses (Holtain) Circumferences: mid-upper arm, hip, neck (SECA 200) Heel ultrasonography (optional; lunar achilles insight)	Marfell-Jones et al. (2006), Kondolot et al. (2017), Zebaze et al. (2003); Barba et al. (2014), Kettaneh et al. (2005)
Face-to-face interview on medical history		Questionnaire containing information on chronic diseases of the child and family and medication of the child	

[a]For more information we refer to Chap. 4 of this book

guardian, e.g. because the examinations take place in a school setting, the child itself was asked about his/her fasting status. In any case, the parents obtain written instructions that the examinations require that the child may consume nothing else than water within 8 h prior to the examinations.

Leg-to-leg bioelectrical impedance analysis (BIA) is an alternative to the somewhat burdensome arm-to-leg BIA, although resulting in higher measurement error (see, e.g. Kettaneh et al. 2005). The company TANITA specifically adapted their scale with leg-to-leg BIA for use in small children. This adapted scale is based on the model TANITA BC 420 SMA and returns body weight and resistance.

Only underwear and T-shirts should be worn for measurement. All other clothing including diapers has to be taken off. For children not able to stand on the scale, a child–parent weighing procedure is foreseen where the parent is weighed with and without the child on his/her arm. In these cases, the BIA measurement is skipped.

Waist circumference is measured using a flexible SECA 200 tape at the mid-point between the top of the iliac crest and the lower coastal border (10th rib). Both reference points and the mid-point are landmarked with a pen directly on the skin. The tape is placed laterally on the marked mid-point, and waist circumference is measured at the end of a gentle expiration (Marfell-Jones et al. 2006).

Fasting venous blood is collected from each consenting child after a local anaesthetic (EMLA patch) was applied to the skin. In the IDEFICS/I.Family surveys, the venous blood draw is limited to 1% of the estimated total blood volume for ethical reasons. According to a review on safe limits of blood sampling volumes for children by Howie (2011), paediatric guidelines allow for 1–5% of total blood volume (TBV) that can safely be sampled over a 24-h period. The TBV of a child amounts to around 75–80 ml per kg body weight. A table is provided to the field staff where the maximum volume to be drawn can be conveniently read off. If venous blood cannot be obtained, capillary blood is taken from the fingertip. The set of blood samples generally includes two tubes of venous blood: one native tube for serum collection and one ethylenediaminetetraacetic acid (EDTA) tube. Additionally, a PAXgene tube containing ribonucleic acid (RNA)-stabilising agent is drawn from a subsample of children for gene expression analysis. Blood lipids and glucose as metabolic markers are measured on-site with a point-of-care analyser (Cholestech LDX, Inverness Medical) from the first drop of venous or capillary blood (Whitehead et al. 2014). Such on-site analysis allows for immediate feedback to the parents. Another drop of blood applied to a collection kit is used for fatty acid (FA) analysis (Sigma-Aldrich cod. 11312-1KT) of circulating lipids. It involves measurement of FA profiles in a single drop of blood dried on a strip of chromatography paper and trans-methylation for gas chromatography analysis. This method has shown several advantages in terms of applicability, time and costs (Marangoni et al. 2005, 2007; Wolters et al. 2017).

All measurement readings and details on the collection of blood have to be documented on the recording sheet for physical examinations A (for access see Sect. 3.7).

3.4   Physical Examination B (Fasting Status not Required)

Module B of the physical examination comprises a series of measurements, a face-to-face interview of the parents on the medical history of the child and the inspection of drug packages (see also Sect. 3.5).

Resting blood pressure is measured preferably at the right arm at heart level using the automated oscillometric Welch Allyn 4200B-E2 device. First, the adequate cuff size has to be determined by measuring the mid-upper arm circumference and reading the appropriate cuff from a table abstracted from the General Survey Manual (for access see Sect. 3.7) for use by field staff. One measurement consists of three blood pressure readings with 2-min rest between them. The third measurement can be omitted, if systolic and diastolic blood pressure of the second measurement differ less than 5% from those of the first measurement. For this purpose, a table that contains 5% tolerance intervals for a large range of measurements is provided to the field staff. Especially for younger children, it can be very helpful to perform the measurement with the child sitting on the lap of a parent with a pillow supporting his/her arm. The blood pressure monitor returns the heart rate during measurement, which is also recorded.

The measurement of body height is restricted to children who are able to stand. The stadiometer SECA 225 is used to measure standing height with shoes and hair ornaments removed and the head positioned in the Frankfort plane.

Neck, hip and mid-upper arm circumferences are measured with a flexible SECA 200 tape. The decision for neck circumference was made, since it is a quick measurement. Moreover, it seems to be well accepted, especially in obese children (Ben-Noun et al. 2001). The neck circumference is measured with the head in Frankfort plane at the point just above the larynx perpendicular to the long axis of the neck. Hip circumference is measured at the maximum extension of the buttocks in a horizontal plane. Mid-upper arm circumference is measured at the mid-point between acromiale and radiale along the lateral side of the arm. Both of these points including mid-point have to be marked with a pen on the skin of the child.

Skinfold thickness is measured twice, using manual Holtain callipers. To lower burden to survey centres and to study subjects and because some of the IDEFICS survey centres have lesser experience with skinfold measurements, only two sites (triceps and subscapular) are mandatory; two additional sites (biceps and suprailiac) are optional to the centres. All skinfold measurements are performed with extensive prior landmarking (Marfell-Jones et al. 2006), and two measurement cycles of all defined skinfolds. Biceps, triceps and subscapular skinfold sites have been defined according to the International Standards for Anthropometric Assessment published by the International Society for the Advancement of Kinanthropometry (ISAK) (Marfell-Jones et al. 2006), whereas the suprailiac skinfold site has been defined according to Lohman and colleagues (Lohman et al. 1988).

Bone stiffness is determined by ultrasonography of the calcaneus with the Lunar Achilles Insight device (Gluer et al. 2004; Herrmann et al. 2014). Both heel bones of a child are measured successively. Heels need to be amply dampened with isopropyl alcohol to ensure precision of the measurement. Readings are automatically transferred to a computer via an interface. Subjects should be asked which leg is their dominant leg in the medical interview.

All measurement results have to be documented in the recording sheet for physical examinations B (for access see Sect. 3.7).

3.5 Medical History

Medical information about the child is assessed by a parental interview done face to face by a medically trained person, preferably by a physician. The questionnaire on medical history (for access see Sect. 3.7) assesses diseases in the family (biological parents, grandparents, siblings); diseases, medications and hospital stays during pregnancy with the child; and diseases, disabilities, hospital stays and specific therapies of the child.

Parents are asked to have all drug packages (prescribed, over-counter drugs and nutritional supplements) of current medications (week preceding the interview) of the child available for the interview on medical history. Medications are recorded using a drug inspection sheet, including drug name and purpose of medication, dose and duration of intake and information whether the drug was prescribed by a physician or not. For nutritional supplements, the type of supplement, respectively the main ingredients (e.g. vitamin C), is also recorded. If the parent forgets to have the packages of current medications available, this is made up at another appointment or the information is assessed from the parent's memory. In addition to current medications, parents are asked to report any other drugs taken by their child for at least two weeks during his/her lifetime. Drugs are coded according to the Anatomical Therapeutic Chemical (ATC) Classification System and diseases according to the International Classification of Diseases and Health-Related Problems (ICD-10 for diagnoses and procedures).

3.6 Practical Experiences Gained

In general, acceptance of the physical examination modules was high among the children with only few rare exceptions. Very small children were sometimes afraid of the stadiometer and, therefore, refused height measurement. Unexpectedly, quite some children experienced the measurement of neck circumference as unpleasant, especially since a hooked-in device was used. In some countries, several of the children complained about the landmarking with a pen and the observers had to clean all landmarks meticulously after performing the measurements. This was, however, the exception. In most countries, children were proud of the landmarks ("tattoos") and liked the measurement procedures in general. Also, applying the skinfold calliper was usually not a problem when the children were shown the calliper and were allowed to try it out before the actual measurement.

Nevertheless, anthropometric measurements are not easy to perform in very young children. One reason is that most children try to look at the procedure, thus not maintaining the proper posture for the measurement. Therefore, a second observer who also can note down the results is very helpful when measuring children. In some countries, e.g. Cyprus, and in certain age groups (beginning of puberty), removal of clothes for the examinations was an issue. To enhance compliance, privacy at the examination site has to be ensured, e.g. by curtains or screens.

Blood pressure measurement was mostly rather boring for the children, and it was sometimes hard for the field staff to keep the children calm and quiet. Here, standard operating procedures (SOP) as laid down in the General Survey Manuals seem to be of limited use. Sometimes, the fieldworkers talked quietly with the child, when they had the impression that this would help keeping the child calm although the SOP is asking for not talking to the child.

Since it is recommended that the pain-reducing EMLA patch is applied 1 h before blood drawing, in some survey centres the parents were asked to apply the EMLA patch at home prior to the visit. This was partly a problem, when the patch was put on the wrong spot, or it turned out that the other arm was better suited for blood drawing. After these experiences, most survey centres altered the procedure such that the patches were applied on-site, sometimes with shortened waiting time before blood drawing. In these cases, EMLA cream offers a cheaper alternative to the patches. The response proportion for venous blood drawing in the IDEFICS baseline survey was 56.6%. In cases where venous blood drawing was refused, capillary blood was asked for. By this approach, an additional 20% of blood samples was obtained.

The ultrasonography of the heel bone was well liked by most of the children. The measurement duration was short, and the children were able to observe the measurement without obstructing it. The automated measuring process included the swelling of two elastic membranes ("balloons") filled with warm water, nestling up against the children's feet; creating a comfortable feeling on the skin. As the calcaneal bone density measurement also could serve as indicator for bone mineral density (Babaroutsi et al. 2005) and may be predictive of fractures and osteoporosis, some centres invited mothers to have measurements performed as incentive to increase their willingness to participate.

3.7 Provision of Instruments and Standard Operating Procedures to Third Parties

All instruments described in this chapter including the General Survey Manuals that provide among others all standard operating procedures can be accessed on the following website: www.lcibniz-bips.de/ifhs after registration.

Each third partner using the instruments provided in this chapter is kindly requested to cite this chapter as follows:

Bammann K, Peplies J, Mårild S, Molnár D, Suling M, Siani A, on behalf of the IDEFICS and I.Family consortia. Physical examinations. In: Bammann K, Lissner L, Pigeot I, Ahrens W, editors. Instruments for health surveys in children and adolescents. Cham: Springer Nature Switzerland; 2019. p. 47–55.

Acknowledgements The development of instruments, the baseline data collection and the first follow-up work as part of the IDEFICS study (www.idefics.eu) were financially supported by the European Commission within the Sixth RTD Framework Programme Contract No. 016181 (FOOD). The most recent follow-up including the development of new instruments and the adaptation of previously used instruments was conducted in the framework of the I.Family study (www.ifami-lystudy.eu) which was funded by the European Commission within the Seventh RTD Framework Programme Contract No. 266044 (KBBE 2010–14).

We thank all families for participating in the extensive examinations of the IDEFICS and I. Family studies. We are also grateful for the support from school boards, headmasters and communities.

References

Babaroutsi E, Magkos F, Manios Y, Sidossis LS. Body mass index, calcium intake, and physical activity affect calcaneal ultrasound in healthy Greek males in an age-dependent and parameter-specific manner. J Bone Miner Metab. 2005;23(2):157–66.

Bammann K, Huybrechts I, Vicente-Rodriguez G, Easton C, De Vriendt T, Marild S, et al. IDEFICS consortium. Validation of anthropometry and foot-to-foot bioelectrical resistance against a three-component model to assess total body fat in children: the IDEFICS study. Int J Obes (Lond). 2013;37(4):520–6.

Barba G, Buck C, Bammann K, Hadjigeorgiou C, Hebestreit A, Marild S, et al. IDEFICS consortium. Blood pressure reference values for European non-overweight school children: the IDEFICS study. Int J Obes (Lond). 2014;38(Suppl 2):S48–56.

Ben-Noun L, Sohar E, Laor A. Neck circumference as a simple screening measure for identi-fying overweight and obese patients. Obes Res. 2001;9(8):470–7.

Gibson RS. Principles of nutritional assessment. 2nd ed. Oxford: Oxford University Press; 2005.

Gluer CC, Eastell R, Reid DM, Felsenberg D, Roux C, Barkmann R, et al. Association of five quantitative ultrasound devices and bone densitometry with osteoporotic vertebral fractures in a population-based sample: the OPUS study. J Bone Miner Res. 2004;19(5):782–93.

Herrmann D, Intemann T, Lauria F, Marild S, Molnar D, Moreno LA, et al. IDEFICS consortium. Reference values of bone stiffness index and C-terminal telopeptide in healthy European children. Int J Obes (Lond). 2014;38(Suppl 2):S76–85.

Howie SR. Blood sample volumes in child health research: review of safe limits. Bull World Health Organ. 2011;89(1):46–53.

Kavey RE, Daniels SR, Flynn JT. Management of high blood pressure in children and adolescents. Cardiol Clin. 2010;28(4):597–607.

Kettaneh A, Heude B, Lommez A, Borys JM, Ducimetiere P, Charles MA. Reliability of bioimpedance analysis compared with other adiposity measurements in children: the FLVS II Study. Diabetes Metab. 2005;31(6):534–41.

Kondolot M, Horoz D, Poyrazoglu S, Borlu A, Ozturk A, Kurtoglu S, et al. Neck circumference to assess obesity in preschool children. J Clin Res Pediatr Endocrinol. 2017;9(1):17–23.

Labayen I, Moreno LA, Blay MG, Blay VA, Mesana MI, Gonzalez-Gross M, et al. Early programming of body composition and fat distribution in adolescents. J Nutr. 2006;136(1):147–52.

Lohman TG, Roche AF, Martorell R. Anthropometric standardization reference manual. Champaign, IL: Human Kinetics Publishers; 1988.

Marangoni F, Colombo C, Galli C. A method for the direct evaluation of the fatty acid status in a drop of blood from a fingertip in humans. World Rev Nutr Diet. 2005;94:139–43.

Marangoni F, Colombo C, Martiello A, Negri E, Galli C. The fatty acid profiles in a drop of blood from a fingertip correlate with physiological, dietary and lifestyle parameters in volunteers. Prostaglandins Leukot Essent Fatty Acids. 2007;76(2):87–92.

Marfell-Jones M, Olds T, Stewart A, Carter L. International standards for anthropometric assessment. Potchefstroom, South Africa: International Society for the Advancement of Kinanthropometry; 2006.

Moayyeri A, Adams JE, Adler RA, Krieg MA, Hans D, Compston J, et al. Quantitative ultrasound of the heel and fracture risk assessment: an updated meta-analysis. Osteoporos Int. 2012;23(1):143–53.

Whitehead SJ, Ford C, Gama R. A combined laboratory and field evaluation of the Cholestech LDX and CardioChek PA point-of-care testing lipid and glucose analysers. Ann Clin Biochem. 2014;51(Pt 1):54–67.

Wolters M, Dering C, Siani A, Russo P, Kaprio J, Rise P, et al. IDEFICS and I. Family consortia. The role of a FADS1 polymorphism in the association of fatty acid blood levels, BMI and blood pressure in young children-analyses based on path models. PLoS ONE. 2017;12(7): e0181485.

Zebaze RM, Brooks E, High M, Duty E, Bronson W. Reproducibility of heel ultrasound measurement in prepubescent children: lack of influence of ethnicity, sex, or body size. J Ultrasound Med. 2003;22(12):1337–40.

Chapter 4
Biological Samples—Standard Operating Procedures for Collection, Shipment, Storage and Documentation

Jenny Peplies, Kathrin Günther, Andrea Gottlieb, Annette Lübke, Karin Bammann and Wolfgang Ahrens

Abstract The collection of morning urine, stool, capillary and venous blood was a central component of the IDEFICS/I.Family studies to investigate the metabolic health of children, to assess gene expression of related genes, to determine correlates of bone health and to validate nutritional intake with biochemical markers. Saliva samples were used as a source of deoxyribonucleic acid (DNA) for genetic analyses but also to measure cortisol levels as an indicator of chronic stress. Stool samples were collected to assess the association of health outcomes like obesity with the gut microbiome. Considerable efforts were undertaken to ensure standardisation of sample collection procedures as well as pre-analytics, shipment, storage and laboratory analysis across all eight countries. Sample collection and processing were usually done outside a clinical setting, often in temporary recruitment centres set up for the study in schools or kindergartens. In order to

On behalf of the IDEFICS and I.Family consortia.

J. Peplies (✉) · K. Bammann
Working Group Epidemiology of Demographic Change,
Institute for Public Health and Nursing Research (IPP),
University of Bremen, Bremen, Germany
e-mail: jenny.peplies@uni-bremen.de

K. Günther · W. Ahrens
Leibniz Institute for Prevention Research and Epidemiology—BIPS,
Bremen, Germany

A. Gottlieb
Unit 12 "Research Services", Academic Affairs, University of Bremen,
Bremen, Germany

A. Lübke
Zentrum Für Netze (ZfN), University of Bremen, Bremen, Germany

W. Ahrens
Faculty of Mathematics and Computer Science, University of Bremen,
Bremen, Germany

© Springer Nature Switzerland AG 2019
K. Bammann et al. (eds.), *Instruments for Health Surveys in Children and Adolescents*, Springer Series on Epidemiology and Public Health,
https://doi.org/10.1007/978-3-319-98857-3_4

ensure a fail-safe fieldwork and to optimise compliance by participating children, robust and minimally invasive procedures were deployed despite their higher costs as compared to procedures commonly used in a clinical setting, e.g. a point-of-care analyser requiring only one drop of capillary blood. Quality management included the provision of detailed standard operating procedures (SOPs) to the field staff, central training, several quality control measures including site visits, establishment of a central biorepository, choice of a central certified clinical laboratory and documentation of all process steps from collection to analysis in a central laboratory information system. By collecting and analysing biological samples in a large and diverse group of small children from all over Europe, the study did not only provide important insights into the aetiology of diet- and lifestyle-related disorders and it also generated population-based, age-specific reference values obtained from healthy children that will help to improve paediatric practice in the future.

4.1 Introduction

One of the main objectives of the IDEFICS/I.Family studies was to assess the distribution of diet- and lifestyle-related health conditions and to understand the causal pathways leading there. The main emphasis of the study was put on three conditions: obesity/overweight, metabolic health and impaired bone health. Obesity/overweight was defined by age-dependent body mass index (BMI) (Cole et al. 1995), metabolic health covered all components of the metabolic syndrome (Ahrens et al. 2014a) including blood lipids (De Henauw et al. 2014), blood pressure (Barba et al. 2014), markers of insulin resistance (Peplies et al. 2014) and waist circumference (Nagy et al. 2014, 2016). Impaired bone health was defined by a low stiffness index of the heel bone assessed by ultrasonography (Herrmann et al. 2014).

Each of these health conditions is associated with a set of biological markers or is even partly defined by them, as it is the case for insulin resistance (Peplies et al. 2014). Therefore, a whole work package of the IDEFICS/I.Family studies was dedicated to biological mechanisms including the analysis of biochemical disease markers.

Fasting blood levels of glucose and insulin were used to calculate the homoeostasis model assessment (HOMA) index. Glycated haemoglobin (HbA1c) representing the average plasma glucose concentration over the last two or three months was included to verify the fasting glucose measurement since determination of fasting status was based on self-reports of the children. Blood lipids (cholesterol, high-density lipoprotein (HDL) cholesterol, triglycerides) were measured as important cardiovascular risk factors (De Henauw et al. 2014). C-reactive protein (CRP) was analysed as a marker of inflammation (Schlenz et al. 2014) which was found to be a predictor of metabolic syndrome in later life (Devaraj et al. 2009; Skinner et al. 2010).

Several minerals were included as markers of dietary habits (calcium, sodium, potassium, magnesium, phosphorus). Dietary habits were also shown to correlate well with the fatty acid (FA) composition of circulating lipids (Marangoni et al. 2007). Cortisol measured in hair, urine, saliva and serum was included in the set of markers as an indicator of chronic stress which is believed to be one of the causal factors for overweight/obesity (Vanaelst et al. 2012, 2013; Michels et al. 2013; Charmandari et al. 2003). Leptin was examined as an important regulator of body weight (Erhardt et al. 2014). It may serve to identify children at risk of obesity and also act as a factor to determine the success of an intervention programme in paediatric obesity (Venner et al. 2006). Adiponectin was analysed as an indirect regulator of glucose metabolism (Erhardt et al. 2014). It increases insulin sensitivity, improves glucose tolerance and inhibits inflammation (Jeffery et al. 2008).

Three markers were taken into account for bone health as the third main outcome (Herrmann et al. 2014; Sioen et al. 2012): serum vitamin D as the key player in bone development and bone mineral density, urinary and serum calcium and phosphate as the essential minerals for bone development and serum carboxy-terminal collagen crosslinks (CTX) as a specific marker for bone resorption (Szulc et al. 2000). In addition to the above biochemical markers, selected candidate genes were analysed in DNA obtained from mouth mucosal cells, since genetic factors are believed to play a significant role in all the health problems of interest (Gianfagna et al. 2017; Lauria et al. 2016). To provide a better insight into the pathways leading to disease development, gene expression was analysed in blood samples of a small subsample of children (Sánchez et al. 2012; Priego et al. 2014, 2015; Iacomino et al. 2016).

Most of the parameters of interest required the provision of blood serum (glucose, insulin, CRP, hormones and markers of bone health), but anticoagulated blood from tubes coated with ethylenediaminetetraacetic acid (EDTA) was also needed for HbA1c and fatty acid analysis. Minerals were measured in urine, as were albumin and glucose. Ribonucleic acid (RNA) was analysed in blood samples but DNA was extracted from saliva samples to minimise the discomfort for the children and thus also to increase the compliance. The complete set of biological markers analysed during the IDEFICS surveys and the biological materials collected for the analyses are depicted in Table 4.1.

4.2 Standardised Procedures

The standardised collection of biological samples in epidemiological multi-centre studies is a challenging task, especially in children. During the first preparatory year of the IDEFICS study, a quality management system was set up and applied to the IDEFICS survey (Peplies et al. 2010). Standardisation across different environmental conditions and settings was ensured by a set of SOPs giving detailed instructions on the collection of biological samples itself and on procedures for

Table 4.1 Overview of biological markers analysed in the IDEFICS study

Biological marker	Sample type	Remarks
Point-of-care analyses		
Blood glucose	Whole venous blood or capillary blood	Core marker
Blood lipids (cholesterol, triglycerides, HDL/LDL*)	Whole venous blood or capillary blood	Core marker
Analyses in central laboratories		
HbA1c	EDTA whole blood	Core marker
Insulin	Serum	Core marker
C-reactive protein (CRP)	Serum	Core marker
Urinary glucose	Morning urine	Core marker
Urinary albumin	Morning urine	Core marker
Urinary creatinine	Morning urine	Core marker
Selected minerals (Na, K, Mg, P, Ca)	Morning urine	Core marker
Cortisol	Morning urine	Core marker
Fatty acid profiles	Whole venous blood or capillary blood	In case–control study on overweight/obesity
Fatty acid profiles (for validation study)	EDTA plasma, RBC	In small subsample of children
Genetic markers	Saliva samples	In case–control study on overweight/obesity
Gene expression	Whole blood collected in RNA stabilising PAXgene tubes	In small subsample of children
Hormones of energy metabolism (leptin, adiponectin)	Serum	In case–control study on overweight/obesity
Markers of bone metabolism (vitamin D, Ca, β-crosslaps)	Serum	In case–control study on bone health

LDL Low-density lipoprotein; *RBC* Red blood cells; *Na* Sodium; *K* Potassium; *Mg* Magnesium; *P* Phosphorus; *Ca* Calcium

sample processing, shipment, storage and documentation. These were part of the General Survey Manual of the IDEFICS study (for access see Sect. 4.5).

In clinical research, SOPs are defined as "detailed written instructions to achieve uniformity of the performance of a specific function" (ICH 1996). We created study-specific SOPs for each type of biological sample on the following aspects:

- Collection: consent, time of collection, materials, devices, temperatures, and necessary preconditions like, e.g., fasting status.
- Processing: laboratory devices, calibration procedures, time intervals and temperature ranges allowed for processing steps.

- Shipping: conditions, intervals.
- Storage: temperatures, sorting conditions, documentation.

Biochemical analyses were carried out in a central laboratory accredited according to ISO 15189, an international standard by the International Organisation for Standardisation (ISO) for the quality management system requirements particular to medical laboratories. The IDEFICS survey manual did thus not include SOPs on laboratory procedures.

4.3   General Considerations on Practical Aspects

Study participants were only subjected to a study procedure if both the children and their parents had given their informed consent. Study subjects and their parents could consent to single components of the study while refraining from others. For ethical reasons, the amount of blood drawn varied by age, weight and height of a child and were not allowed to exceed 1% of the estimated blood volume of the child (about 10–25 ml blood can be taken from 2 to 10-year-old children).

Children were asked to donate fasting venous blood, morning urine and saliva samples. Patches with local anaesthetics (EMLA, Aspen Pharmacare Australia Pty Ltd) were offered to the children who agreed to donate venous blood to allow for a painless blood withdrawal (Shaikh et al. 2009). If venous blood could not be obtained, capillary blood was taken where possible by fingerprick. The set of blood samples generally included two tubes of venous blood: one native tube for serum collection and one EDTA tube for HbA1c analysis and the separation into plasma and red and white blood cells. Additionally, a PAXgene Blood RNA tube (PreAnalytiX GmbH, Hombrechtikon, Switzerland) containing an RNA stabilising agent was drawn from a subsample of children for gene expression analysis (Rainen et al. 2002). Morning urine was collected by the parents at home and carried to the survey centres for freezing. Saliva was collected for DNA extraction. The collection procedure for saliva differed by the children's ability to spit the required amount of saliva: Oragene DNA Collection Kit OG-250 with saliva sponges (DNA Genotek Inc., Ottawa, Ontario, Canada) was used for younger children who were usually not yet able to spit (see Table 4.2 for a description of the procedure).

Oragene DNA Self-Collection Kit OG-300 (DNA Genotek Inc., Ottawa, Ontario, Canada) was used otherwise (the application is depicted in Table 4.3).

The kits are user-friendly and provide a high amount of good quality DNA (Rogers et al. 2007). Stool samples were collected from a subsample of children for analysis of the gut microbiome. Parents collected their child's stool sample at home using a paper stool collector and tubes including a measuring spoon that were pre-filled with 8 ml of stool DNA stabiliser (PSP Spin Stool DNA Plus Kit from STRATEC Molecular, Berlin, Germany; see Table 4.4).

Samples of all types were processed at the local survey centres and shipped to the central biorepository and to the clinical laboratory for analysis at regular intervals.

Table 4.2 Saliva collection in the younger age group with OG-250 and saliva sponges

1.	Place the saliva sponge into the child's mouth in the cheek pouch (the space between the gums and the inner cheek). Gently move the saliva sponge around the upper and lower cheek pouches on both sides of the mouth to soak up as much saliva as possible. There is no need to "scrape" the inner cheek with saliva sponges— simply collect as much saliva as possible from the cheek pouches. The sponge will absorb more saliva if it is left in the child's mouth for a longer time (up to 60 s).
2.	Cut the sponge into the blue base of the Oragene kit as follows. Place the sponge firmly against the bottom of the kit between the tooth and the kit wall. This will ensure that the sponge tip remains in the container during the cutting action. Using scissors cut the narrow part of the handle just above the sponge

(continued)

Table 4.2 (continued)

3.	Collect up to five saliva sponges from the same child. A resting period of about 5 min between each collection of two sponges is helpful. To prevent the saliva samples from drying out, cap the vial (see step 4) within 15 min of the first collection If you have not had a chance to collect all 5 sponges within 15 min, you may carefully reopen the kit. If you remove the cap, be sure that the inside is facing upwards when putting it on any surface. Do not spill the contents. Follow these steps for collecting multiple sponges: 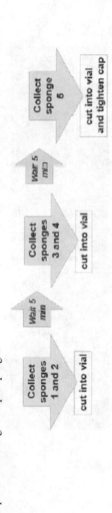
4.	Carefully cap the kit and tighten it firmly. Once the Oragene liquid is released from the cap, it will preserve the DNA collected by the sponge(s) 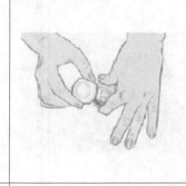

(continued)

Table 4.2 (continued)

5.	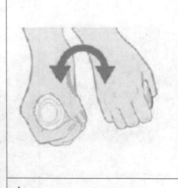	Invert gently five times to ensure that the sponge tips are covered with the Oragene solution The scissors should be rinsed with tap water and wiped dry with a disposable paper towel between donors

Pictures and instructions printed with the permission of Alere (Abbott)

Table 4.3 Saliva collection in the older age group (with OG-300)

Before use, rinse your mouth with drinking water. After rinsing, discard or swallow drinking water. Then wait 5 min before spitting saliva sample in Step 1

1	2	3	4	5
Spit until the amount of liquid saliva (not bubbles) reaches the level shown in first picture Finish spitting within 15 min	Hold tube upright Close funnel with big white cap When closed, liquid in the big white cap will be released to mix with saliva	Hold tube upright Unscrew funnel from tube (by twisting counterclockwise)	Close tube with small cap	Mix five times Throw out funnel and big white cap

Pictures and instructions printed with the permission of Alere (Abbott)

Table 4.4 Stool collection with the PSP® Spin Stool DNA Plus Kit

1 Please fix the stool collector on your toilet bowl above the surface of the water	2 Open the stool collection tube and collect a spoon of the stool sample **Attention**: Please take only one spoon of the middle of the stool sample	3 Transfer the spoon with the stool sample back into the stool collection tube and close the tube very tight	4 Mix the sample for a short time by shaking. That will lead to homogenisation of the stool sample

Avoid temperatures of more than 40 °C and direct sunlight. Keep the tube at ambient temperature (15–30 °C). Under these conditions, a cooled transport is not necessary and the DNA is protected from degradation for up to 3 days

Pictures reprinted with kind permission by Süsse Labortechnik (1), STRATEC molecular (2 and 3), and Alere/Abbott (4)

A couple of measures were aimed at increasing the response proportion for biological samples. As blood lipids and blood glucose represent the most essential markers for metabolic syndrome, these were assessed on-site by point-of-care analysis with the Cholestech LDX analyser (Panz et al. 2005). This rather expensive method was chosen as an easy-to-use and a very convenient method because one drop of either venous or capillary blood was sufficient for this procedure, and thus, the threshold for consenting to this measurement module was minimised. The immediate feedback on fasting glucose and blood lipids provided by this analyser also served as an incentive for the parents.

A description of sample analysis with this device is given in Table 4.5. The blood sample for fatty acid analysis of circulating lipids was collected via a simple kit (see Fig. 4.1) which again only needed one drop of either venous or capillary blood (Sigma-Aldrich cod. 11312-1KT).

Venous blood was collected from the blood tube by pipette; capillary blood was directly absorbed with a strip of prepared filter paper from the pricked fingertip. The method was developed by Marangoni et al. (2004) as an alternative to the conventional procedure which is rather complex regarding sample collection, storage, shipment and preparation for analysis (Wolters et al. 2014).

In order to maximise compliance, morning urine was collected at home by the parents, who received a corresponding collection kit with detailed instructions in advance to the examination.

To ensure that all study centres used exactly the same technical equipment and thus to enhance comparability, all sampling kits and processing materials were purchased centrally even though this entailed higher shipping costs, which could rise to 10% of the material costs depending on the type of consumables affected.

All procedures were centrally trained. Participation was mandatory for all survey centres. The whole set of instruments was tested during a pretest (Suling et al. 2011). During the survey, a central telephone hotline was established for the field staff to answer questions regarding collection and processing of biological samples. Survey site visits were conducted by a central quality control unit where the practical fieldwork was inspected and deviations from SOPs were corrected directly if possible, or else further actions were initiated.

Barcoded labels were used for quick and easy sample registration in the central laboratory information system (LIMS) that allowed tracking of each single aliquot from collection to laboratory analysis. Each biological sample was labelled with an unambiguous 10-digit identification number (ID) with the last two digits clearly defining the type of aliquot. The LIMS supported recording of detailed information on the pre-analytical conditions (collection, processing and storage) of each sample (e.g. cryotube or vial). Each centre used the LIMS to keep an overview of the locally collected material. The storage location for every sample (aliquot) was registered down to the position in the cryobox so that retrieval of samples for further use or withdrawal of samples could be done easily. The database also facilitated the shipping of samples to the central laboratories by an automated generation of delivery notes.

Table 4.5 Point-of-care analysis with the Cholestech LDX Analyser

1. Open the drawer Press the RUN button on the Analyser. The cassette drawer will open, and the screen will display: ``` Load cassette and press RUN. ```	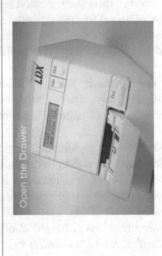
2a. **For venous blood**: Dispense the sample Draw up 35 μl of native venous blood into a standard pipette with a pipette tip. Make sure that no air bubbles are in the pipette tip Place the end of the pipette into the sample well of a test cassette and dispense 35 μl of native venous blood. Keep the cassette level after the sample has been applied Cassettes should sit at room temperature for at least 10 min before opening the pouch. They should be used as soon as the pouch is opened!	2b. **For capillary blood**: Perform a fingerstick, collect the sample and dispense the sample After cleaning the selected site with alcohol and drying it thoroughly, firmly prick the site with a lancet. Gently squeeze the finger to obtain a large drop of blood. **Wipe off the first large drop of blood** Squeeze the finger gently again until a large drop of blood forms. Hold the capillary tube horizontally by the end with the plunger. Touch it to the drop of blood without touching the skin. Fill the capillary tube within 10 s. **Do not allow any bubbles to enter the capillary tube** Place the end of the capillary tube into the sample well of a test cassette and dispense the sample by pushing down on the plunger. Keep the cassette level after the sample has been applied

(continued)

(continued)

Table 4.5 (continued)

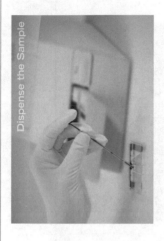

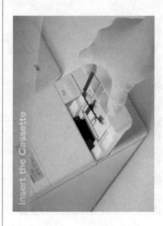

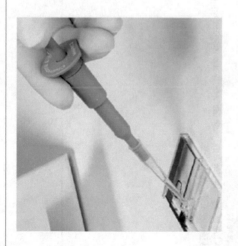

3. Insert the cassette
Immediately place the cassette into the Analyser drawer with the black reaction bar towards the Analyser and the brown magnetic stripe on the right

Table 4.5 (continued)

4. Run the test

Press RUN. The drawer will close. When the test is finished, the Analyser will beep and the drawer will open. **Put everything that touched the blood sample into a biohazardous waste container**

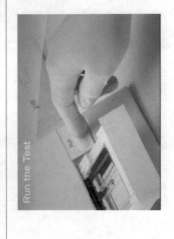

5. View the results

Press the DATA button on the Analyser once or twice (depending on the test cassette) to view remaining results

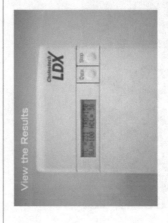

(continued)

Table 4.5 (continued)

6. Results automatically print The results will be printed when the test is finished. One, two or three labels may be printed. Additionally, data should be transferred to a computer	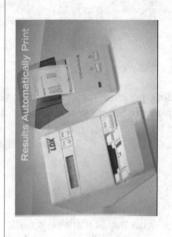

Pictures reprinted with kind permission by Alere/Abbott

Fluka //
Sigma-Aldrich Chemie GmbH
Industriestrasse 25, CH-9471 Buchs

_____Specimen Collection Paper_____

Sample Source: _____

Date: _____

Note:
• Do not touch specimen area
• Wear powder-free gloves when handling device
• Follow instructions provided with product
Notices:
• Ne pas toucher la zone d'échantillon
• Utiliser des gants non poudrés
• Suivre les instructions d'utilisations fournies
  avec le produit

Hinweis:
• Proben Bereich nicht berühren
• Pulverreie Handschuhe benützen
• Beiliegende Arbeitsanleitung einhalten
Nota:
• Non toccare l'area di raccolta
• Usare guanti "powder-free"
• Seguire le istruzioni incluse

Sigma-Aldrich Chemie GmbH
Riedstrasse 2, D-89555 Steinheim
http://www.sigma-aldrich.com

IVD LOT 6242906/51   REF 10535141 CE

2008-09

Fig. 4.1 Collection kit for fatty acid analysis

Parents were asked for their permission to store possible remaining biological samples beyond the termination of the study for subsequent research activities. A central biobank of all remaining samples was built up for future analyses.

4.4   Practical Experiences

As verified by the site visits, overall compliance with the SOPs was good in all survey centres, although some difficulties occurred concerning the standardised collection and processing of biological samples. These showed up in measures of sample quality like, e.g., problems with the fasting status, cooling of first morning urine until freezing or the failure to comply with the permitted times between collection and processing of blood samples. The varying sample quality in different survey centres is described elsewhere in detail (Peplies et al. 2010). The first version of the in-house programmed biosample database proved to be too complicated during the first IDEFICS survey. Survey centres complained about the complexity of this tool, leading to a considerable delay in data entry. Therefore, the database was replaced by a commercial web-based LIMS. However, although the original database showed limitations for monitoring the sample processing during the ongoing baseline survey, it was useful for retrospective quality control. The new commercial LIMS was introduced for the follow-up surveys and the use of a barcode scanner became mandatory to aid storage documentation.

Response proportions varied for different types of biological samples. At baseline, urine samples were provided by 85.6% of the children. Blood samples were collected from 79.7% of the children in total (capillary or venous blood) and were thus eligible for point-of-care analysis. Venous blood could be collected from 56.6% of children across all countries. The choice of a non-invasive procedure for the collection of genetic material raised the compliance by more than 50% (86.4% of children gave saliva samples compared to about 57% of children who gave venous blood) (Peplies et al. 2010). Response proportions for invasive sample collection seemed to be influenced by national characteristics, whereas differences in sample quality seemed to depend on survey logistics, e.g. allocated manpower or geographical distance between the place of sample collection and the place of pre-analytic sample processing. When two separate survey teams were employed in the two regions of a country, comparability within the country usually suffered, unless a special emphasis was put on internal quality control including the occasional exchange of personnel.

Decisions made for user-friendly solutions generally improved compliance like, e.g., point-of-care analysis of the main biological markers for metabolic syndrome (glucose, total cholesterol, HDL, triglycerides), DNA collection with saliva kits that did not need to be processed or cooled, and FA test strips that only needed one drop of blood for the analysis of complete fatty acid profiles in whole blood. These solutions were associated with high response proportions and ensured standardised quality. For example, the point-of-care analysis that was used for blood glucose and lipid analyses in a drop of blood increased participation by about 23% as compared to venipuncture. These robust and user-friendly solutions implied, however, increased costs: the price for point-of-care analysis, for example, was seven times higher compared to the laboratory analysis of the respective metabolic markers.

In order for biomarkers to be useful in accurately diagnosing and treating disorders in children and adolescents, age-specific reference values are needed. When the study began, only few age-specific reference values were available for children (Mansoub et al. 2006). The IDEFICS/I.Family studies closed this gap for several markers of clinical relevance in generating population-based, age-specific reference values obtained from healthy children for paediatric practice (Ahrens et al. 2014b).

4.5 Provision of Instruments and Standard Operating Procedures to Third Parties

All standard operating procedures (SOPs) described in this chapter are provided by the General Survey Manuals that can be accessed on the following website: www. leibniz-bips.de/ifhs after registration.

Each third partner using the SOPs provided in this chapter is kindly requested to cite this chapter as follows:

Peplies J, Günther K, Gottlieb A, Luebke A, Bammann K, Ahrens W, on behalf of the IDEFICS and I.Family consortia. Biological samples—standard operating procedures for collection, shipment, storage and documentation. In: Bammann K, Lissner L, Pigeot I, Ahrens W, editors. Instruments for health surveys in children and adolescents. Cham: Springer Nature Switzerland; 2019. p. 57–76.

Acknowledgements The development of instruments, the baseline data collection and the first follow-up work as part of the IDEFICS study (www.idefics.eu) were financially supported by the European Commission within the Sixth RTD Framework Programme Contract No. 016181 (FOOD). The most recent follow-up including the development of new instruments and the adaptation of previously used instruments was conducted in the framework of the I.Family study (www.ifamilystudy.eu) which was funded by the European Commission within the Seventh RTD Framework Programme Contract No. 266044 (KBBE 2010–14).

We thank all families for participating in the extensive examinations of the IDEFICS and I. Family studies. We are also grateful for the support from school boards, headmasters and communities.

We greatly appreciate the input of the following colleagues: Dr. Robert Scott and Dr. Yannis Pitsiladis from the Faculty of Biomedical and Life Sciences, University of Glasgow, Scotland, Dr. Alfonso Siani from Institute of Food Sciences, CNR, Avellino, Italy, and Dr. Arno Fraterman from Laboratoriumsmedizin Dr. Eberhard und Partner, Dortmund, Germany.

References

Ahrens W, Moreno LA, Mårild S, Molnár D, Siani A, De Henauw S, et al. IDEFICS consortium. Metabolic syndrome in young children: definitions and results of the IDEFICS study. Int J Obes (Lond). 2014a;38(Suppl 2):S4–14.

Ahrens W, Moreno LA, Pigeot I. Filling the gap: international reference values for health care in children. Int J Obes (Lond). 2014b;38(Suppl 2):S2–3.

Barba G, Buck C, Bammann K, Hadjigeorgiou C, Hebestreit A, Mårild S, et al. IDEFICS consortium. Blood pressure reference values for European non-overweight school children: the IDEFICS study. Int J Obes (Lond). 2014;38(Suppl 2):S48–56.

Charmandari E, Kino T, Souvatzoglou E, Chrousos GP. Pediatric stress: hormonal mediators and human development. Horm Res. 2003;59(4):161–79.

Cole TJ, Freeman JV, Preece MA. Body mass index reference curves for the UK, 1990. Arch Dis Child. 1995;73:25–9.

De Henauw S, Michels N, Vyncke K, Hebestreit A, Russo P, Intemann T, et al. IDEFICS consortium. Blood lipids among young children in Europe: results from the European IDEFICS study. Int J Obes (Lond). 2014;38(Suppl 2):S67–75.

Devaraj S, Singh U, Jialal I. Human C-reactive protein and the metabolic syndrome. Curr Opin Lipidol. 2009;20(3):182–9.

Erhardt E, Foraita R, Pigeot I, Barba G, Veidebaum T, Tornaritis M, et al. IDEFICS consortium. Reference values for leptin and adiponectin in children below the age of 10 based on the IDEFICS cohort. Int J Obes (Lond). 2014;38(Suppl 2):S32–8.

Gianfagna F, Grippi C, Ahrens W, Bailey ME, Börnhorst C, De Henauw S, et al. IDEFICS consortium. The role of neuromedin U in adiposity regulation. Haplotype analysis in European children from the IDEFICS cohort. PLoS ONE. 2017;12(2):e0172698.

Herrmann D, Intemann T, Lauria F, Mårild S, Molnár D, Moreno LA, et al. IDEFICS consortium. Reference values of bone stiffness index and C-terminal telopeptide in healthy European children. Int J Obes (Lond). 2014;38(Suppl 2):S76–85.

Iacomino G, Russo P, Stillitano I, Lauria F, Marena P, Ahrens W, et al. Circulating microRNAs are deregulated in overweight/obese children: preliminary results of the I.Family study. Genes Nutr. 2016;11:7.

International Conference on Harmonization of Technical Requirements for Registration of Pharmaceuticals for Human Use (ICH) (1996) ICH harmonised tripartite guideline—guideline for good clinical practice E6(R1), current step 4 version. https://www.ich.org/fileadmin/Public_Web_Site/ICH_Products/Guidelines/Efficacy/E6/E6_R1_Guideline.pdf. Accessed: 06 Apr 2018.

Jeffery AN, Murphy MJ, Metcalf BS, Hosking J, Voss LD, English P, et al. Adiponectin in childhood. Int J Pediatr Obes. 2008;3(3):130–40.

Lauria F, Siani A, Picó C, Ahrens W, Bammann K, De Henauw S, et al. IDEFICS consortium. A common variant and the transcript levels of MC4R gene are associated with adiposity in children: the IDEFICS study. J Clin Endocrinol Metab. 2016;101(11):4229–36.

Mansoub S, Chan MK, Adeli K. Gap analysis of pediatric reference intervals for risk biomarkers of cardiovascular disease and the metabolic syndrome. Clin Biochem. 2006;39(6):569–87.

Marangoni F, Colombo C, Galli C. A method for the direct evaluation of the fatty acid status in a drop of blood from a fingertip in humans: applicability to nutritional and epidemiological studies. Anal Biochem. 2004;326:267–72.

Marangoni F, Colombo C, Martiello A, Negri E, Galli C. The fatty acid profiles in a drop of blood from a fingertip correlate with physiological, dietary and lifestyle parameters in volunteers. Prostaglandins Leukot Essent Fatty Acids. 2007;76(2):87–92.

Michels N, Sioen I, Braet C, Huybrechts I, Vanaelst B, Wolters M, et al. Relation between salivary cortisol as stress biomarker and dietary pattern in children. Psychoneuroendocrinology. 2013;38(9):1512–20.

Nagy P, Kovacs E, Moreno LA, Veidebaum T, Tornaritis M, Kourides Y, et al. IDEFICS consortium. Percentile reference values for anthropometric body composition indices in European children from the IDEFICS study. Int J Obes (Lond). 2014;38(Suppl 2):S15–25.

Nagy P, Intemann T, Buck C, Pigeot I, Ahrens W, Molnar D. Percentile reference values for anthropometric body composition indices in European children from the IDEFICS study. Int J Obes (Lond). 2016;40(10):1604–5 [Erratum for "Nagy et al. Percentile reference values for anthropometric body composition indices in European children from the IDEFICS study. Int J Obes (Lond) 2014;38(Suppl 2):S15–25."].

Panz VR, Raal FJ, Paiker J, Immelman R, Miles H. Performance of the CardioChek PA and Cholestech LDX point-of-care analysers compared to clinical diagnostic laboratory methods for the measurement of lipids. Cardiovasc J S Afr. 2005;16(2):112–7.

Peplies J, Fraterman A, Scott R, Russo P, Bammann K. Quality management for the collection of biological samples as applied in the European multicentre study IDEFICS. Eur J Epidemiol. 2010;25:607–17.

Peplies J, Jiménez-Pavón D, Savva SC, Buck C, Günther K, Fraterman A, et al. IDEFICS consortium. Percentiles of fasting serum insulin, glucose, HbA1c and HOMA-IR in pre-pubertal normal weight European children from the IDEFICS cohort. Int J Obes (Lond). 2014;38(Suppl 2):S39–47.

Priego T, Sánchez J, Picó C, Ahrens W, Bammann K, De Henauw S, et al. IDEFICS consortium. Influence of breastfeeding on blood-cell transcript-based biomarkers of health in children. Pediatr Obes 2014;9(6):463–70.

Priego T, Sánchez J, Picó C, Ahrens W, De Henauw S, Kourides Y, et al. IDEFICS and I.Family consortia. TAS1R3 and UCN2 transcript levels in blood cells are associated with sugary and fatty food consumption in children. J Clin Endocrinol Metab. 2015;100(9):3556–64.

Rainen L, Oelmueller U, Jurgensen S, Wyrich R, Ballas C, Schram J, et al. Stabilization of mRNA expression in whole blood samples. Clin Chem. 2002;48(11):1883–90.

Rogers NL, Cole SA, Lan HC, Crossa A, Demerath EW. New saliva DNA collection method compared to buccal cell collection techniques for epidemiological studies. Am J Hum Biol. 2007;19(3):319–26.

Sánchez J, Priego T, Picó C, Ahrens W, De Henauw S, Fraterman A, et al. IDEFICS consortium. Blood cells as a source of transcriptional biomarkers of childhood obesity and its related metabolic alterations: results of the IDEFICS study. J Clin Endocrinol Metab. 2012;97(4):E648–52.

Schlenz H, Intemann T, Wolters M, González-Gil EM, Nappo A, Fraterman A, et al. IDEFICS consortium. C-reactive protein reference percentiles among pre-adolescent children in Europe based on the IDEFICS study population. Int J Obes (Lond). 2014;38(Suppl 2):S26–31.

Shaikh FM, Naqvi SA, Grace PA. The influence of a eutectic mixture of lidocaine and prilocaine on minor surgical procedures: a randomized controlled double-blind trial. Dermatol Surg. 2009;35(6):948–51.

Sioen I, Mouratidou T, Kaufman JM, Bammann K, Michels N, Pigeot I, et al. IDEFICS consortium. Determinants of vitamin D status in young children: results from the Belgian arm of the IDEFICS (Identification and prevention of dietary- and lifestyle-induced health effects in children and infants) study. Public Health Nutr. 2012;15(6):1093–9.

Skinner AC, Steiner MJ, Henderson FW, Perrin EM. Multiple markers of inflammation and weight status: cross-sectional analyses throughout childhood. Pediatrics. 2010;125(4):e801–9.

Suling M, Hebestreit A, Peplies J, Bammann K, Nappo A, Eiben G, et al. IDEFICS consortium. Design and results of the pretest of the IDEFICS study. Int J Obes (Lond). 2011;35(Suppl 1): S30–44.

Szulc P, Seeman E, Delmas PD. Biochemical measurements of bone turnover in children and adolescents. Osteoporos Int. 2000;11(4):281–94.

Vanaelst B, Huybrechts I, Bammann K, Michels N, de Vriendt T, Vyncke K, et al. Intercorrelations between serum, salivary, and hair cortisol and child-reported estimates of stress in elementary school girls. Psychophysiology. 2012;49(8):1072–81.

Vanaelst B, Michels N, De Vriendt T, Huybrechts I, Vyncke K, Sioen I, et al. Cortisone in hair of elementary school girls and its relationship with childhood stress. Eur J Pediatr. 2013;172 (6):843–6.

Venner AA, Lyon ME, Doyle-Baker PK. Leptin: a potential biomarker for childhood obesity? Clin Biochem. 2006;39(11):1047–56.

Wolters M, Schlenz H, Foraita R, Galli C, Risé P, Moreno LA, et al. IDEFICS consortium. Reference values of whole-blood fatty acids by age and sex from European children aged 3–8 years. Int J Obes (Lond). 2014;38(Suppl 2):S86–98.

Chapter 5
Web-Based 24-h Dietary Recall: The SACANA Program

Antje Hebestreit, Maike Wolters, Hannah Jilani, Gabriele Eiben
and Valeria Pala

Abstract In research, dietary intake data are mainly assessed using food frequency questionnaire (FFQ) (semi-, quantitative), 24-h dietary recall (repeated, 24HDR) or food diary/records (repeated). In the USA, a Web-based automated, self-administered 24HDR was shown to be a low-cost method for collecting accurate dietary intake information, but no such instrument was available for Europe. In I.Family, we developed a Web-based automated, self-administered 24HDR for large scale assessment of dietary intake data in children, adolescents and their families across Europe. The Self-Administered Children, Adolescents and Adults Nutrition Assessment (SACANA) program used in the I.Family study is able to assess the absolute nutrient and energy intake, the per cent contribution from foods and drinks to total energy and nutrient intake, as well as portion sizes and food groups among the children and their families. Further, place and time of all eating and snacking occasions during the past 24 h as well as eating in company and simultaneous eating activities (e.g., reading, TV watching) can be reported. The program collects self-reported dietary data in individuals from 11 years of age and above, with parental assistance at younger ages. In order to reduce errors in portion size estimation, in food composition tables and incomplete recalls the program offers features such as photo-assisted correct portion size estimation, multiple plausibility checks and reminding questions. The instrument was found to collect reproducible and valid data. SACANA is a reproducible, validated and suitable

On behalf of the IDEFICS and I.Family consortia.

A. Hebestreit (✉) · M. Wolters · H. Jilani
Leibniz Institute for Prevention Research and Epidemiology—BIPS,
Bremen, Germany
e-mail: hebestr@leibniz-bips.de

G. Eiben
University of Gothenburg, Gothenburg, Sweden

V. Pala
Fondazione IRCCS Istituto Nazionale Dei Tumori, Milan, Italy

© Springer Nature Switzerland AG 2019
K. Bammann et al. (eds.), *Instruments for Health Surveys in Children and Adolescents*, Springer Series on Epidemiology and Public Health,
https://doi.org/10.1007/978-3-319-98857-3_5

self-administered instrument for obtaining Web-based 24HDR data from children, adolescents and adults in large-scale studies across Europe.

5.1   Dietary Assessment: The 24-h Dietary Recall (24HDR)

Dietary intake assessment research presents many challenges. Over the course of days and weeks, individuals can consume hundreds of foods, exceeding the limits of most respondent's memories. The choice of the most appropriate method is important though very ambitious too, since there is no absolute reference measure of the true dietary intake. The most optimal method depends mainly on the purpose and the foreseen outcome level, e.g. groups or individuals. However, other factors are also influencing the choice of method, including time, personnel and financial resources, target population and population size. The 24-h dietary recall (24HDR) method has been used in different large-scale surveys (e.g. European Prospective Investigation into Cancer and Nutrition (EPIC) calibration study, the National Health and Nutrition Examination Survey (NHANES) and different national food consumption surveys) and has been recommended as a dietary assessment method for the use in multi-country food consumption surveys (De Henauw et al. 2002). In the I.Family study, two retrospective methods have been chosen, a 24HDR called SACANA (Self-Administered Children, Adolescents and Adult Nutrition Assessment) and a food frequency questionnaire (FFQ) (Lanfer et al. 2011; Bel-Serrat et al. 2014), which have been used in the IDEFICS study and were modified for data collection in I.Family. For detailed description of the I.Family FFQ, please see Chap. 6 of this book. The challenge in I.Family was to assess dietary habits in a multi-centre setting, where large differences in available foods and dietary patterns were to be expected. In order to get broad information about eating habits and nutrient and energy intake in the participating countries with their particular cultures, the 24HDR was implemented in combination with the FFQ. For this purpose, food groups of the FFQ are identical with 24HDR food groups (see Sect. 5.6). As any recalled day could be exceptional, the collection of data on one single day provides the dietary intake primarily on the group level, less relevant on the individual level. Thus, multiple 24HDRs are better suited for estimating long-term food intake and for taking into account large day-to-day variation of the diet. The I.Family study protocol required the assessment of three 24HDRs during a time frame of 4 weeks in a first wave and an additional triplet after 6 months in all participants, in order to capture the day-to-day variation on individual level (Willett 1998; Jahns et al. 2005; Hoffmann et al. 2002). However, if only one 24HDR per participant is available, statistical procedures can be used for estimating individual usual dietary intake using the National Cancer Institute Method (Tooze et al. 2006;

Kipnis et al. 2009) accounting for the daily variation in diet and adjusting for weekend days/weekdays, interview sequence, age and sex. Also exclusion of recalls with implausible energy reporting or stratified analysis considering plausible and misreporters may help to correct for reporting bias (Börnhorst et al. 2013).

5.2   Overview

The SACANA program was developed to assess absolute nutrient and energy intakes, the per cent contribution from foods and drinks to total energy and nutrient intake as well as portion sizes and food groups among the children and their families in the I.Family study (for access see Sect. 5.9). The software was based on the offline Self-Administered Children and Infants Nutrition Assessment (SACINA) system used during the IDEFICS study. Previous publications using SACINA data have investigated food intake, energy intake, carbohydrate intake and dietary energy density in relation to body mass index (BMI) (Hebestreit et al. 2014a, b, 2016; Hunsberger et al. 2015), daily breakfast consumption in childhood (Papoutsou et al. 2014), European children's sugar intake on weekdays and weekends (Svensson et al. 2014) and Mediterranean diet score (Tognon et al. 2014). The program has been updated from SACINA to SACANA to reflect typical food choices of older age groups (e.g. alcoholic drinks had to be added). The program was developed to collect self-reported dietary data in individuals from 11 years of age and above. As children aged 10–12 years have been proven to be reliable reporters of their food intake (Livingstone and Robson 2000), and children below 11 years were advised to ask their parents for help. Using the SACANA Web version, participants entered their dietary intake during the previous 24 h: the type and amount of all foods and drinks consumed during the previous day, starting with the first intake after waking up on the previous day. Further, place and time of all eating and snacking occasions during the past 24 h as well as eating in company and simultaneous eating activities (e.g. reading and TV watching) can be reported. The time required for one interview was 20–30 min, which was a relatively low participant burden compared to a food record. The 24HDR method as described above can be administered in different ways (e.g. as face-to-face interview or as telephone interview). In some situations (e.g. on Saturdays, holidays), it can be difficult to collect data describing intake of the previous day. In I.Family, it was decided to use an online self-reported 24HDR method, as it allows highest flexibility to enter dietary data for participants outside survey centres.

5.3   Application

5.3.1   Data Entry in Future 24HDRs

The program aims to be self-explanatory and user-friendly. Instructions are given in the program before starting the first recall to facilitate its use even by children or adult participants with low computer literacy skills, and additional instructions are available where needed (Annex 5.1). Eight country-specific SACANA versions are in use, with local as well as age-adapted food items and pictures. The program collects data for one single day (24 h) at a time and is structured according to three main meal occasions (breakfast, lunch and evening meal) plus various flexible snacks and drinks in between. Participants may complete the first 24HDR at the survey centre after provision of their login details that contains user IDs and password. Subsequent 24HDRs can be completed from home or elsewhere. Consecutive questions take the participant through a range of sequential activities (e.g. 'When did you wake up yesterday in the morning?', 'What time did you go to sleep?', 'Did you take a nap during the recorded day?', 'Where did you eat?', 'What did you do while eating?', 'Was the reported day a special day?'). These questions were intended to provide a context, which helps to recall all foods and drinks. For every meal occasion, participants are invited to select all food items eaten at that particular occasion beginning with either (a) choosing the food group displayed in the centre of the screen or (b) using a 'search' function (Fig. 5.1). The 'search' function helps particularly younger or more computer skilled individuals to track

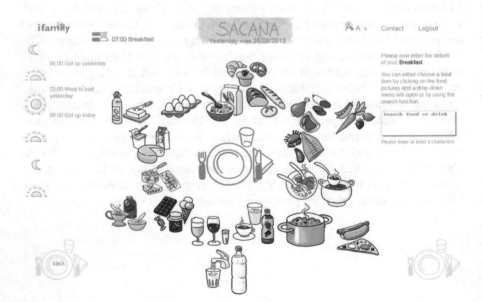

Fig. 5.1 I.Family food groups to choose from and the 'search' function

foods/drinks faster and more directly. Individuals with less computer skills may prefer to select food groups using the vignettes.

Further specification of type of food, e.g. milk plain or skimmed milk, can be entered using a systematic guide in a drop-down menu. Quantities can be assessed using standardised photos of serving sizes, standard portions, customary packing size and foods in pieces or slices. Standardisation required that the pictures were taken from a 42° angle. The food was presented on white plates with a diameter of 24 cm. If the food was presented in a bowl, the bowl was placed on the plate. A tablecloth covered the table under the place setting; knife and spoon flanked the plate with 2.9 cm distance. In addition, a spoon had to lie above the plate and a glass was placed on the upper right side.

These standardised photos assist accurate estimation of portion size: the participant can increase or decrease the portions or fluid level according to the consumed portions (see Figs. 5.2 and 5.3). The first photo displays an empty standard plate. By ticking the button 'more', the first standardised amount of food was displayed on the plate. With every tick on the button 'more', the amount of food on the plate increases, and ticking the 'less' button, the amount reduces. Up to 17 photos per food item or beverage help to estimate and enter the correct amount and thus facilitate the precise estimation of the portion size consumed. Alternatively, amounts that are known can be entered directly, e.g. 100 g of bread. Foods with commonly static amounts, such as eggs, croissants or bananas are displayed with one photo only. Other pictures display diverse filling levels of glasses and cups (Figs. 5.4 and 5.5), cans and bowls. Spreads are displayed in varying thickness on a standard slice of bread (Fig. 5.6). Corresponding pictures can be chosen by ticking the respective picture.

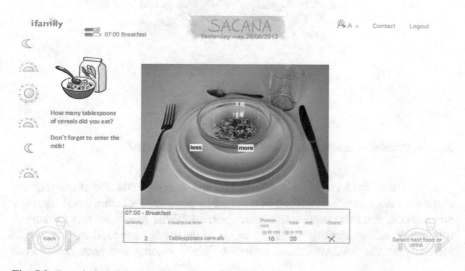

Fig. 5.2 Description and quantification of a food item (here cereals) in SACANA

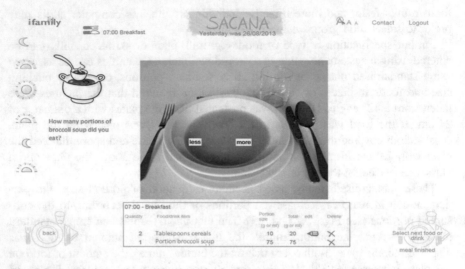

Fig. 5.3 Description and quantification of a food item (here soup) in SACANA

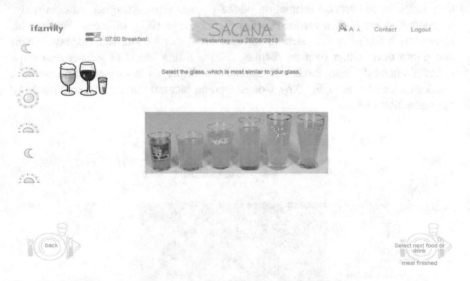

Fig. 5.4 Description and quantification of cold beverages in SACANA

If a certain food is not in the food list and consequently not displayed, the participant may describe the food as detailed as possible, including name, quantity and amount. For this purpose, the open question 'What food item was missing in the menu?' allows capturing missing foods. Afterwards, that food may be added manually to the SACANA food item list. When amount and quantity of each

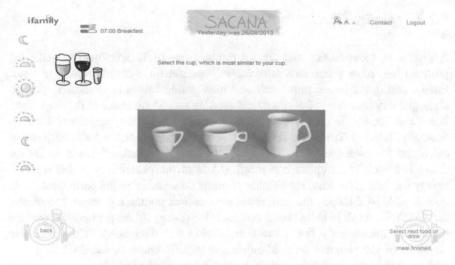

Fig. 5.5 Description and quantification of hot beverages in SACANA

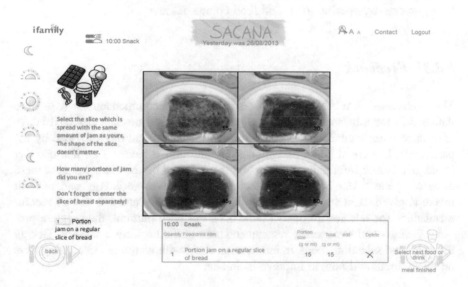

Fig. 5.6 Description and quantification of spreads (here jam) in SACANA

reported food are available, calculation of all nutrient values and total energy for the complete 24HDR is possible and the food is available in future 24HDRs. This extra information can be used, to regularly update the food item list with new pictures, standard amounts and food groups.

5.3.2   Quality Checks

A system of cross-checks and control routines has been developed to make the program less error prone and safer for self-assessment without expert guidance. Firstly, during the recall, impossible and implausible values (e.g. amount (portion size), quantity (numbers of portions) and missing meals) are checked for single food items and for single recalls and are re-confirmed with the participant directly. Secondly, internal checks for reliability are programmed with a 'reliability score' calculated for each interview. The reliability score is calculated based on (a) the duration it took to complete one recall, (b) from the plausibility of the reported energy intake and (c) from the number of corrections made by the participant. With each SACANA 24HDR, the participant may collect points, e.g. when completing the SACANA recall in more than 5 min, or if the energy intake is plausible, or if the participant makes only few corrections during the data entry. This game-like character of the program aims at enhancing attractiveness of the 24HDR recall, while gaining more and more points. Lastly, cross-checks have been programmed, and a system of probing for frequent and easily forgettable foods has been prepared based on country-specific foods and food combinations.

5.3.3   Feedback

The Web-based SACANA offers a feedback with recommendations (e.g. fibre Annex 5.2) for a balanced diet for the participants based on their personal intake after three completed 24HDRs. If there is only one recalled day provided by the participant, this could be an exceptional day and thus a feedback of just one day could give biased information to the participant. Based on the dietary data of these three complete SACANA recalls, feedback on the average energy and nutrient intake is given. It includes percentage fulfilment of daily national dietary recommendations for selected nutrients (Table 5.1). For each nutrient, the program provides the age- and sex-specific recommendation of the respective country. Ticking the nutrients' selection opens an information sheet with additional interesting facts on this nutrient and how to improve its intake.

5.4   Application Architecture

The Web application consists of a so-called N-tier architecture which is a client–server architecture. The SACANA software consists of three layers in which presentation, logic and data are separated in different layers, known as 'three-tier architecture':

Table 5.1 Nutrients displayed in the SACANA feedback

Nutrients	Recommendations (local)
Energy (kcal)	No recommendation
Carbohydrates (g and energy%)	Carbohydrates (as energy%)
Protein (g and energy%)	Protein (as energy%)
Fat (g and energy%)	Fat (as energy%)
Simple sugars (g and energy%)[a]	Simple sugars (as energy%)[a]
Fibre (g)	Fibre (g/d)
Calcium (mg)	Calcium (mg/d)
Iron (mg)	Iron (mg/d) (missing)
Folate (μg)[b]	Folate (μg/d)[b]
Vitamin C (mg)	Vitamin C (mg/d)

[a]Not available in Cyprus
[b]Not available in Cyprus and Belgium

- Presentation tier is a user interface of the application, and the main purpose of this layer is the interaction with the user. It represents and accepts data by sending and getting to and from the browser.
- Logic tier is a logic layer of the application also called middle tier, and the main function of this layer is implementing logic of a domain and perform calculations regarding this domain. It is a connection layer between the presentation and data tier.
- Data tier is a data layer of the application, and the main responsibility of this layer is to store and retrieve data from a database or another data repository. Data in this layer are used by the logic tier.

Required system software on the server side is a Web server like *Apache Web Server,* which is an open-source server that processes HTTP requests, the basic network protocol to distribute information on the World Wide Web.

Furthermore, *PHP* and *MySQL*, both open-source software projects, are used to develop the system. The *PHP* programming language is a server-side scripting language which is utilised to implement the business logic of the application, and *MySQL* is an open-source relational database management system to persist the data of the application.

On the client side, a simple browser is needed to access the application. We strongly recommend *Firefox* as a client browser for security and reliability reasons.

To run SACANA, an operating system like *Linux* or *Windows* (minimum *Windows XP*) is necessary. The server should have a minimum of 4 GB of RAM and 100 GB of free disk space.

5.5   SACANA and Its Databases

The program consists of two major components: a central editing tool called the 'basis menu' that contains all food and drink items with national pictures and standardised portion sizes for the country-specific SACANA and eight country-specific European Food Composition Tables (FCTs). The latter combines the national FCTs that were used to code the items of the basis menu with the respective nutrients. Both components are provided on one central data server at the coordinating institute. The collected data of SACANA are stored in a *MySQL* database including entries of the 24HDR and answers of the questions given under Sect. 5.3.1. Detailed information on the single components is given below.

5.5.1   Basis Menu

Every centre (country) maintains its own database of foods and drinks that are provided by the program; it is named the country-specific 'basis menu'. Prior to data collection, all food and drink items are coded with food item codes from country-specific FCTs that provide energy and nutrient contents of the food items (in 100 g standard portions). Additionally, all items of the FCTs are coded with one food group out of a set of food groups that was developed for I.Family (see Sect. 5.6). The previous linkage is important to enable direct feedback for participants after completing three SACANA recalls.

One database application that includes the configuration tool of SACANA to work on the local basis menu was provided for all centres. This database application is called 'EditBasismenu' and was developed in *Microsoft Access*. The EditBasismenu contains the forms and functions to edit the local basis menu table. The centres can enter new food items, delete food items, assign food items to FCT codes (food item codes) as well as to food group codes and improve existing food items, e.g. to include photos. Figure 5.7 shows an overview of the functions of EditBasismenu.

The applications can be used as follows:

- For editing menu data, please select Browse Menu Data. This is the editing tool for the basis menu and supports:

  - coding of food items (assigning food item codes if missing),
  - changing pre-questions, questions and remarks to 'direct addressing',
  - changing the check amount,
  - changing the response fields and the menu string total,
  - correcting food items (e.g., typos, including pictures, changing food type).

- For editing the menu structure, please select Menu Management (e.g. add new food items, change 'tree structure' of the food groups).

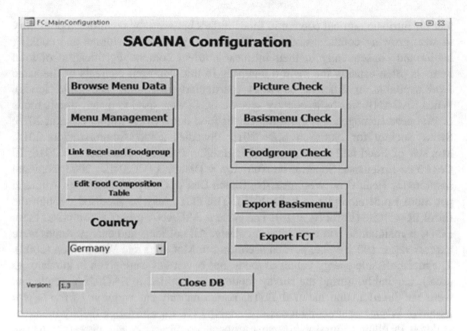

Fig. 5.7 Overview of EditBasismenu functions and choice of country

- For assigning a food group code to all food item codes of the FCT, please select Link Becel and Food group.
- Nutrient contents of food items in the local FCT (that will be necessary when assigning food group codes) can be found, and new food items/recipes can be added to the local FCT under Edit Food Composition Table.
- For receiving a report of missing pictures, please select Picture Check.
- A report of errors (missing food item codes, etc.) in the basis menu table can be extracted in Basismenu Check.
- Selecting Food group Check will provide a report of missing food group codes.
- For generating a file of the local basis menu after editing, please select Export EditBasismenu. This file is the base for the import in Web SACANA (management tool).

5.5.2   European Food Composition Tables Used in I.Family

Not only the accuracy and completeness of the reported foods but also the food composition information is an important determinant of the quality of dietary data. This requires an updated comprehensive and extensive database with nutrient values for all European foods consumed by the target population. When computing nutrient intake from information on food consumption, it was important to consider that the intrinsic nutrient content in foods differs between the countries. Foods vary in size, growing conditions, degree of maturity, processing, storage and cooking habits and consequently in their intrinsic nutrient content. Fortification of food items is often causing the main differences in micronutrient contents of the same food available in different countries (particularly for baby and child foods). When SACANA was built, country-specific FCTs were used to match simple foods or European homogeneous multi-ingredient food items (Max Rubner-Institut 2016; Swiss Society for Nutrition SSN 2015; Swedish Food Administration 2016; Minister of Food and Agriculture 2015; Belgian Federal Public Service 2016; El Centro de Enseñanza Superior de Nutrición y Dietética (CESNID) 2003; National Institute for Health and Welfare 2016; Banca Dati di Composizione degli Alimenti per Studi Epidemiologici in Italia 2015). The FCTs may be accessed through the EuroFIR website (EuroFIR 2018). The current SACANA program comprises these FCTs, is maintained and is updated regularly. All nutrients and energy values were expressed per 100 g edible portion according to McCance and Widdowson (2002). The metabolisable energy values of foods and beverages were given in kilocalories (kcal). Inevitably, during the survey foods were reported in SACANA recalls that were not listed in the national FCTs, hence subsequent addition of foods was required. While constructing a comprehensive FCT for estimating dietary intake of children in eight culturally diverse European countries, it was necessary to use multiple sources of information (Cameron and van Staveren 1988). If a particular food was not in the country FCT, a comparable food item could be used from other European FCTs according to standardised criteria. Specifically, the most comparable food item (in fat content, energy density, etc.) from another European FCT in the same food group must be chosen or the most similar food item (in fat content, energy density, etc.) from another European FCT in the same food group must be chosen. Digital versions of the country-specific FCTs were provided from all I.Family countries and are now available in SACANA for calculating nutrient intake. The completeness in nutrient values is important, because missing values in the database count as zero when calculating intake of that nutrient (with missing values). Not all countries have the advantage of a comprehensive FCT with nutrient values for all foods included. Hence, the following nutrients were chosen with respect to their relevance for dietary risk estimation and for comparing dietary intake across countries. This minimum set of thirteen nutrients for all centres are recommended and in use. The water content was not considered as a main exposure variable, but may be an important marker for the energy density of diet.

The I.Family minimal nutrient set

1. Energy
2. Total protein
3. Total fat
4. Saturated fatty acids
5. Mono-unsaturated fatty acids

6. Poly-unsaturated fatty acids
7. Total carbohydrates
8. Sugars (sum of mono-disaccharides)
9. Starch
10. Total dietary fibre
11. Calcium
12. Iron
13. Water

Additionally, an extended set of nutrients is available, for those countries with a more comprehensive FCT. Therefore, the list of nutrients was completed with nutrients that were available in all local FCTs and had reasonably compatible definitions of nutrients:

The I.Family additional set of nutrients

14. Alcohol
15. Total retinol equivalent
16. Vitamin B1—thiamine
17. Vitamin D2—riboflavin
18. Vitamin B7—total folic acid
19. Vitamin C—ascorbic acid
20. Sodium
21. Potassium
22. Magnesium
23. Phosphor
24. Zinc
25. Cholesterol

5.5.3   Minimal Requirements and Harmonisation Procedure of the FCTs

Different nutrient databases were used, varying in structure, content and reliability. It was important to harmonise the nutrient databases across countries by adopting common guidelines and procedures to prevent and minimise bias. First, all nutrient data were expressed in 100 g standard portion per food 'as consumed'. Second, all units of nutrients and energy were harmonised when expressed differently (Table 5.2). Reference units were taken from McCance and Widdowson standard units (McCance and Widdowson 2002).

As nutrient intake can only be compared when the same method was used to determine the nutrient values for all foods, nutrient values were harmonised using the documentation of the country-specific food components. Energy including dietary fibres was harmonised in order to attain total energy without energy from

Table 5.2 Standard units used in common nutrient database

Nutrient definition	Variable name	Unit (g)
Energy (kcal)	e_kcal	kcal/100
Energy (kJ)	e_kj	kJ/100
Water	water	g/100
Protein	protein	g/100
Fat	fat	g/100
Saturated fatty acids	sfa	g/100
Mono-unsaturated fatty acids	mufa	g/100
Poly-unsaturated fatty acids	pufa	g/100
Cholesterol	chol	mg/100
Total carbohydrates (digestible)	carb	g/100
Starch	starch	g/100
Total sugars—sum of mono—and disaccharides	sugars	g/100
Dietary fibre	fibre	g/100
Alcohol	alcohol	g/100
Total retinol equivalent	retinol_eq	µg/100
Vitamin B1—thiamine	thiamine	mg/100
Vitamin B2—riboflavin	riboflavin	mg/100
Vitamin B7—total folic acid	folate	µg/100
Vitamin C—ascorbic acid	vitamin C	mg/100
Sodium	na	mg/100
Potassium	k	mg/100
Calcium	ca	mg/100
Magnesium	mg	mg/100
Phosphorous	p	mg/100
Iron	fe	mg/100
Zinc	zn	mg/100

fibres. Finally, total energy was calculated in kilocalories (kcal) and kilojoules (kJ). Carbohydrate components were recalculated in grams versus monosaccharide equivalents. The analytic method was used for the estimation (sum of analysed fractions versus 'by difference' method) and if the dietary fibres were included or not. Starches were classified including or excluding dextrin and glycogen. For some FCTs, nutrient content information was missing for starch and total sugar. For these countries, the missing information was calculated from other available carbohydrate information within the respective FCT (Table 5.3). As a result, SACANA provides harmonised nutrient data for eight European countries.

Table 5.3 Calculation for missing nutrient information

Nutrient definition	Missing variable	Calculation formula
Energy (kcal)	Energy excluding fibre	Energy (kcal) incl. fibre (g)—fibre (g) $\times$ 2[a]
Energy (kJ)	Energy	Energy (kcal) $\times$ 4.1868
Carbohydrates (g)	Digestible carbohydrates (g) without fibres as glucose equivalents	Starch (g) + sugars (g)
Starch (g)	Starch	Carbohydrates (g)—sugars (g)
	Starch as glucose equivalents	Starch (in MSEQ[b])/1.1
Sugar (g)	Total sugar	Glucose + fructose + sucrose + maltose + lactose
	Total sugar	Monosaccharide + disaccharide
	Total sugar	Carbohydrates (soluble) (in MSEQ[b])/1.05

[a]We estimated missing energy excluding fibre values from interviews containing full information on energy including fibre, energy excluding fibre and total fibre using the following linear regression model: energy excl. fibre = energy incl. fibre + total fibre. The result (energy excl. fibre = 0.0037 + energy incl. fibre—4.0624 total fibre) was brought to a round figure yielding to the formula energy excl. fibre (kcal) = energy incl. fibre (kcal)—2 total fibre (g)
[b]Monosaccharide equivalents

5.5.4 Procedure in the Case of Inconsistency in Raw/Cooked Status

In general, food quantity was estimated 'as consumed' as presented in the food pictures to allow comparison of food to food group consumption, and also to relate raw to cooked food quantities in the FCTs for the calculation of nutrient data. As the majority of food items in the Italian FCT did not provide nutrient data for cooked but only for raw foods, a raw/cooked coefficient was applied when large raw/cooked deviations were expected after preparation (>20% variation due to boiling or steaming). Raw/cooked coefficients were calculated by Italian dieticians through cooking experiments (unpublished) that were conducted for the 24HDR program EPICSOFT (Pala et al. 2003). These raw/cooked coefficients (describing the weight change after preparation) were mainly applied for dried cereals (pasta, rice) and dried legumes. The raw/cooked coefficient for vegetables (e.g. for potatoes) was 0.95. Each raw ingredient was assigned to a raw/cooked coefficient. In case of no change in energy through preparation (e.g. oil) or in case that ingredients were already cooked (e.g. tinned beans), the coefficient was 1.0. It is important to note that here, only a change in weight was taken into account. This procedure did not account for any loss of vitamins and minerals during preparation.

5.6   I.Family Food Grouping Standards

The analysis of food group consumption compared to single nutrients had advantages: including the creation of eating habit scores based on relative frequencies of two or more food groups and the potential to identify common dietary patterns. This may be especially challenging in a multi-centre study design. Creation of the food grouping standard was accomplished as follows. The major target for each centre was the assignment of one of the 145 food groups to each of the SACANA food items from the 24HDRs. Since it was sometimes difficult to distinguish between a food item/dish with a single food code ID and a dish from a mixed recipe (from diverse food code IDs), an extra food group 'L' for mixed dishes was created. Here, recipes were classified based on their main ingredient. Complex baby foods were also assigned to this food group; a specific group for baby food was not provided as baby foods were often based on different ingredients. Moreover, an option was given to classify foods as 'not found' or 'invalid entry'. An overview of the current version of the food grouping standards that was used to classify the consumed foods is given in Annex 5.3. Entry of dietary supplements was not supported through the SACANA program. Hence, supplement use was recorded in an extra questionnaire of the 'health and medical history interview'. This interview collects information on therapies and medications during the past seven days prior to the examination of the child. In this way, information on supplement use during the past 24 h (SACANA reporting period) was available for later inclusion in the 24-h recall nutrient information.

5.7   Coordination, Data Cleaning and Plausibility Checks

The data flow consists of different steps: data collection, data cleaning and plausibility checks. The data which are entered by the participants in the SACANA Web tool is directly submitted to the coordinating centre. There, all previously described plausibility checks are conducted. Implausible data are identified and submitted to a data correction database. The centres have access to this data correction database and conduct corrections or deletion if necessary. Multiple steps for plausibility checks and data cleaning are recommended, since recall and reporting bias may affect data quality. Additionally, programming errors through incorrect data entry, incorrect coding or incorrect standard amounts may occur but have been found to play an almost minor role. For example, the SACANA tool does not allow missing or zero amounts and quantities which was a problem in the previous version SACINA. Therefore, missing or zero intakes do not occur in the SACANA data.

Nevertheless, solutions for varying problems have to be considered not only to data quality and data comprehensiveness but also to time and financial resources, target population and population size. The plausibility checks were item-specific (e.g. if the intake of a single item exceeds 1500 g or if the intake of a nutrient from one food item exceeds an upper cut-off) and day-specific (e.g. if the intake of daily energy exceeds an age- and sex-specific cut-off).

Experience gained during I.Family showed that after correction from the SACANA database in 0.18% of all recall days more than 5 or more implausible intakes occur. In I.Family, those recall days were excluded from following analyses. The remaining implausible intakes were imputed by sex-, age- and country-specific means. This was the case for 0.14% of all food item entries.

5.8   Validation

Measurement errors in self-reported dietary intake may explain the lack of consistency in epidemiological research of the association between diet and disease risk. Measurement error is especially challenging in studies of children where in addition to other sources of error, we also have to cope with the relative unreliability of children when self-reporting their diet (Livingstone and Robson 2000). Previously, the absolute validity of proxy-reported energy intakes from the SACINA 24HDR has been investigated based on comparison with total energy expenditure measured using the doubly-labelled water technique. The instrument was found to be valid to assess energy intake on group level rather than on individual level (Börnhorst et al. 2014).

The SACANA instrument has been validated twice (publications in progress). In a first approach, SACANA was analysed for its internal (repeatability) and external (plausibility) validity on a sample of 395 children aged 8–17 years. Participants were requested to recall their previous day's food intake twice in one day, once with the assistance of a dietician/interviewer and once without assistance in randomised order. Repeatability was examined by comparison of energy intake (EI) estimated on the first (EI1) and on the second (EI2) recall and was seen high for children which were assisted during the first recall (group 1) and moderate in children in which the first recall was unassisted (group 2). The plausibility of estimated EI was evaluated by categorising the children in under- and plausible reporters depending on their ratio of EI to basal metabolic rate (BMR): providing assistance to the child during the dietary recall significantly increased the chance to have a plausible EI report, compared to the unassisted.

To conclude, SACANA completed by children from the age of 8 years showed a good repeatability and enabled children to self-report their diet with a frequency of implausible EI reports that was similar to those of adults. The still non-negligible number of implausible recalls (about 40%) points out the need for feasible approaches to account for misreporting. Median values of energy intake were below the BMR requirement in this validation sample (data not shown), which is not surprising since under-reporting is known to be a major problem in children's self-reported dietary assessments.

In a second validation analysis, sugar intake reported by children using SACANA was compared with urinary sugars (urinary fructose and urinary sucrose) as objective marker measured in spot morning urine collected the morning after the recall day. Biomarkers that measure concentrations of specific compounds in urine, blood or other tissues may substitute or complement dietary assessment but do not necessarily have the same quantitative relationship with intake for every individual in a given study population (Jenab et al. 2009). Urinary levels of sucrose and fructose are concentration biomarkers associated with dietary intake of simple sugars. In the 1970s, it was observed that in healthy subjects a small amount of dietary fructose and sucrose are excreted in urine commensurate with their dietary intake (Menzies 1972; Nakamura and Tamura 1972). We observed that urinary sugars not only correlated with short-term total sugar intake but also with medium-term total sugar intake and usual sugar density (g/kcal) assessed by SACANA. The analysis supports the relative validity of SACANA as a self-reporting instrument for assessing sugar intake in children (Intemann et al. 2018).

These findings have important implications for the design of new studies that employ Web-based assessment tools, viz. that children can complete them by themselves if appropriate guidance is provided the first time by an instructor. In the I.Family study, at the time of the first recall, dieticians and other field personnel were available to answer any questions or doubts raised by the child during the self-assessment process.

5.9 Provision of SACANA and Standard Operating Procedures to Third Parties

The program SACANA (test version) including the General Survey Manual that provides among other all standard operating procedures can be accessed on the following website: www.leibniz-bips.de/ifhs after registration. The full program can be provided upon request.

Each third partner using SACANA or the corresponding SOPs, respectively, is kindly requested to cite this chapter as follows:

Hebestreit A, Wolters M, Jilani H, Eiben G, Pala V, on behalf of the IDEFICS and I.Family consortia. Web-based 24-hour dietary recall: the SACANA program. In: Bammann K, Lissner L, Pigeot I, Ahrens W, editors. Instruments for health surveys in children and adolescents. Cham: Springer Nature Switzerland; 2019. p. 77–102.

Acknowledgements The development of instruments, the baseline data collection and the first follow-up work as part of the IDEFICS study (www.idefics.eu) were financially supported by the European Commission within the Sixth RTD Framework Programme Contract No. 016181 (FOOD). The most recent follow-up including the development of new instruments and the adaptation of previously used instruments was conducted in the framework of the I.Family study (www.ifamilystudy.eu) which was funded by the European Commission within the Seventh RTD Framework Programme Contract No. 266044 (KBBE 2010–14).

We thank all families for participating in the extensive examinations of the IDEFICS and I. Family studies. We are also grateful for the support from school boards, headmasters and communities.

We greatly appreciate the input of the following colleagues: Markus Modzelewski from Technologie-Zentrum Informatik und Informationstechnik, Bremen, Germany, Selim Cici, Claudia Brünings-Kuppe, and Timm Intemann from the Leibniz Institute for Prevention Research and Epidemiology—BIPS, Bremen, Germany.

Annex 5.1: Instructions for Participants

How to Complete SACANA

- You are welcome to ask family members for help with filling out SACANA.
- Fill out three SACANAs on three non-consecutive days, including 2 weekdays and 1 weekend day (e.g. Monday, Wednesday and Saturday).
- Please try to complete the three SACANAs within 4 weeks.
- After completing all three SACANAs, you will receive feedback on your diet.
- It's only possible to enter the data of the day before.
- You will need about 30 min for your first SACANA and less time for the second and third.
- You can choose food or drink items either by ticking on the respective food picture or using the search function on the right side of the screen.
- Please enter everything you ingested, even a snack or drink of water.
- When you enter food items where the portion size is chosen by clicking on 'more' and a plate or a jar is filled, it may be necessary to add the item again if you need to enter a higher portion size.

Instructions for PC

- The screen size of the PC can easily be changed by pressing 'CTRL' and using the scroll wheel of the mouse. Please do not use SACANA on PCs with very small screens such as netbooks, tablets, iPads.
- You will be logged off after being non-active for 10 min. The data will be stored.
- If the computer stops responding while completing SACANA, it may be necessary to log out and to log in again afterwards. The data will be stored.
- If you need a break you can log out and continue later. The data will be stored.
- Don't react too fast, SACANA sometimes needs some time.

Annex 5.2: Example Recommendation Sheet for Fibre

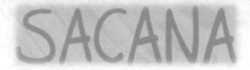

Information on dietary fibre

The term dietary fibre is used to describe a special type of plant substances in our diet that is not digested in the small intestine. In contrast to other food compounds, dietary fibres arrive at the colon undigested. Most fibres can be decomposed by the bacteria that live in the gut and are then converted to small fats and gases. From the mouth to the colon, fibres cause different physiological effects that are important for health and the prevention of certain diseases.

Tips

- Prepare vegetables like carrots and [*Please add other country specific vegetables like kohlrabi, fennel, cherry tomatoes, celery, peppers*] as a snack for between meals.

- Crisp vegetables that are ready to eat are a popular snack and will help in reducing less healthy choices like chips and snack food.

- Whole fruits, dried fruits and nuts are also fibre filled snacks. Eat fruits like apples with their skin.

Annex 5.3: I.Family Food Grouping Standards

Code	Description
A	Cereals and cereal products and starchy snacks not specified
A01	Bread, rolls and similar—not specified
A01a	Bread, crisp bread, rusks, roll (refined, fibre <5%)
A01b	Bread, crisp bread, rusks, roll (wholemeal fibre ≥ 5%)
A02	Breakfast cereals, corn flakes, muesli not specified
A02a	Complete breakfast cereals/flakes unsweetened, (sugar <15%), wholemeal (fibre ≥ 5%)
A02b	Complete breakfast cereals/flakes sweetened (sugar ≥ 15%), wholemeal (fibre ≥ 5%)
A02c	Refined breakfast cereals/flakes, unsweetened (sugar <15%, fibre <5%)
A02d	Refined breakfast cereals/flakes, sweetened, sugar added (sugar ≥ 15%, fibre <5%)
A03	Flour meals and creamed cereals without milk and sugar
A04	Pasta (any kind)
A05	Rice and other cereal grains (not ready to eat)—not specified
A05a	Rice and other cereals—white, refined
A05b	Rice and other cereals—complete, unrefined
A06	Sweet bakery, biscuits, pies (sweet), cakes, sweet fritters and other confectionery
A06a	With fat ≥ 20%
A06b	With fat <20%
A07	Savoury-fatty snacks (crisps, chips and other little snacks)
B	Sugar and sugar products
B08	Sugar, honey, jam and sweet sauces or dessert sauces
B09	Confectionery (non chocolate)
B09a	Sugar-free candies, chewing gum
B09b	Candies, candy bars, chewing gum, (with sugar)
B10	Chocolate—not specified
B10a	Chocolate bars, chocolate-coated nuts, confetti, twix, lion, mars
B10b	Chocolate spread, paste, powder, sauce
B11	Other sugar product—not specified
B11a	Marzipan, sugar-coated peanuts/almonds, nut spread
B11b	Water ice, sorbet (excluding ice cream)
B11c	No milk-based puddings
C	Fats, oils and sauces (excluding dessert sauces)
C12	Vegetable oils not specified
C12a	Olive oil
C12b	Other vegetable oils
C13	Margarine and lipids of mixed origin
C14	Butter and animal fats
C15	Sauces, dressing and condiments—not specified
C15a	Cold sauces ≥ 40% fat

(continued)

(continued)

Code	Description
C15b	Cold sauces <40% fat
C15c	Very low/no calorie condiments and other minor ingredients
C15d	Based on meat
C15e	Based on vegetables
C15f	Based on dairy
C15g	Based on fish products
C15h	Based on meat, cheese, eggs, vegetables
D	Fruits and vegetables
D16	Nuts, seeds and olives—not specified
D16a	Nuts and seeds
D16b	Olives, avocado
D17	Pulses not specified
D18	Vegetables not specified
D18a	Vegetables raw
D18b	Vegetables cooked or preserved (not deep fried)
D18c	Vegetable cooked (deep fried)
D18d	Maize all kind
D19	Potatoes and other starchy vegetables
D19a	Potatoes cooked (not deep fried)
D19b	Potatoes cooked (deep fried)
D20	Fruit not specified
D20a	Fresh fruit
D20b	Preserved fruit
D20c	Fruit and dairy
E	Non-alcoholic beverages and soups
E21	Bouillon—meat/fish/vegetable
E22	Water
E23	Coffee, tea, coffee surrogate, decaff, herbal—not specified
E24	Fruit, vegetable juices and smoothies—not specified
E24a	Fruit (and vegetable) juices—fresh-made squeezed
E24b	Fruit (and vegetable) juices—manufactured
E24c	Vegetable juices
E25	Soft and sweetened drinks
E25a	Carbonated drink (sweetened)
E25b	Carbonated drink low calorie, sugar reduced
E25c	Other drinks normally sweetened
E25d	Other drinks sugar free, reduced sugar
E25e	Energy drinks
F	Alcoholic beverages not specified
F26	Beer and cider

(continued)

(continued)

Code	Description
F27	Wine
F28	Other alcoholic drinks not specified
F28a	$\geq 20\%$ alcoholic drinks
F28b	<20% alcoholic beverages
G	Meat and meat products
G29	Meat (other than poultry)—not specified
G29a	Meat—very fatty cut/fatty preparation (fat $\geq 10\%$)
G29b	Meat—low fat preparation/lean cut and (fat <10%)
G30	Poultry not specified
G30a	Poultry fatty preparation (fat $\geq 10\%$)
G30b	Poultry non-fatty preparation (fat <10%)
G31	Rabbit and game
G32	Offal
G33	Processed meat, salami, processed poultry products, meat salad—not specified
G33a	Fatty/very fatty items (fat $\geq 20\%$)
G33b	Lean/very lean items (fat <20%)
G33c	Liver, blood and derived processed meats
H	Finfish, shellfish and their products
H34	Fish and seafood
H34a	Fish, fatty preparation
H34b	Fish, lean preparation
H35	Processed fish products
I	Eggs not specified
I36	Eggs and simple egg recipes (not fried)
I37	Eggs and simple egg recipes (fried, stir-fried)
J	Dairy products and similar
J37	Milk, yogurt and similar—not specified
J37a	Milk, plain whole
J37b	Milk, plain reduced fat
J37c	Chocolate milk, vanilla milk and similar
J37d	Yogurt, probiotic and other fermented milk unsweetened, full fat
J37e	Yogurt, probiotic and other fermented milk unsweetened, low fat
J37f	Sweet yogurt, probiotic and other fermented milk, full fat
J37g	Sweet yogurt, probiotic and other fermented milk, low fat
J38	Cheese not specified
J38a	Cheese low fat and curd (unsweetened)
J38b	Cheese medium fat/full fat (unsweetened)
J38c	Sweetened cheese and curd
J39	Other milk products—not specified
J39a	Milk-based ice creams, desserts, (chocolate) pudding

(continued)

(continued)

Code	Description
J39b	Milk-based dishes, no sugar added
J39c	Cream
K	Special products
K40	Soya products and meat and dairy substitutes not specified
K40a	Vegetarian burgers, tempeh, tofu, seitan
K40b	Vegetal milk (soya milk, rice milk etc.)
K40c	Soya-based dessert, cakes and similar
K41	Products for special nutritional use
L	Mixed dishes
L42	Based on meat not specified
L43	Based on cereals not specified
L43a	Pasta/rice/cereals + meat/fish/eggs/cheese
L43b	Pasta/rice/cereals + legumes/vegetables/potatoes
L43c	Dressed bread, pizza (Italian) and other bread-based recipes (fat <12%)
L43d	Salty pies, quiches, any kind
L43e	Fritters, yeast dough fried, fast food sandwiches, hot dog, Doner kebab and similar (fat ≥ 12%)
L44	Legumes/vegetables not specified
L44a	Soup, veloutè, LIQUID
L44b	Legumes/vegetables NOT LIQUID
L44c	Mixed salad (as a final recipe)
L45	Based on eggs or/and dairy not specified
L45b	With meat/fish
L45c	With vegetables/potatoes/cereals
L46	Based on fish not specified
L46a	Fish and vegetables/legumes
L46b	Fish and potatoes pasta/rice
L47	Based on potatoes
Z88	Item not found
Z99	Invalid entry

References

Banca Dati di Composizione degli Alimenti per Studi Epidemiologici in Italia (BDA). Food composition database for epidemiological studies in Italy. Milan, Italy: European Institute of Oncology. 2015. http://www.bda-ieo.it/. Accessed 27 Mar 2018.

Bel-Serrat S, Mouratidou T, Pala V, Huybrechts I, Börnhorst C, Fernandez-Alvira JM, et al. Relative validity of the children's eating habits questionnaire-food frequency section among young European children: the IDEFICS study. Public Health Nutr. 2014;17(2):266–76.

Belgian Federal Public Service. La Table Belge de composition des aliments. Nubel. 2016. http://www.nubel.com/fr/table-de-composition-des-aliments.html. Accessed 27 Mar 2018.

Börnhorst C, Bel-Serrat S, Pigeot I, Huybrechts I, Ottavaere C, Sioen I, et al. IDEFICS consortium. Validity of 24-h recalls in (pre-)school aged children: comparison of proxy-reported energy intakes with measured energy expenditure. Clin Nutr. 2014;33(1): 79–84.

Börnhorst C, Huybrechts I, Hebestreit A, Vanaelst B, Molnar D, Bel-Serrat S, et al. IDEFICS consortium. Diet-obesity associations in children: approaches to counteract attenuation caused by misreporting. Public Health Nutr. 2013;16(2):256–66.

Cameron ME, van Staveren WA. Manual on methodology for food consumption studies (Oxford Medical Publications). New York: Oxford University Press; 1988.

De Henauw S, Brants HA, Becker W, Kaic-Rak A, Ruprich J, Sekula W, et al. EFCOSUM Group. Operationalization of food consumption surveys in Europe: recommendations from the European food consumption survey methods (EFCOSUM) project. Eur J Clin Nutr. 2002;56 (Suppl 2):S75–88.

El Centro de Enseñanza Superior de Nutrición y Dietética (CESNID). Tablas de composición de alimentos del CESNID. Barceolona: Edicions Universitat de Barcelona; 2003.

European Food Information Resource (EuroFIR). Food composition databases. 2018. http://www.eurofir.org/food-information/food-composition-databases-2/. Accessed 6 Apr 2018.

Hebestreit A, Barba G, De Henauw S, Eiben G, Hadjigeorgiou C, Kovacs E, et al. IDEFICS consortium. Cross-sectional and longitudinal associations between energy intake and BMI z-score in European children. Int J Behav Nutr Phys Act. 2016;13(1):23.

Hebestreit A, Börnhorst C, Barba G, Siani A, Huybrechts I, Tognon G, et al. Associations between energy intake, daily food intake and energy density of foods and BMI z-score in 2-9-year-old European children. Eur J Nutr. 2014a;53(2):673–81.

Hebestreit A, Börnhorst C, Pala V, Barba G, Eiben G, Veidebaum T, et al. IDEFICS consortium. Dietary energy density in young children across Europe. Int J Obes (Lond). 2014b;38(Suppl 2): S124–34.

Hoffmann K, Boeing H, Dufour A, Volatier JL, Telman J, Virtanen M, et al. Estimating the distribution of usual dietary intake by short-term measurements. Eur J Clin Nutr. 2002;56: S53–62.

Hunsberger M, Mehlig K, Börnhorst C, Hebestreit A, Moreno L, Veidebaum T, et al. Dietary carbohydrate and nocturnal sleep duration in relation to children's BMI: findings from the IDEFICS study in eight European countries. Nutrients. 2015;7(12):10223–36.

Intemann T, Pigeot I, De Henauw S, Eiben G, Lissner L, Krogh V, et al.; I.Family consortium. Urinary sucrose and fructose to validate self-reported sugar intake in children and adolescents: results from the I.Family study. Eur J Nutr. 2018. (Epub 2018 Mar 6). https://doi.org/10.1007/s00394-018-1649-6.

Jahns L, Arab L, Carriquiry A, Popkin BM. The use of external within-person variance estimates to adjust nutrient intake distributions over time and across populations. Public Health Nutr. 2005;8(1):69–76.

Jenab M, Slimani N, Bictash M, Ferrari P, Bingham SA. Biomarkers in nutritional epidemiology: applications, needs and new horizons. Hum Genet. 2009;125(5–6):507–25.

Kipnis V, Midthune D, Buckman DW, Dodd KW, Guenther PM, Krebs-Smith SM, et al. Modeling data with excess zeros and measurement error: application to evaluating relationships between episodically consumed foods and health outcomes. Biometrics. 2009;65(4):1003–10.

Lanfer A, Hebestreit A, Ahrens W, Krogh V, Sieri S, Lissner L, et al. IDEFICS consortium. Reproducibility of food consumption frequencies derived from the children's eating habits questionnaire used in the IDEFICS study. Int J Obes (Lond). 2011;35(Suppl 1):S61–8.

Livingstone MB, Robson PJ. Measurement of dietary intake in children. Proc Nutr Soc. 2000;59 (2):279–93.

Max Rubner-Institut. Bundeslebensmittelschlüssel des Bundesministeriums für Ernährung, Landwirtschaft und Verbraucherschutz. Federal Ministry of Food and Agriculture. 2016. https://www.mri.bund.de/de/service/datenbanken/. Accessed 27 Mar 2018.

McCance RA, Widdowson EM. The composition of foods, vol. 6. Cambridge, London: The Royal Society of Chemistry and the Food Standards Agency; 2002.

Menzies IS. Urinary excretion of sugars related to oral administration of disaccharides in adult coeliac disease. Clin Sci. 1972;42(4):18P.

Minister of Food and Agriculture. The Norwegian food composition table. 2015. http://www.matportalen.no/. Accessed 27 Mar 2018.

Nakamura H, Tamura Z. Gas chromatographic analysis of mono- and disaccharides in human blood and urine after oral administration of disaccharides. Clin Chim Acta. 1972;39(2):367–81.

National Institute for Health and Welfare. Fineli, national food composition database in Finland. 2016. https://fineli.fi/fineli/en/index. Accessed 27 Mar 2018.

Pala V, Sieri S, Palli D, Salvini S, Berrino F, Bellegotti M, et al. Diet in the Italian EPIC cohorts: presentation of data and methodological issues. Tumori. 2003;89(6):594–607.

Papoutsou S, Briassoulis G, Hadjigeorgiou C, Savva SC, Solea T, Hebestreit A, et al. The combination of daily breakfast consumption and optimal breakfast choices in childhood is an important public health message. Int J Food Sci Nutr. 2014;65(3):273–9.

Svensson A, Larsson CL, Eiben G, Lanfer A, Pala V, Hebestreit A, et al. IDEFICS consortium. European childrens's intake of sugars and sugar-rich foods and drinks on weekdays versus weekends - the IDEFICS study. Eur J Clin Nutr. 2014;68(7):822–8.

Swedish Food Administration. The Swedish food composition database. National Food Agency. 2016. http://www.livsmedelsverket.se/en/food-and-content/naringsamnen/livsmedelsdatabasen/. Accessed 27 Mar 2018.

Swiss Society for Nutrition SSN. Swiss food composition table. Federal Food Safety and Veterinary Office FSVO. 2015. http://www.naehrwertdaten.ch/. Accessed 27 Mar 2018.

Tognon G, Moreno LA, Mouratidou T, Veidebaum T, Molnar D, Russo P, et al. IDEFICS consortium. Adherence to a Mediterranean-like dietary pattern in children from eight European countries. The IDEFICS study. Int J Obes (Lond). 2014;38(Suppl 2):S108–14.

Tooze JA, Midthune D, Dodd KW, Freedman LS, Krebs-Smith SM, Subar AF, et al. A new statistical method for estimating the usual intake of episodically consumed foods with application to their distribution. J Am Diet Assoc. 2006;106(10):1575–87.

Willett WC. Nutritional epidemiology, monographs in epidemiology in biostatistics. 2nd ed. New York: Oxford University Press; 1998.

Chapter 6
Dietary Behaviour in Children, Adolescents and Families: The Eating Habits Questionnaire (EHQ)

Valeria Pala, Lucia A. Reisch and Lauren Lissner

Abstract The Eating Habits Questionnaire (EHQ) was used in the IDEFICS and I.Family studies to investigate dietary behaviour, family food environments and the frequency of consumption of food items likely to be associated with overweight and general health in children, teenagers and adults. This chapter describes the rationale for developing the EHQ, as well as its methodological basis and structure. The children's version (Children's Eating Habits Questionnaire, CEHQ) is completed by a proxy reporter (usually a parent), on behalf of a child aged 2–11 years. The teenager's version (Teenagers' Eating Habits Questionnaire, TEHQ) is a self-reporting instrument for persons between 12 and 18 years. The adult version (Adult's Eating Habits Questionnaire, AEHQ) is a self-reporting instrument for respondents of 19 years and over. Most of the questions and the overall structure are closely similar in the three versions. The novelty of the EHQ is that it is a brief instrument assessing simultaneously a few dimensions of eating habits of children, teenagers and adults from the perspective of obesity-related food patterns. The EHQ has been tested and validated in eight culturally diverse European populations that participated in the IDEFICS and I.Family studies. It is expected to be useful in future studies concerned with obesity in children and their families.

On behalf of the IDEFICS and I.Family consortia

V. Pala (✉)
Fondazione IRCCS Istituto Nazionale dei Tumori, Milan, Italy
e-mail: valeria.pala@istitutotumori.mi.it

L. A. Reisch
Copenhagen Business School, Frederiksberg, Denmark

L. Lissner
Section for Epidemiology and Social Medicine (EPSO),
Department of Public Health and Community Medicine, Sahlgrenska Academy,
University of Gothenburg, Gothenburg, Sweden

© Springer Nature Switzerland AG 2019
K. Bammann et al. (eds.), *Instruments for Health Surveys in Children and Adolescents*, Springer Series on Epidemiology and Public Health,
https://doi.org/10.1007/978-3-319-98857-3_6

6.1 Introduction to the Eating Habits Questionnaire (EHQ)

Assessing dietary behaviours in multi-centre epidemiological studies is a considerable challenge. Detailed dietary assessment can be time-consuming and burdensome to participants and research staff and may adversely affect compliance. Briefer instruments, such as screeners (Golley et al. 2017; Kolodziejczyk et al. 2012), make use of a limited number of questions that assess key dietary habits and food types of concern for public health, rather than the exhaustive list of foods that characterises the classic energy-nutrient approaches to dietary assessment. However, with shorter instruments there is the problem that food types (which should include items having closely similar nutritional content in all countries) may be too generic and not easily understood by people in countries with differing cultural backgrounds and eating habits.

Diet is more than a list of foods consumed and includes eating times, places and dining companions. For instance, family eating occasions involve dimensions besides the foods put on the table, namely attitudes and behaviours, the people eating together and, in the case of our study, the attitudes and behaviours of children, siblings, parents and caregivers.

Assessing diet in children presents several additional problems. Very young children may not have sufficiently well-developed recall skills, and children under the age of 12 may have limited knowledge of what they are eating (Garcia-Dominic et al. 2010). Proxy reports (by parents, caregivers, etc.) are a solution but such reports are unlikely to be complete because some eating patterns (e.g. snacking or school meals) may be unknown to the reporter (Livingstone et al. 2004). Accounting for this requires inserting specific questions for proxy responders and in particular enquiring which of the child's eating occasions during the day the proxy was present at. For our purposes, it was also important to be able to compare food choices by members of the same family, e.g. to investigate the influence of parents' dietary choices on children's eating. We therefore had to design questions that were age-sensitive but also sufficiently similar to permit comparisons between family members.

To meet these requirements, the IDEFICS and I.Family studies developed the Eating Habits Questionnaire (EHQ), with three versions: for children, for teenagers (teens) and for adults. This questionnaire was designed to (a) assess dietary behaviour, (b) investigate the family food environment, (c) estimate the frequency of consumption of foods likely to be associated with weight status and general health in all family members. The EHQ was developed in English and translated into the languages of the participating countries (including the languages of ethnic minorities). Each language version contains descriptions of culture-specific food items The CEHQ for 2–11-year-old children is completed by a proxy reporter, usually a parent. The teenager version (TEHQ) is a self-reporting instrument for persons between 12 and 18 years. The adult version (AEHQ) is a self-reporting instrument for persons of 19 and above. For access to all three versions see Sect. 6.7.

Section 6.2 is a detailed description of the procedures and methods for questionnaire development, together with methodological issues. Section 6.3 presents the part of the questionnaire designed to elicit information on various aspects of dietary behaviours like time, place, setting and company during the meals. Section 6.4 describes a part of the questionnaire that is only present in the CEHQ, which is concerned with eliciting parental feeding practices and beliefs. Section 6.5 describes the part of the questionnaire concerned with the frequency of consumption and nutritional characteristics of selected foods. Section 6.6 examines the performance of the questionnaires during the I.Family and IDEFICS surveys and assesses their strengths and limitations.

6.2   Methods of Questionnaire Development

6.2.1   Development, Pretesting and Data Collection Procedure

The EHQ questionnaires were developed to be simple and easy to answer and without illustrations, so that they could also be completed by telephone.

They were designed for use in families and adapted in such a way that the respondent could be a proxy for the child (CEHQ), a teenager (TEHQ) or an adult (AEHQ). It was important to provide an instrument that was easily understood by parents and guardians irrespective of their educational level and cultural background, and which produced unambiguous responses. The number of items necessary to provide answers to the research questions had to be balanced against the need to keep the questionnaire as short as possible so as to ensure highest possible response proportions and data quality.

Before starting the study a beta version of the EHQ was prepared, translated into each of the study languages and sent to each survey centre for adaptation and pretesting on the parents of local children. Following a standardised training period of all the staff in all centres regarding procedure and instrumentation (Suling et al. 2011), a two-month pretest was carried out by all centres. Between ten and thirty dietary assessment tests were conducted at each centre. During this time, in-person meetings and conference calls between centre nutritionists and the study diet panel participants were held weekly to discuss problems and propose changes or amendments to the EHQ. The main aims of this pretesting phase were to determine whether the food groups included were adequate to capture the foods and food preparation methods used by the children's parents, and to check that all EHQ questions were clearly understood.

Suggestions to change wording to improve clarity and modify food groups to accommodate local dietary habits were made at this stage and were incorporated into the final version. To ensure, as far as possible, that questions were understood correctly and that food items could be recognised by respondents of different backgrounds, questions were accompanied by explanations and specific local examples. The questions were short and couched in simple language, avoiding professional jargon and abbreviations.

Once the EHQ was translated from English and adapted and tested in the eight local EHQ versions, they were back translated into English and sent to the coordinating centre. These reverse translations were useful for highlighting discrepancies between the versions of the different countries and to standardise the questions between countries. At the end of the process, all centres in the eight countries participating in the study had EHQ versions in the local language and in major immigrant languages.

The CEHQ was usually completed at school by the child's parent or caregiver. Study personnel at the schools helped parents to complete the questionnaires and also checked for completeness. At some centres, parents could take home their copy of the questionnaire and return it completed by mail or at the next scheduled visit.

The AEHQ was self-completed by parents and the TEHQ was self-completed by teenagers. Yet, as for the CEHQ, study personnel were available to help complete the questionnaires and to check for completeness.

The time taken to complete the EHQ was also tested. It is relevant since in general, questionnaire length affects response proportion reliability (Thompson and Subar 2013); moreover, in our study, an overly long time for completion of the questionnaire could interfere with other survey activities. Average compilation times for the CEHQ, TEHQ and AEHQ were each less than 20 min, with an inter-quartile range of 10–25 min, in all countries.

6.2.2 Quantification Issues

The EHQ assesses both the quality of food eaten and the frequency of intake without attempting to quantify portion sizes. The reason is that most items on the EHQ are not single and precisely defined items of food but rather food groups that are nutritionally similar but not the same. For example, the question enquiring about "*Nuts and seeds*" includes different types of foods that cannot be quantified in a consistent way (e.g. by means of number of items). Moreover, in an international multi-centre study such as ours, defining standard portions is problematic. To address the question of food quantities and portion sizes, an additional dietary assessment method—the repeated 24-h recall—was included in the survey in which portion sizes and quantities consumed are assessed by means of the food-specific multi-function quantification system: the 24-h recall assessment is discussed in detail elsewhere (see Chap. 5 of this book). For the EHQ, the previous month was chosen as the reference period and frequencies of consumption were asked from the following, close-ended, mutually exclusive list of options:

- Never/less than once a week
- 1–3 times per week
- 4–6 times per week
- Once per day
- Twice per day
- Three times per day or more.

This list of frequency categories was applied to all foods as it was found to be easily understandable and quick to use. A possible disadvantage of the list is that the highest frequencies are contained in a single category. For example, eating bread four times a day is indistinguishable from eating bread ten times a day. This does not seem to be a major problem, however, since the food frequency questions (FFQ) were not designed to detect extreme patterns of consumption but to distinguish habitual consumers from occasional consumers from those who eat the item rarely.

6.2.3 Period Investigated

When completing the EHQ, participants were asked to base their answers on "*in a typical week in the preceding month*". The previous month was chosen as the reference period as opposed to longer periods often used in dietary assessment tools for adults, in order to take into account the child's and teenager's rapidly changing diet and make it easier to give accurate estimates. The date of completion was recorded with a view to taking the season of the year into account when analysing food habits.

6.2.4 Checking Procedures and Quality Assurance

As in the pretesting stage, weekly meetings and conference calls between the principle investigators of the survey centres were held in order to ensure uniform procedures over all countries and a thorough understanding of the EHQ's purpose and administration procedures in the centres. A manual was given to local nutritionists and staff explaining how to interpret questions if a respondent did not understand. All questionnaires were checked after being completed by study personnel in order to minimise missing data.

6.3   Eating Behaviour Questions

6.3.1   Usual Meal Patterns

The usual meal pattern is investigated by the question "*How often does your child/ do you usually eat (breakfast, lunch, etc.)*"?

This question is included in all three versions, CEHQ, TEHQ and AEHQ. There is growing interest in meal pattern behaviours as the frequency and timing of food consumption occasions may influence appetite control, dietary intake and composition, activity of the gastrointestinal system and several aspects of glucose and lipid metabolism (Stenvers et al. 2012). For example, regular consumption of breakfast has been associated with a healthier diet and better health status (Hallstrom et al. 2013; Hunsberger et al. 2015) and the substitution of a skipped main meal with a snack has been pointed out as a possible cause of overeating and overweight (Dykstra et al. 2016; Karatzi et al. 2017). In addition, it has been suggested that lack of clear rules about food consumption is associated with unhealthy eating behaviour for adolescents (Holubcikova et al. 2016).

The question on usual meal patterns asks how many times in a typical week in the preceding month a meal or a snack was consumed. The frequencies of the following meals are requested: breakfast, morning snack(s), lunch, afternoon snack (s), dinner and evening snack(s). Possible replies to this question and transforming of frequencies are shown in Table 6.1.

6.3.2   Frequency of Meals Eaten with Parents' Knowledge

In addition, the proportion of the child's meals eaten under parental control is investigated by the question "*How often does your child usually eat a meal or a snack in your presence*"? Therefore, it only appears in the CEHQ and is not included in the teenager's (TEHQ) or the adult's (AEHQ) questionnaires. The parent is asked to state how many times in a typical week in the preceding month

Table 6.1 Coding of EHQ frequency categories

Reply entered in the EHQ	Frequency (*times per week*)
Never	0
On fewer occasions than once a week	0.2
1–2 times per week	1.5
3–6 times per week	4.5
Daily	7

the child ate each of the meals in their presence or under their control: breakfast, morning snack(s), lunch, afternoon snack(s), dinner and evening snack(s). Possible replies to this question and corresponding imputed frequencies are the same as those shown in Table 6.1.

There has been a marked increase in eating meals away from home together with a decrease in the number of occasions when the family eats together (Devine et al. 2009; Kant and Graubard 2004; Orfanos et al. 2009). These trends, together with changes in dietary habits during the transition from infancy to childhood, effectively reduce the amount of control that parents have on their children's diet in terms of quality and quantity. Findings from several studies suggest that parental control of meals is associated with a healthier diet in children, and that regular family meals during childhood and early adolescence may contribute to the formation of healthy eating habits (Burgess-Champoux et al. 2009; Valdes et al. 2013). In one study, adolescents who ate more frequently with their families reported a lowered risk of disordered eating behaviours (Neumark-Sztainer et al. 2008). Also, it has been suggested that lack of parental clear rule-setting on food consumption is associated with unhealthy eating behaviour in boys and girls (Holubcikova et al. 2016).

However, other studies suggest that excessive parental control over children's eating habits may interfere with the children's ability to regulate their food intake, potentially resulting in overweight (Birch and Fisher 1998) and that parental control is not always associated with a healthier diet in children (Fisher et al. 2002; Wardle et al. 2005; Robinson et al. 2001). Responses to this question will make it possible to investigate the complex relationships between parental control of children's food intake, parental feeding styles/food behaviour and children's dietary habits. Parental responses also tell us about the completeness of the information obtained and make it possible to adjust the food intake estimation derived from the food frequency sections of the EHQ (see Sect. 6.5).

6.3.3 Eating While Doing Something Else

The habit of performing other activities during meals is enquired by the question "*How often does your child/do you eat while doing something else*"? This question is included in CEHQ, TEHQ and AEHQ versions and enquires about the daily frequency of meals that are eaten while distracted by performing other activities (e.g. TV, computer, smartphone or reading). The aim is to investigate whether performing other activities while eating is independently associated with one's food quality and health status. Consuming meals while watching TV or with attention on other activities like video games has been associated with the children's poor dietary quality (Avery et al. 2017) and development of obesity in several epidemiological studies (Gortmaker et al. 1996; Monasta et al. 2010; Robinson 1998, 2001) and various mechanisms by which television viewing patterns are thought to affect children's weight have been discussed (Reisch et al. 2013). TV and other media may influence children's dietary choices as they are regularly exposed to advertising of energy-dense nutrient-poor foods (Boyland et al. 2011; Harris and Bargh 2009). The cognitive immaturity of children increases their receptiveness to advertisements for foods of poor nutritional quality, which are typically broadcast during children's television programmes and are believed to lead to unhealthy food preferences and dietary imbalances associated with obesity. Another mechanism by which TV could promote obesity is reduction of time spent doing physical activity, which results in lower energy expenditure. However, this suggestion is not supported by American (Epstein et al. 2008) and European (Manios et al. 2009) studies which found that the effect of TV time on childhood obesity was independent of the amount of physical activity they engaged in.

Answers to this question enable investigation of a third, understudied possible mechanism leading to childhood obesity, i.e. the effect of attention being elsewhere during food intake. Early studies of children and later studies of adults (Bellisle and Dalix 2001; Bellisle et al. 2009), adolescents (Stroebele and de Castro 2004) as well as children (Dubois et al. 2008; MacFarlane et al. 2009) suggest that the normal internal cues regulating food intake are less effective while watching TV (or when one's attention is elsewhere).

6.3.4 Food Restrictions

The question "*Does your child/do you typically exclude any of the following food items*"? is included in CEHQ, TEHQ and AEHQ versions and aims to capture special dietary patterns such as those practised by particular religious, cultural or other subgroups and which would not be easily identified from food frequency questions. This question focuses on those classes of foods sourced from animals that are typically avoided such as meat, fish, dairy and eggs. By integrating this information with the food frequency section of the EHQ and with dietary data from the 24 h dietary recall (see Chap. 5 of this book), it will be possible to determine whether important sources of nutrients are missing from these diets or whether they are available from alternative sources. Feeding patterns related to conditions such as allergies and intolerance are investigated through a specific question asked of parents as part of the child's medical history.

It is important to enquire about foods that are avoided and the extent to which these are substituted by others that are nutritionally equivalent in order to formulate culturally acceptable advice to reduce the risk of obesity in children from ethnic or religious minorities (Maynard et al. 2009). Studies from the USA and UK, i.e. countries with long-established ethnic minority groups, have shown that ethnicity is a consistent correlate of childhood obesity (Dubois et al. 2008; Ogden et al. 2006, 2010; Saxena et al. 2004; Taylor et al. 2005). However, little is known to date about obesity in children belonging to minority groups in other European countries.

According to the 2016 International Migration Outlook (IMO) by the Organisation for Economic Co-operation and Development (OECD) (IMO 2016) permanent migration flows increased sharply in the OECD area in 2015. Around 4.8 million people migrated permanently to OECD countries in 2015, about ten per cent more than in 2014, and numbers are expected to increase in the coming years. Thus, the variety of dietary styles is likely to increase in Europe and it will be a challenge to monitor these styles, their modifications and their correlations with the health of the new citizens.

6.3.5   Fast Food Restaurants and Street Vendors

The question *"How many times does your child/do you eat in a fast food restaurant or at stands or kiosk"*? is included in CEHQ, TEHQ and AEHQ versions and is concerned with how often a full meal is eaten at a fast food outlet (i.e. how often fast food substitutes a "normal" meal) and how often fast food is eaten between meals. There are several definitions of fast food restaurants; some of them focus on the way the food is eaten, i.e. quickly, often while standing, in crowded areas inside or outside the premises where the food is bought (Wang et al. 2016). Other definitions consider what is eaten and refers to foods that are high in fat and refined carbohydrate with a low-nutrient/energy ratio (Fleischhacker et al. 2011).

Both fast-eating and eating high-calorie, low-nutrient foods have been associated with overweight in children (Larson and Story 2009; Sugimori et al. 2004). Some fast food chains have acknowledged this and have turned to offer healthier foods and the possibility of consuming them more slowly in a more convivial environment. It has been shown that obese and overweight children eat faster than normal weight children and do not slow down towards the end of meal as normal weight children do (Barkeling et al. 1992). Fast food restaurants and menus provide environmental cues that may trigger overeating (Garber and Lustig 2011). For example, children who often eat in a hurry and in fast food settings might be distracted from noticing satiety signals by such environments and therefore tend to overeat. By means of question 6.3.5, the *place/setting* effect of fast food consumption can be distinguished from the effect of high-calorie, low-nutrient food per se (investigated in the food frequency section of the EHQ) to determine whether place/setting has an independent effect on children's health. Another possible mechanism whereby fast food is linked with obesity could be via the increase in portion sizes. The association of fast food consumption with portion sizes will be investigated by comparing replies to this question with quantification of portion sizes by means of the 24-h dietary recall instrument used in the I.Family study (SACANA) (see Chap. 5 of this book).

6.4   Family Food Environment Questions

6.4.1   The Family Food Environment

Questions on food environment are only included in the children's version of the questionnaire (CEHQ) that was completed by a proxy reporter (usually a parent). These questions aim to measure parental eating- and weight-related attitudes as well as parental worries towards their child's food style. The underlying hypothesis is that parents' eating and weight-related attitudes and their worries about their children's eating patterns directly and indirectly influence their pedagogic approach as regards family food styles and food management—and ultimately, their children's eating behaviour. Worries might lead to tensions around eating and meals, power struggles with the child, more or less stressful family meals as well as specific reward and punishment strategies, all in the effort to gain more control over the child's diet. Also, parents of overweight children who are not worried about their child's body mass index (BMI) might equally be problematic. Either interest in their child's health could be low or their sense of the appropriate weight and BMI departs from official norms. Some of the questions are included to reveal whether the parent has a realistic view of the child's weight status, since the child's BMI and the parental perception of the child's weight status are both assessed in this study.

The questions were compiled by a group of experts within the IDEFICS project in 2007/8. The topics were collected from the literature on parent–child food styles and were inspired by different existing instruments available a decade ago. Of particular, influence was the work by Diehl (1999). Questions on parental feeding practices originated from the maternal feeding questionnaire for pre-schoolers by Baughcum et al. (2001). For the IDEFICS study, only those items with the highest factor loadings were chosen from this questionnaire and both parents were addressed. The ten chosen items (see Sects. 6.4.2–6.4.11) cover five constructs: difficulty on child feeding; concern about children overeating and becoming overweight; pushing the child to eat more; the situation and structure during feeding; age-inappropriate feeding.

The questions were included in the pretesting of the overall questionnaire. Answer categories are provided on a five-point Likert scale (never–rarely–sometimes–often–always).

6.4.2   Struggling with Child's Food Intake

The question asked in the CEHQ is: "*Is it a struggle to get your child to eat*"? The item should reveal whether the parent thinks that the child is a difficult or picky eater. Potentially, meals might be conceived as stressful and there might be a power struggle and debates over food and eating styles going on.

6.4.3   Self-Feeding Versus Parental Feeding

The question asked is: "*Do you feed your child yourself if he/she does not eat enough*"*?* When parents think that their child does not eat enough, they might try to feed the child by either forcing him/her ("feed") or by other means of convincing such as bribes or rewards. The question should also reveal, when assessed against the reported actual diet and BMI of the child, whether parents' perception of what is "enough" is justified. This question is more relevant for younger children who are largely under the food control of their parents. It might be less appropriate for older children.

6.4.4   How to Stop Overeating

The question asked is "*Do you have to stop your child from eating too much*"*?* This item reveals whether the parent thinks that the child is eating too much (which can be cross-checked with the reported diet) and additionally, whether the parent takes action or not. Again, this item is about recognising real or assumed problem behaviour and about having control and taking action.

6.4.5   Thinks Child Should Be Put on Diet

The question asked is: "*Do you think about putting your child on a diet to keep him/her from becoming overweight*"? The item reveals whether the parent thinks that the child is overweight and whether he/she thinks that a diet is a useful and feasible strategy. Traditional weight loss diets have increasingly been criticised as because of the "Yo-yo effect", particularly in adults (Lowe et al. 2013). Diets come with rigid rules for "healthy eating" that are disconnected from internal cues like hunger or emotional issues such as stress.

6.4.6   Making Children Finish All Food

The question asked is: "*Do you make your child eat all the food on his/her plate*"? Forcing children to finishing all the food on their plate has been a long-standing parental rule. However, it might prevent children from developing their own sense of being full and to stop eating when they are not hungry any longer. Hence, this parental routine might be conducive for becoming overweight.

6.4.7   Thinks Child Eats Too Much

The question asked is: "*Do you worry that your child is eating too much*"? If the parent worries that the child eats too much, expectations regarding the ideal weight have been violated and the parent might be afraid of the child being/becoming overweight.

6.4.8   Thinks Child Doesn't Eat Enough

The question asked is: "*Do you worry that your child is not eating enough*"? If the parent worries that the child isn't eating enough, expectations regarding the ideal weight might have been violated and the parent might be afraid of the child being/becoming underweight.

6.4.9   Use of Favourite Foods as Rewards for Healthy Food Intake

The question asked is: "*Do you use foods that your child likes as a way to get your child to eat 'healthy' foods he/she does not like?*" A common parental practice is to "bribe" children by rewarding them with their favourite food if they also eat "healthy" food. In this way, the child might learn that healthy foods are not likeable but only acceptable if they come together with rewards. Potential liking of the healthy food might be inhibited by this pedagogic strategy. In other words, the child's intrinsic motivation might be displaced by an extrinsic stimulus (i.e. the food reward).

6.4.10   Child Has Poor Appetite

The question asked is: "*Does your child have a poor appetite*"? If parents perceive the child as a poor eater with low appetite, they might adapt their food strategy accordingly and might potentially offer more nutritious food and/or food strongly preferred by the child. Parents might also worry about the general health of their child if he/she has poor appetite.

6.4.11   Sitting Down with Child at Meals

The question asked is: "*Do you sit down with your child when he/she eats meals*"? Having a meal together seems to be a family activity that might promote healthy eating in a positive way. Parents who take the time to share a meal with their children might act as role models and transfer knowledge and positive attitudes, both directly and indirectly (see also Sect. 6.3.2).

6.5   Food Frequency Questions

6.5.1   Introduction to Food Frequency Questions

The question "*In the last month, how many times did your child/you eat or drink the following food items*"? enquires about the frequency of intake of selected food items. In the CEHQ, the parents were asked to indicate only foods and drinks they knew about, i.e. what their child ate in their presence.

A questionnaire enquiring about the frequency of intake of specific foods is one of the most common tools used in large-scale population-based studies to examine the relation between diet and disease, owing to easy administration and low cost. The EHQ part that enquires about food frequency, referred to here as food frequency questions (FFQ), is specifically designed to investigate the consumption of foods shown by consistent evidence to be related, either positively or negatively, to overweight and obesity in children. The FFQ from the adult, teen and proxy child versions of the EHQ have the same structure and enquire about the same food items, except for the question regarding alcohol consumption, which, for ethical reasons, is not present in the proxy child version.

In the FFQ special emphasis is placed on foods (e.g. olive oil, raw and fresh non-processed vegetables and deep-fried foods) that could represent typical dietary patterns in many countries and thereby facilitate international comparisons. Frequency of food groups that are the main ingredients of mixed dishes should be reported separately, e.g. "chilli con carne" should be considered part of two different food groups; once under "meat" and again under "legumes".

The FFQ was not designed to estimate total energy intake or total food intake but aims to distinguish healthy from unhealthy food forms (e.g. white vs. wholemeal bread).

The food frequency questions are grouped into 15 food groups, namely vegetables; fresh fruits; drinks; breakfast cereals; milk; yoghurt; fish; meat and meat products; eggs and mayonnaise; meat replacement products and soy products; cheese; spreadable products; olive oil; cereal products; and snacks.

The 15 food groups have a variable number of food items (questions) for a total of 60 food items in TEHQ and AEHQ and 59 in the CEHQ (no question on alcohol consumption). The sequence of food items queried for each food group was designed to avoid confusion and to minimise the risk of double reporting for the same food. The list of food items and food groups was developed in English translated into eleven languages, namely Estonian, Flemish, French, German, Greek, Hungarian, Italian, Russian, Spanish, Swedish and Turkish, i.e. the languages spoken by majority or minority study groups within the study's community settings. For the local versions, it was important to minimise departures from the original format in order to obtain comparable data on eating behaviour across all participating centres. The rationale governing the choice and wording of the foods/food groups investigated by the FFQ are presented in the following sections.

6.5.2   Vegetables

Dietary energy density can be reduced by increasing intake of water- and fibre-rich foods such as vegetables, which also induce satiation (Rolls 2009). Starting a meal with a vegetable course and increasing the proportion of vegetables in the main course has been found to reduce hunger and to moderate energy intake (Flood and Rolls 2007; Rolls et al. 2004). Data from several clinical trials have shown that reducing dietary energy density by increasing the proportion of vegetables is an effective strategy for moderating children's (Leahy et al. 2008) and adult's (Ello-Martin et al. 2005) energy intake, resulting in substantial weight loss, even though participants ate greater quantities of food.

Vegetables are divided into five subgroups in the FFQ: legumes; potatoes divided into fried and not fried; all other cooked vegetables; and all raw vegetables.

Legumes (dietary pulse), defined as non-oilseed legumes harvested solely for their grain (e.g. beans, peas, chickpeas, broad beans and lentils), are high in fibre and protein and low in glycaemic index, which are properties that have been shown to reduce appetite (Li et al. 2014) and chronic disease risk (Bazzano et al. 2001). The protein and carbohydrate of legumes are absorbed slowly, and legume protein is known to increase glucagons release, which enhances fat oxidation and inhibits lipogenesis by down-regulating lipogenic enzymes (McCarty 2000).

A separate question is asked about the consumption of fried potatoes/French fries/croquettes. These foods have high energy content [163 kcal/100 g, fried potatoes, 223 kcal/100 g, croquette potatoes and 276 kcal/100 g, French fries according to the United States Department of Agriculture (USDA)] and are a major component of the Western diet. High consumption of these foods has been associated with overweight and obesity in children (Fox et al. 2009; Receveur et al. 2008). French fries and similar foods are the most commonly consumed vegetable by children who eat a school lunch in the USA (Condon et al. 2009). Reduction in consumption of French fries is one of the first changes parents say they make to the diets of their overweight children, so the reporting of their consumption is likely to be biased by social desirability.

Potatoes (not fried) are documented separately from other cooked vegetables because of their high starch content and consequently higher energy density compared to other vegetables. However, non-fried potatoes could be considered to belong to the same pattern as other cooked vegetables and may help to identify children who usually consume a hot meal with one or more vegetables. This type of meal is likely to be at home and served at the table and is more likely to have a good nutrient density/energy density ratio. Regular consumption of raw vegetables is known to improve insulin sensitivity and body weight control (Song et al. 2005). A recent analysis conducted in I. Family (Pala et al. 2013) based on CEHQ data suggests that children with the highest vegetable consumption, especially raw vegetables, had the lowest risk of becoming overweight/obese. Raw vegetables seem to exert a greater and more prolonged satiety effect than cooked vegetables (Gustafsson et al. 1995a, b). From the nutritional point of view, raw vegetables have nutrient density scores (NDS) that are among the highest of any food group. NDS is defined as the ratio of nutrient density to energy density of a food (Drewnowski and Fulgoni III 2008; Maillot et al. 2008). A low NDS diet (e.g. low in raw vegetables) may be an indirect correlate of obesity if excessive calories are necessarily consumed in order to achieve the recommended daily intake of vitamins and micronutrients. Unfortunately in many developed countries, fresh vegetables are fairly expensive. A national survey in the UK on low income and diet showed that the most deprived 15% of the population were less likely to consume fresh vegetables (Nelson et al. 2010). Several other studies in European (North and Emmett 2000; Ruxton et al. 1996) and non-European countries (Beydoun and Wang 2008; Lorson et al. 2009; Kirkpatrick and Tarasuk 2008; Kettings et al. 2009) reported similar findings. Cultural factors and a city environment (Pala et al. 2002) might also be important in influencing the consumption of raw vegetables and can interact with socio-economic factors limiting their consumption. In the USA, dietary recommendations directed at low-income groups make a point of suggesting less costly fresh vegetables with a favourable nutrient to price ratio (Hampson et al. 2009; Drewnowski 2010).

For hypertension, coronary heart disease, stroke and several cancer sites, there is convincing evidence that increasing the consumption of vegetables reduces the risk of disease (Boeing et al. 2012). Therefore, from a scientific point of view, national campaigns to increase vegetable and fruit consumption are justified. That eating more vegetables will result in lower risk of weight gain is a commonly espoused proposition as a person presumably will eat less of other foods, and the resulting reduction in calories will be greater than the increase in calories from vegetables. However, this fact has neither been proved nor clearly disproved (Casazza et al. 2013), so the collection of solid data from this and other studies will help to clarify the subject.

6.5.3 Fresh Fruits

The FFQ does not attempt to assess different kinds of fruits; instead, it classifies them together with fresh-squeezed fruit juices. The only additional question is about adding sugar to fruit, which provides information about simple sugar intake as well as about taste preferences.

Fruits, like vegetables, have high nutrient and vitamin density and low-energy density and their consumption helps prevent overweight in children and adults (Hampson et al. 2009; Epstein et al. 2001; Roblin 2007; Silva-Sanigorski et al. 2010). In pre-adolescent children, breakfast and morning snacks based on fruit and low glycaemic index (GI) food have been shown to have a significant impact on the reduction of food intake at lunch (Warren et al. 2003). The high palatability and the sweet taste of fresh fruit make it suitable and ideal for children's dietary intervention aimed at increasing diet quality. It has been reported that dietary intervention based on fruit is more effective (Overby et al. 2012) and sustained over time (Bere et al. 2007) compared with vegetables in reducing the frequency of unhealthy snack consumption in schoolchildren.

6.5.4   Drinks

It is recognised that the increasing use of sweetened drinks with a concomitant reduction in water consumption is strongly associated with obesity in children (Ludwig et al. 2001) and adolescents (Berkey et al. 2004). Sugar-rich drinks like fruit juices that may have some nutrient and fibre content and sweetened drinks (particularly sugar-sweetened beverages) with very high GI (Foster-Powell et al. 2002) are also likely to have a very low-nutrient content. The beneficial effect on body weight of reducing consumption of sweetened drinks is compelling (Brownell et al. 2009; Ebbeling et al. 2006; Council on School Health 2015).

The FFQ distinguishes between water, packaged fruit juices, carbonated sugar drinks (regular and sugar-reduced) and other sweetened drinks (regular and sugar-reduced). Consumption of hot beverages like coffee, tea or herbal teas is also captured with details about sugar content.

Consumption of reduced sugar and artificially sweetened drinks may indicate an attempt by the parents to reduce the energy intake of the child. It has been observed that parents of high (as opposed to low) socio-economic status are more likely to use this strategy to control obesity (Lopez-Alvarenga et al. 2007). Regarding the effectiveness of artificially sweetened drinks, there is some evidence that they may help adults to maintain weight loss if used to replace sugar-sweetened beverages (Phelan et al. 2009; Raben et al. 2002). However, the sparse evidence available for children from cross-sectional (O'Connor et al. 2006) and prospective studies (Johnson et al. 2007) does not clearly support consumption of low-energy beverages as part of an effective weight-control programme.

As explained above, consumption of alcoholic beverages is only asked of teens (TEHQ) and adults (AEHQ) and is not included in the CEHQ.

6.5.5   Breakfast Cereals

Feedback from centres during the pilot phase indicated that breakfast cereals are among the most common foods eaten by children at breakfast time. In many areas, they are displacing bread and biscuits as products to eat with milk or yoghurt. Breakfast cereal consumption has been associated with enhanced diet quality and nutritional profile in children and adults (van den Boom et al. 2006) and lower BMI in children (Barton et al. 2005); but the "protective" effect might have been driven by the indirect "protective" effect of having breakfast as a meal (Song et al. 2006; Szajewska and Ruszczynski 2010; MacFarlane et al. 2009). To ensure a simple but meaningful classification comprehensible to participants in all countries, we distinguished ready-to-eat, sweetened cereals (usually with high GI) from unsweetened products (ready-to-eat or requiring cooking, usually with fairly low GI) (Foster-Powell et al. 2002).

6.5.6   Milk and Yoghurt

Rising childhood obesity rates have coincided with a secular decline in dairy consumption (Nicklas et al. 2004). Some studies (Carruth and Skinner 2001; Barba et al. 2005; Moore et al. 2006; Kral et al. 2008) but not all (Bradlee et al. 2010; Moore et al. 2008; Warren et al. 2003; O'Connor et al. 2006; Huh et al. 2010; Gunther et al. 2007; Fiorito et al. 2006; St Onge et al. 2009; Ghayour-Mobarhan et al. 2009) have suggested an inverse association between milk or dairy intake and children's adiposity. Most studies point out the substitution effect of milk (Keller et al. 2009; Kral et al. 2008; Linardakis et al. 2008; Fiorito et al. 2009) as an alternative to sugar-sweetened beverages and fruit juice, all directly associated with adiposity in children. The consumption of dairy foods and calcium in dairy foods has been suggested to be beneficial in the regulation of body weight in adults (Teegarden 2005; Major et al. 2008); however, there is a considerable controversy about whether high intakes of dairy products are necessary. Milk and dairy products can be a source of exogenous steroid hormones and the interaction of exogenous dietary intake with daily endogenous production in pre-pubertal children could have a role in regulation of body composition at this critical age. Early US studies suggested exogenous components of dairy products like estrone cause weight gain (Wolford and Argoudelis 1979). A more recent study showed that children who drank the most milk gained more weight, but the added calories and not estrone milk content appeared responsible (Berkey et al. 2005). To our knowledge, there is no large prospective study that has investigated effects of milk or yoghurt on weight status in European children.

The FFQ makes it possible to assess the extent to which milk and yoghurt are being replaced by other drinks or snacks of lower nutrient content (e.g. soft drinks) and to determine whether obesity/overweight is also involved. The question whether milk fat content could play a role in the milk-obesity association in children is still debated (Huh et al. 2010; Wang et al. 2009) and a specific question on the kind of milk/yoghurt consumed based on the fat content is investigated by the FFQ.

Several European countries like Denmark (Miljø- og fødevareministeriet 2018) and Italy (INRAN 2018) have started public health programmes to encourage reduction in dairy fat consumption, and a switch from full-fat to low-fat milk was part of a successful school intervention (Hollar et al. 2010) on reducing prevalence of childhood overweight. Additional questions in the FFQ ask about sugar added to milk and yoghurt in order to contribute to the sugar intake score and provide information about taste preferences.

6.5.7 Fish

Fish is a food of high-nutrient density (high in protein, retinol, vitamin D and vitamin E, iodine and selenium and often omega 3 fatty acids). In addition, fish is low in saturated fatty acids.

As component of Mediterranean diet, fish has been associated with reduction of visceral adiposity (Mar Bibiloni et al. 2011) and lower risk of major types of atherosclerosis-related cardiovascular diseases (Tektonidis et al. 2015). A few studies from different geographical socio-economic contexts suggest that consuming fish may play a part in preventing overweight in children (Oellingrath et al. 2011; Morshed et al. 2016), and adolescents (St-Jules et al. 2014) but this is not confirmed by other studies (Dong et al. 2015; Nicklas et al. 2004; Boniecka et al. 2009; Villa et al. 2007). There may be several reasons for inconsistent results on fish-overweight association, such as interaction with other protein sources, or an influence of socio-economic status (Aranceta et al. 2006). Also, fish preparation methods, e.g. deep-fried fish or canned fish, can be very different in terms of nutrient content (Fillion and Henry 1998; Dong et al. 2015) but were rarely considered in the previous studies. The present instrument addresses these unknowns regarding the consumption of fish by asking separate individual questions about fresh, canned/preserved and deep-fried fish.

6.5.8 Meat and Meat Products

High consumption of meat in Western countries has been associated with overweight (Paradis et al. 2009; Wang et al. 2009) and abdominal obesity (Romaguera et al. 2009) in adults. More recently, an ecological study of countries at different stages of the nutrition transition showed that high meat availability is correlated with increased prevalence of obesity and other diseases (You and Henneberg 2016). In children, evidence suggests that meat consumption is directly associated with adiposity (Friedman et al. 2009; Bradlee et al. 2010; Kleiser et al. 2009; Shin et al. 2007; Sugimori et al. 2004) and that high intake of protein from meat in children of 2–8 years is associated with high BMI later in life (Skinner et al. 2004).

The FFQ distinguishes fresh meat from processed/ready-to-eat/convenience meat products since the latter are often high in energy density and likely to be less nutrient-dense and higher in salt and fat content. Distinguishing these two categories will also provide information on consumption habits and preparation methods in the families. The questionnaire also asks about high-fat cooking (deep-fried, etc.) for meats, which may be related to overweight/obesity because of the higher energy content due to the cooking method (Fillion and Henry 1998).

In the original IDEFICS questionnaire, all meats were considered together in one question. In the new version of the FFQ used in I.Family, the meats have been split into two categories, poultry and red meats, each of which is then further subdivided by cooking method or preparation. Although there is no evidence of the differences in effect of poultry compared to other meats on obesity risk (Vergnaud et al. 2010), there is evidence of the diverging effect of poultry compared to red meat on some chronic diseases such as colon rectal and stomach cancer (World Cancer Research Fund/American Institute for Cancer Research 2007). Another rationale for this change from the original version was the need to clarify whether poultry should be considered as meat.

6.5.9 Eggs and Mayonnaise

Eggs are a convenient source of high-quality protein and ingredients in a wide variety of dishes in European countries. Adding eggs to the diet can effectively correct the problem of protein malnutrition in developing countries (Mayurasakorn et al. 2010). However, there is no evidence of association with overweight/obesity in well-nourished European children, neither in cross-sectional studies (Villa et al. 2007; Aranceta et al. 2006) nor prospectively. Because nutritional characteristics of egg dishes may vary widely depending on cooking/frying method (Fillion and Henry 1998) the FFQ distinguishes between fried/scrambled eggs and boiled eggs. There is also a separate question on the use of eggs in sauces, such sauces being very high in fat, similar in composition and popular in all European countries.

6.5.10 Meat Replacements and Soy Products

This food group includes a variety of products of widely varying nutritional content and is indicative of a consumer preference based on a desire for a typically non-animal source of protein. This may occur in the presence or absence of special (e.g. culture-related or religion-related) dietary practices (see Sect. 6.3.4).

The evidence base that links vegetarian food with overweight is limited, as most studies on this topic are fraught with methodological limitations, including cross-sectional designs or inadequate adjustment for potential confounders (Newby 2009). The aims of this question are to identify parents interested in new ways of feeding their families and to investigate the overall consequences of this attitude on children's diet and health. In addition, it is important to better understand if plant foods/meat-alternative are affordable and accessible to children of all income levels, knowledge of socio-economic and cultural norms that affect consumption is crucial. The present question will make it possible to identify associations between this "alternative" behaviour and overall dietary patterns, socio-economic status, nutritional beliefs, etc.

6.5.11 Cheese

Cheeses and cheese products vary markedly in energy density, from the 4.1 kcal/g of cream cheese to 1.4 kcal/g of ricotta cheese (USDA 2010). Cheese consumption by US children has increased over the last 20 years in parallel with the increase in adiposity (Nicklas et al. 2004). However, no studies so far have associated high cheese consumption with overweight/obesity, neither among US (Bradlee et al. 2010) nor among European (Friedman et al. 2009; Weker 2006; Gunther et al. 2006) children. Because the types of cheese consumed differ widely across Europe, and dishes containing cheese are even more varied, an extremely detailed questionnaire would have been necessary to capture this variety.

The aim of the question used in the FFQ was to distinguish two ways of using cheese that is easily recognised in all European countries: an alternative to other protein-rich dishes (like meat and fish); and in spreadable products on bread instead of products that are high in sugar (jam, honey), high in fat (butter) or high in both (chocolate spread). We added a question about grated cheese added to dishes, since the practice of adding small quantities of grated cheese to pasta dishes is very common in some countries (e.g. Italy, Spain). If the question had not been included, reporting of cheese consumption from these countries would have been flawed and inconsistent. The FFQ also asks about consumption of reduced fat cheeses.

6.5.12 Spreadable Products

Spreads on bread are used in a variety of ways in Europe. Butter or margarine on bread may be part of breakfast, lunch, evening meal or home snacks. However, an obesity promoting effect of using of jam, butter or chocolate spread might be difficult to detect. While these products are usually energy dense, nutrient dilute or both, they might be a less obesogenic alternative to bakery products and biscuits. This section seeks to obtain information about the use of bread with fat (butter, margarine), high sugar products (honey, jam) and products high in both fat and sugar (nut spreads, chocolate spreads). There is a specific question on reduced fat spreads, which have been suggested to be effective in intervention studies on childhood obesity prevention (Marcus et al. 2009). A separate question also enquires about the use of ketchup in sandwiches and as a topping for French fries and other fast food items.

6.5.13   Olive Oil for Cooking and Salads

Enquiring about intake of oils and fat in general is difficult in a food questionnaire as these are most likely "hidden" in prepared or cooked food (Schaefer et al. 2000). Nevertheless, we felt it important to ask this question, as the response is more likely to be associated with a general pattern rather than specific food behaviour. Olive oil is an important component of the Mediterranean diet, a dietary pattern that was associated with a decreased risk of obesity and other chronic diseases (Tognon et al. 2014; Buckland and Gonzalez 2015). In addition, the use of oil for cooking, dressing or preparation implies that the food was prepared and consumed at home (and therefore presumably healthier) as opposed to "convenience" ready-to-eat foods. Again, using olive oil for cooking may reflect a generalised rather than a specific dietary behaviour.

6.5.14   Cereal Products

The increasing rates of overweight in children continued through the end of the twentieth century notwithstanding reduction or stasis in fat consumption. One suggested reason for this is that the consumption of high GI carbohydrates has increased (Ball et al. 2003). A low-GI carbohydrate diet, rich, for example, in whole-grain products, seems to be a promising alternative to standard dietary treatment for obesity in children (Spieth et al. 2000), as such foods are slowly absorbed and have high power to satiate. The questions on cereal products were designed to distinguish hot dishes typically eaten at home and at the table from other fast food preparations (e.g. sandwiches). With regard to bread on the table, we sought to distinguish quickly absorbed (high GI) white bread from slowly absorbed (low GI) wholemeal bread. With regard to hot main course or side dish cereals eaten during family meals, the questions sought to distinguish three categories: pasta/rice, milled cereals (e.g. porridges, Mămăligă, "polenta", semolina) and pizza.

6.5.15　Snacks

Snacks may be defined according to composition (often high in fats or/and sugars, low in nutrients and energy-dense) or according to mode of consumption (fast and/ or between main meals) (Gregori and Maffeis 2007). Both food composition and mode of consumption may be involved in the development of overeating behaviour and obesity (Guthrie et al. 2002; Rosenheck 2008).

It is noteworthy that, according to the latter definition of snacks, even fruit, "crudités" or a glass of milk could be defined as "snack" if eaten between main meals. However, this type of healthier snacking is captured in other parts of the FFQ (see Sects. 6.5.2, 6.5.3 and 6.5.6).

For salt-rich snacks like crisps and other savoury foods, a possible reason for a link with obesity could be because of increased intake of sugar-sweetened drinks to quench salt-induced thirst (He et al. 2008). This and other hypotheses can be examined by means of questions about energy-dense snacks classified as high-fat/ high-nutrient density (nuts and seeds), high-fat/low-nutrient density (crisps, "potato chips") and high-fat and refined sugars/low-nutrient density (chocolate bars, candy bars).

6.6　Validation, Limitations and Adaptation of EHQ

6.6.1　Repeatability and Validity

The EHQ was shown to give reproducible estimates of consumption frequencies in European children by re-administering it a second time to a sample of 331 parents from between 13 days to eight months later. Differences in season, time between the two compilations and whether the second respondent was or was not the same parent as in the first round, were also recorded (Lanfer et al. 2011).

The EHQ was also found valid against objective biomarkers: frequency of milk consumption as estimated by the CEHQ was associated with higher urinary potassium and calcium excretion (Huybrechts et al. 2011).

6.6.2　Limitations and Adaptation for Use in Other Populations

The EHQ is a screening instrument designed to investigate the characteristics of diet and dietary behaviour that are relevant to childhood obesity. Dietary screening instruments are alternatives to more detailed methods of investigating dietary behaviour. Because only foods or behaviours that are strictly pertinent to the study question are investigated, these instruments are not comprehensive or exhaustive.

Dietary screening instruments cannot be used to measure energy intake, and so it is not possible to normalise EHQ results by energy-adjustment procedures (Willett et al. 1997). The present version of the instrument was not designed to capture dietary variations throughout Europe as it was only tested in the eight countries participating in the IDEFICS and I.Family studies.

The validity of a food frequency instrument depends on whether it can accurately assign persons to different intake groups. Several validated food questionnaires for adults are already available in Europe. However, they are usually country-specific. Although the EHQ can be used in various contexts to capture a wide variety of dietary habits, it will need to be adapted to make it applicable to those other than populations on which it has been specifically tested. As an example, to adapt it for use with adults and teens (AEHQ and TEHQ) some alcoholic drinks have been added to the previous children's version. In future implementations, it is likely that other items will be added, always after checking the performance by pilot studies and open-ended interviews.

The EHQ was originally designed to be completed by telephone interview although this was not done in the IDEFICS and I.Family studies. It has not been specifically validated for administration by remote methods.

6.6.3 Concluding Remarks

The novelty of the EHQ is that it investigates dietary habits from the perspective of obesity-related food behaviours and dietary patterns, in contrast to the classic energy-nutrient approach. Moreover, it has been developed and tested in a wide variety of culturally diverse European populations participating in the IDEFICS and I.Family studies. It promises to lend itself well to future applications in other populations.

6.7 Provision of Instruments and Standard Operating Procedures to Third Parties

All instruments described in this chapter including the General Survey Manuals that provide among other all standard operating procedures can be accessed on the following website: www.leibniz-bips.de/ifhs after registration.

Each third partner using the instruments provided in this chapter is kindly requested to cite this chapter as follows:

Pala V, Reisch LA, Lissner L, on behalf of the IDEFICS and I.Family consortia. Dietary behaviour in children, adolescents and families: the Eating Habits Questionnaire (EHQ). In: Bammann K, Lissner L, Pigeot I, Ahrens W, editors. Instruments for health surveys in children and adolescents. Cham: Springer Nature Switzerland; 2019. p. 103–133.

Acknowledgements The development of instruments, the baseline data collection and the first follow-up work as part of the IDEFICS study (www.idefics.eu) were financially supported by the European Commission within the Sixth RTD Framework Programme Contract No. 016181 (FOOD). The most recent follow-up including the development of new instruments and the adaptation of previously used instruments was conducted in the framework of the I.Family study (www.ifamilystudy.eu) which was funded by the European Commission within the Seventh RTD Framework Programme Contract No. 266044 (KBBE 2010–14).

We thank all families for participating in the extensive examinations of the IDEFICS and I. Family studies. We are also grateful for the support from school boards, headmasters and communities.

References

Aranceta BJ, Serra-Majem L, Perez-Rodrigo C, Ribas-Barba L, Delgado-Rubio A. Nutrition risk in the child and adolescent population of the Basque country: the enKid study. Br J Nutr. 2006;96(Suppl 1):S58–66.

Avery A, Anderson C, McCullough F. Associations between children's diet quality and watching television during meal or snack consumption: a systematic review. Matern Child Nutr. 2017. https://doi.org/10.1111/mcn.12428.

Ball SD, Keller KR, Moyer-Mileur LJ, Ding YW, Donaldson D, Jackson WD. Prolongation of satiety after low versus moderately high glycemic index meals in obese adolescents. Pediatrics. 2003;111:488–94.

Barba G, Troiano E, Russo P, Venezia A, Siani A. Inverse association between body mass and frequency of milk consumption in children. Br J Nutr. 2005;93:15–9.

Barkeling B, Ekman S, Rossner S. Eating behaviour in obese and normal weight 11-year-old children. Int J Obes Relat Metab Disord. 1992;16:355–60.

Barton BA, Eldridge AL, Thompson D, Affenito SG, Striegel-Moore RH, Franko DL, et al. The relationship of breakfast and cereal consumption to nutrient intake and body mass index: the National Heart, Lung, and Blood Institute growth and health study. J Am Diet Assoc. 2005;105:1383–9.

Baughcum AE, Powers SW, Johnson SB, Chamberlin LA, Deeks CM, Jain A, et al. Maternal feeding practices and beliefs and their relationships to overweight in early childhood. J Dev Behav Pediatr. 2001;22(6):391–408.

Bazzano LA, He J, Ogden LG, Loria C, Vupputuri S, Myers L, et al. Legume consumption and risk of coronary heart disease in US men and women: NHANES I epidemiologic follow-up study. Arch Intern Med. 2001;161:2573–8.

Bellisle F, Dalix AM. Cognitive restraint can be offset by distraction, leading to increased meal intake in women. Am J Clin Nutr. 2001;74:197–200.

Bellisle F, Dalix AM, Airinei G, Hercberg S, Peneau S. Influence of dietary restraint and environmental factors on meal size in normal-weight women. A laboratory study. Appetite. 2009;53:309–13.

Bere E, Veierod MB, Skare O, Klepp KI. Free school fruit–sustained effect three years later. Int J Behav Nutr Phys Act. 2007;4:5.

Berkey CS, Rockett HR, Field AE, Gillman MW, Colditz GA. Sugar-added beverages and adolescent weight change. Obes Res. 2004;12:778–88.

Berkey CS, Rockett HR, Willett WC, Colditz GA. Milk, dairy fat, dietary calcium, and weight gain: a longitudinal study of adolescents. Arch Pediatr Adolesc Med. 2005;159:543–50.

Beydoun MA, Wang Y. How do socio-economic status, perceived economic barriers and nutritional benefits affect quality of dietary intake among US adults? Eur J Clin Nutr. 2008;62:303–13.

Birch LL, Fisher JO. Development of eating behaviors among children and adolescents. Pediatrics. 1998;101:539–49.

Boeing H, Bechthold A, Bub A, Ellinger S, Haller D, Kroke A, et al. Critical review: vegetables and fruit in the prevention of chronic diseases. Eur J Nutr. 2012;51:637–63.

Boniecka I, Michota-Katulska E, Ukleja A, Czerwonogrodzka A, Kowalczyk E, Szczyglowska A. Nutritional behavior of chosen group of school children in aspect of obesity risk. Przegl Lek. 2009;66:49–51.

Boyland EJ, Harrold JA, Kirkham TC, Corker C, Cuddy J, Evans D, et al. Food commercials increase preference for energy-dense foods, particularly in children who watch more television. Pediatrics. 2011;128(1):e93–100.

Bradlee ML, Singer MR, Qureshi MM, Moore LL. Food group intake and central obesity among children and adolescents in the Third National Health and Nutrition Examination Survey (NHANES III). Public Health Nutr. 2010;13(6):797–805.

Brownell KD, Farley T, Willett WC, Popkin BM, Chaloupka FJ, Thompson JW, et al. The public health and economic benefits of taxing sugar-sweetened beverages. N Engl J Med. 2009;361:1599–605.

Buckland G, Gonzalez CA. The role of olive oil in disease prevention: a focus on the recent epidemiological evidence from cohort studies and dietary intervention trials. Br J Nutr. 2015;113(Suppl 2):S94–101.

Burgess-Champoux TL, Larson N, Neumark-Sztainer D, Hannan PJ, Story M. Are family meal patterns associated with overall diet quality during the transition from early to middle adolescence? J Nutr Educ Behav. 2009;41:79–86.

Carruth BR, Skinner JD. The role of dietary calcium and other nutrients in moderating body fat in preschool children. Int J Obes Relat Metab Disord. 2001;25:559–66.

Casazza K, Fontaine KR, Astrup A, Birch LL, Brown AW, Bohan Brown MM, et al. Myths, presumptions, and facts about obesity. N Engl J Med. 2013;368:446–54.

Condon EM, Crepinsek MK, Fox MK. School meals: types of foods offered to and consumed by children at lunch and breakfast. J Am Diet Assoc. 2009;109:S67–78.

Council on School Health. Snacks, sweetened beverages, added sugars, and schools. Pediatrics. 2015;135:575–83.

Devine CM, Farrell TJ, Blake CE, Jastran M, Wethington E, Bisogni CA. Work conditions and the food choice coping strategies of employed parents. J Nutr Educ Behav. 2009;41:365–70.

Diehl JM. Inventar zum Essverhalten und Gewichtsproblemen für Kinder (IEG-Kind). Available upon request from the author as supplementary material to Diehl JM. Einstellungen zu Essen und Gewicht bei 11- bis 16jährigen Adoleszenten. Schweiz Med Wochenschr. 1999;129: 162–75.

Dong D, Bilger M, van Dam RM, Finkelstein EA. Consumption of specific foods and beverages and excess weight gain among children and adolescents. Health Aff (Millwood). 2015;34:1940–8.

Drewnowski A. The nutrient rich foods index helps to identify healthy, affordable foods. Am J Clin Nutr. 2010;91:1095S–101S.

Drewnowski A, Fulgoni V III. Nutrient profiling of foods: creating a nutrient-rich food index. Nutr Rev. 2008;66:23–39.

Dubois L, Farmer A, Girard M, Peterson K. Social factors and television use during meals and snacks is associated with higher BMI among pre-school children. Public Health Nutr. 2008;11:1267–79.

Dykstra H, Davey A, Fisher JO, Polonsky H, Sherman S, Abel ML, et al. Breakfast-skipping and selecting low-nutritional-quality foods for breakfast are common among low-income urban children, regardless of food security status. J Nutr. 2016;146:630–6.

Ebbeling CB, Feldman HA, Osganian SK, Chomitz VR, Ellenbogen SJ, Ludwig DS. Effects of decreasing sugar-sweetened beverage consumption on body weight in adolescents: a randomized, controlled pilot study. Pediatrics. 2006;117:673–80.

Ello-Martin JA, Ledikwe JH, Rolls BJ. The influence of food portion size and energy density on energy intake: implications for weight management. Am J Clin Nutr. 2005;82:236S–41S.

Epstein LH, Gordy CC, Raynor HA, Beddome M, Kilanowski CK, Paluch R. Increasing fruit and vegetable intake and decreasing fat and sugar intake in families at risk for childhood obesity. Obes Res. 2001;9:171–8.

Epstein LH, Roemmich JN, Robinson JL, Paluch RA, Winiewicz DD, Fuerch JH, et al. A randomized trial of the effects of reducing television viewing and computer use on body mass index in young children. Arch Pediatr Adolesc Med. 2008;162:239–45.

Fillion L, Henry CJ. Nutrient losses and gains during frying: a review. Int J Food Sci Nutr. 1998;49:157–68.

Fiorito LM, Ventura AK, Mitchell DC, Smiciklas-Wright H, Birch LL. Girls' dairy intake, energy intake, and weight status. J Am Diet Assoc. 2006;106:1851–5.

Fiorito LM, Marini M, Francis LA, Smiciklas-Wright H, Birch LL. Beverage intake of girls at age 5 y predicts adiposity and weight status in childhood and adolescence. Am J Clin Nutr. 2009;90:935–42.

Fisher JO, Mitchell DC, Smiciklas-Wright H, Birch LL. Parental influences on young girls' fruit and vegetable, micronutrient, and fat intakes. J Am Diet Assoc. 2002;102:58–64.

Fleischhacker SE, Evenson KR, Rodriguez DA, Ammerman AS. A systematic review of fast food access studies. Obes Rev. 2011;12:e460–71.

Flood JE, Rolls BJ. Soup preloads in a variety of forms reduce meal energy intake. Appetite. 2007;49:626–34.

Foster-Powell K, Holt SH, Brand-Miller JC. International table of glycemic index and glycemic load values: 2002. Am J Clin Nutr. 2002;76:5–56.

Fox MK, Dodd AH, Wilson A, Gleason PM. Association between school food environment and practices and body mass index of US public school children. J Am Diet Assoc. 2009;109: S108–17.

Friedman LS, Lukyanova EM, Serdiuk A, Shkiryak-Nizhnyk ZA, Chislovska NV, Zvinchuk AV, et al. Social-environmental factors associated with elevated body mass index in a Ukrainian cohort of children. Int J Pediatr Obes. 2009;4:81–90.

Garber AK, Lustig RH. Is fast food addictive? Curr Drug Abuse Rev. 2011;4:146–62.

Garcia-Dominic O, Wray LA, Ledikwe JH, Mitchell DC, Ventura AK, Hernandez AE, et al. Accuracy of self-reported energy intakes in low-income urban 4th grade minority children. Obesity (Silver Spring). 2010;18:2220–6.

Ghayour-Mobarhan M, Sahebkar A, Vakili R, Safarian M, Nematy M, Lotfian E, et al. Investigation of the effect of high dairy diet on body mass index and body fat in overweight and obese children. Indian J Pediatr. 2009;76:1145–50.

Golley RK, Bell LK, Hendrie GA, Rangan AM, Spence A, McNaughton SA, et al. Validity of short food questionnaire items to measure intake in children and adolescents: a systematic review. J Hum Nutr Diet. 2017;30:36–50.

Gortmaker SL, Must A, Sobol AM, Peterson K, Colditz GA, Dietz WH. Television viewing as a cause of increasing obesity among children in the United States, 1986–1990. Arch Pediatr Adolesc Med. 1996;150:356–62.

Gregori D, Maffeis C. Snacking and obesity: urgency of a definition to explore such a relationship. J Am Diet Assoc. 2007;107:562–3.

Gunther AL, Buyken AE, Kroke A. The influence of habitual protein intake in early childhood on BMI and age at adiposity rebound: results from the DONALD study. Int J Obes (Lond). 2006;30:1072–9.

Gunther AL, Remer T, Kroke A, Buyken AE. Early protein intake and later obesity risk: which protein sources at which time points throughout infancy and childhood are important for body mass index and body fat percentage at 7 y of age? Am J Clin Nutr. 2007;86:1765–72.

Gustafsson K, Asp NG, Hagander B, Nyman M. Satiety effects of spinach in mixed meals: comparison with other vegetables. Int J Food Sci Nutr. 1995a;46:327–34.

Gustafsson K, Asp NG, Hagander B, Nyman M, Schweizer T. Influence of processing and cooking of carrots in mixed meals on satiety, glucose and hormonal response. Int J Food Sci Nutr. 1995b;46:3–12.

Guthrie JF, Lin BH, Frazao E. Role of food prepared away from home in the American diet, 1977–78 versus 1994–96: changes and consequences. J Nutr Educ Behav. 2002;34:140–50.

Hallstrom L, Labayen I, Ruiz JR, Patterson E, Vereecken CA, Breidenassel C, et al. Breakfast consumption and CVD risk factors in European adolescents: the HELENA (Healthy Lifestyle in Europe by Nutrition in Adolescence) study. Public Health Nutr. 2013;16:1296–305.

Hampson SE, Martin J, Jorgensen J, Barker M. A social marketing approach to improving the nutrition of low-income women and children: an initial focus group study. Public Health Nutr. 2009;12:1563–8.

Harris JL, Bargh JA. Television viewing and unhealthy diet: implications for children and media interventions. Health Commun. 2009;24:660–73.

He FJ, Marrero NM, MacGregor GA. Salt intake is related to soft drink consumption in children and adolescents: a link to obesity? Hypertension. 2008;51:629–34.

Hollar D, Messiah SE, Lopez-Mitnik G, Hollar TL, Almon M, Agatston AS. Healthier options for public schoolchildren program improves weight and blood pressure in 6- to 13-year-olds. J Am Diet Assoc. 2010;110:261–7.

Holubcikova J, Kolarcik P, Madarasova GA, van Dijk JP, Reijneveld SA. Lack of parental rule-setting on eating is associated with a wide range of adolescent unhealthy eating behaviour both for boys and girls. BMC Public Health. 2016;16:359.

Huh SY, Rifas-Shiman SL, Rich-Edwards JW, Taveras EM, Gillman MW. Prospective association between milk intake and adiposity in preschool-aged children. J Am Diet Assoc. 2010;110:563–70.

Hunsberger M, Mehlig K, Bornhorst C, Hebestreit A, Moreno L, Veidebaum T, et al. Dietary carbohydrate and nocturnal sleep duration in relation to children's BMI: findings from the IDEFICS study in eight European countries. Nutrients. 2015;7:10223–36.

Huybrechts I, Bornhorst C, Pala V, Moreno LA, Barba G, Lissner L, et al. IDEFICS consortium. Evaluation of the children's eating habits questionnaire used in the IDEFICS study by relating urinary calcium and potassium to milk consumption frequencies among European children. Int J Obes (Lond). 2011;35(Suppl 1):S69–78.

IMO. International migration outlook 2016. OECD Publishing; 2016.

Inran. 2018. http://www.inran.it/servizi_cittadino/stare_bene. Accessed 22 Mar 2017.

Johnson L, Mander AP, Jones LR, Emmett PM, Jebb SA. Is sugar-sweetened beverage consumption associated with increased fatness in children? Nutrition. 2007;23:557–63.

Kant AK, Graubard BI. Eating out in America, 1987–2000: trends and nutritional correlates. Prev Med. 2004;38:243–9.

Karatzi K, Moschonis G, Choupi E, Manios Y. Healthy growth study group. Late-night overeating is associated with smaller breakfast, breakfast skipping, and obesity in children: the healthy growth study. Nutrition 2017;33:141–4.

Keller KL, Kirzner J, Pietrobelli A, St Onge MP, Faith MS. Increased sweetened beverage intake is associated with reduced milk and calcium intake in 3- to 7-year-old children at multi-item laboratory lunches. J Am Diet Assoc. 2009;109:497–501.

Kettings C, Sinclair AJ, Voevodin M. A healthy diet consistent with Australian health recommendations is too expensive for welfare-dependent families. Aust N Z J Public Health. 2009;33:566–72.

Kirkpatrick SI, Tarasuk V. Food insecurity is associated with nutrient inadequacies among Canadian adults and adolescents. J Nutr. 2008;138:604–12.

Kleiser C, Schaffrath RA, Mensink GB, Prinz-Langenohl R, Kurth BM. Potential determinants of obesity among children and adolescents in Germany: results from the cross-sectional KiGGS study. BMC Public Health. 2009;9:46.

Kolodziejczyk JK, Merchant G, Norman GJ. Reliability and validity of child/adolescent food frequency questionnaires that assess foods and/or food groups. J Pediatr Gastroenterol Nutr. 2012;55:4–13.

Kral TV, Stunkard AJ, Berkowitz RI, Stallings VA, Moore RH, Faith MS. Beverage consumption patterns of children born at different risk of obesity. Obesity (Silver Spring). 2008;16:1802–8.

Lanfer A, Hebestreit A, Ahrens W, Krogh V, Sieri S, Lissner L, et al. IDEFICS consortium. Reproducibility of food consumption frequencies derived from the children's eating habits questionnaire used in the IDEFICS study. Int J Obes (Lond). 2011;35(Suppl 1):S61–8.

Larson N, Story M. A review of environmental influences on food choices. Ann Behav Med. 2009;38(Suppl 1):S56–73.

Leahy KE, Birch LL, Rolls BJ. Reducing the energy density of multiple meals decreases the energy intake of preschool-age children. Am J Clin Nutr. 2008;88:1459–68.

Li SS, Kendall CW, de Souza RJ, Jayalath VH, Cozma AI, Ha V, et al. Dietary pulses, satiety and food intake: a systematic review and meta-analysis of acute feeding trials. Obesity (Silver Spring). 2014;22:1773–80.

Linardakis M, Sarri K, Pateraki MS, Sbokos M, Kafatos A. Sugar-added beverages consumption among kindergarten children of Crete: effects on nutritional status and risk of obesity. BMC Public Health. 2008;8:279.

Livingstone MB, Robson PJ, Wallace JM. Issues in dietary intake assessment of children and adolescents. Br J Nutr. 2004;92(Suppl 2):S213–22.

Lopez-Alvarenga JC, Vazquez-Velazquez V, Bolado-Garcia VE, Gonzalez-Barranco J, Castaneda-Lopez J, Robles L, et al. Parental influence in children's food preferences. The ESFUERSO study in two primary schools with different socioeconomic gradients. Gac Med Mex 2007;143:463–9.

Lorson BA, Melgar-Quinonez HR, Taylor CA. Correlates of fruit and vegetable intakes in US children. J Am Diet Assoc. 2009;109:474–8.

Lowe MR, Doshi SD, Katterman SN, Feig EH. Dieting and restrained eating as prospective predictors of weight gain. Front Psychol. 2013;4:577.

Ludwig DS, Peterson KE, Gortmaker SL. Relation between consumption of sugar-sweetened drinks and childhood obesity: a prospective, observational analysis. Lancet. 2001;357:505–8.

MacFarlane A, Cleland V, Crawford D, Campbell K, Timperio A. Longitudinal examination of the family food environment and weight status among children. Int J Pediatr Obes. 2009;4:343–52.

Maillot M, Ferguson EL, Drewnowski A, Darmon N. Nutrient profiling can help identify foods of good nutritional quality for their price: a validation study with linear programming. J Nutr. 2008;138:1107–13.

Major GC, Chaput JP, Ledoux M, St Pierre S, Anderson GH, Zemel MB, et al. Recent developments in calcium-related obesity research. Obes Rev. 2008;9:428–45.

Manios Y, Kourlaba G, Kondaki K, Grammatikaki E, Anastasiadou A, Roma-Giannikou E. Obesity and television watching in preschoolers in Greece: the GENESIS study. Obesity (Silver Spring). 2009;17:2047–53.

Mar Bibiloni M, Martínez E, Llull R, Maffiotte E, Riesco M, Llompart I, et al. Metabolic syndrome in adolescents in the Balearic Islands, a Mediterranean region. Nutr Metab Cardiovasc Dis. 2011;21(6):446–54.

Marcus C, Nyberg G, Nordenfelt A, Karpmyr M, Kowalski J, Ekelund U. A 4-year, cluster-randomized, controlled childhood obesity prevention study: STOPP. Int J Obes (Lond). 2009;33:408–17.

Maynard MJ, Baker G, Rawlins E, Anderson A, Harding S. Developing obesity prevention interventions among minority ethnic children in schools and places of worship: the DEAL (DiEt and Active Living) study. BMC Public Health. 2009;9:480.

Mayurasakorn K, Sitphahul P, Hongto PO. Supplement of three eggs a week improves protein malnutrition in Thai children from rural areas. J Med Assoc Thai. 2010;93:301–9.

McCarty MF. The origins of western obesity: a role for animal protein? Med Hypotheses. 2000;54:488–94.

Miljø- og fødevareministeriet. Altomkost.dk. 2018. www.altomkost.dk. Accessed 22 Mar 2017.

Monasta L, Batty GD, Cattaneo A, Lutje V, Ronfani L, van Lenthe FJ, et al. Early-life determinants of overweight and obesity: a review of systematic reviews. Obes Rev. 2010;11 (10):695–708.

Moore LL, Bradlee ML, Gao D, Singer MR. Low dairy intake in early childhood predicts excess body fat gain. Obesity (Silver Spring). 2006;14:1010–8.

Moore LL, Singer MR, Qureshi MM, Bradlee ML. Dairy intake and anthropometric measures of body fat among children and adolescents in NHANES. J Am Coll Nutr. 2008;27:702–10.

Morshed AB, Becker HV, Delnatus JR, Wolff PB, Iannotti LL. Early nutrition transition in Haiti: linking food purchasing and availability to overweight status in school-aged children. Public Health Nutr. 2016;19:3378–85.

Nelson M, Erens B, Bates B, Church S, Boshier T. Low income diet and nutrition survey, vol. 2. London: The Stationery Office. Food Consumption and Nutrient Intake; 2010.

Neumark-Sztainer D, Eisenberg ME, Fulkerson JA, Story M, Larson NI. Family meals and disordered eating in adolescents: longitudinal findings from project EAT. Arch Pediatr Adolesc Med. 2008;162:17–22.

Newby PK. Plant foods and plant-based diets: protective against childhood obesity? Am J Clin Nutr. 2009;89:1572S–87S.

Nicklas TA, Demory-Luce D, Yang SJ, Baranowski T, Zakeri I, Berenson G. Children's food consumption patterns have changed over two decades (1973–1994): The Bogalusa heart study. J Am Diet Assoc. 2004;104:1127–40.

North K, Emmett P. Multivariate analysis of diet among three-year-old children and associations with socio-demographic characteristics. The Avon Longitudinal Study of Pregnancy and Childhood (ALSPAC) study team. Eur J Clin Nutr. 2000;54:73–80.

O'Connor TM, Yang SJ, Nicklas TA. Beverage intake among preschool children and its effect on weight status. Pediatrics. 2006;118:e1010–8.

Oellingrath IM, Svendsen MV, Brantsaeter AL. Tracking of eating patterns and overweight—a follow-up study of Norwegian schoolchildren from middle childhood to early adolescence. Nutr J. 2011;10:106.

Ogden CL, Carroll MD, Curtin LR, McDowell MA, Tabak CJ, Flegal KM. Prevalence of overweight and obesity in the United States, 1999–2004. JAMA. 2006;295:1549–55.

Ogden CL, Carroll MD, Curtin LR, Lamb MM, Flegal KM. Prevalence of high body mass index in US children and adolescents, 2007–2008. JAMA. 2010;303:242–9.

Orfanos P, Naska A, Trichopoulou A, Grioni S, Boer JM, van Bakel MM, et al. Eating out of home: energy, macro- and micronutrient intakes in 10 European countries. The European prospective investigation into cancer and nutrition. Eur J Clin Nutr. 2009;63(Suppl 4): S239–62.

Overby NC, Klepp KI, Bere E. Introduction of a school fruit program is associated with reduced frequency of consumption of unhealthy snacks. Am J Clin Nutr. 2012;96:1100–3.

Pala V, Berrino F, Vineis P, Palli D, Celentano E, Tumino R, et al. How vegetables are eaten in Italy EPIC centres: still setting a good example? IARC Sci Publ. 2002;156:119–21.

Pala V, Lissner L, Hebestreit A, Lanfer A, Sieri S, Siani A, et al. Dietary patterns and longitudinal change in body mass in European children: a follow-up study on the IDEFICS multicenter cohort. Eur J Clin Nutr. 2013;67:1042–9.

Paradis AM, Godin G, Perusse L, Vohl MC. Associations between dietary patterns and obesity phenotypes. Int J Obes (Lond). 2009;33:1419–26.

Phelan S, Lang W, Jordan D, Wing RR. Use of artificial sweeteners and fat-modified foods in weight loss maintainers and always-normal weight individuals. Int J Obes (Lond). 2009;33: 1183–90.

Raben A, Vasilaras TH, Moller AC, Astrup A. Sucrose compared with artificial sweeteners: different effects on ad libitum food intake and body weight after 10 wk of supplementation in overweight subjects. Am J Clin Nutr. 2002;76:721–9.

Receveur O, Morou K, Gray-Donald K, Macaulay AC. Consumption of key food items is associated with excess weight among elementary-school-aged children in a Canadian first nations community. J Am Diet Assoc. 2008;108:362–6.

Reisch LA, Gwozdz W, Barba G, De Henauw S, Lascorz N, Pigeot I. Experimental evidence on the impact of food advertising on children's knowledge about and preferences for healthful food. J Obes. 2013;2013:408582.

Robinson TN. Does television cause childhood obesity? JAMA. 1998;279:959–60.

Robinson TN. Television viewing and childhood obesity. Pediatr Clin North Am. 2001;48: 1017–25.

Robinson TN, Kiernan M, Matheson DM, Haydel KF. Is parental control over children's eating associated with childhood obesity? Results from a population-based sample of third graders. Obes Res. 2001;9:306–12.

Roblin L. Childhood obesity: food, nutrient, and eating-habit trends and influences. Appl Physiol Nutr Metab. 2007;32:635–45.

Rolls BJ. The relationship between dietary energy density and energy intake. Physiol Behav. 2009;97:609–15.

Rolls BJ, Roe LS, Meengs JS. Salad and satiety: energy density and portion size of a first-course salad affect energy intake at lunch. J Am Diet Assoc. 2004;104:1570–6.

Romaguera D, Norat T, Mouw T, May AM, Bamia C, Slimani N, et al. Adherence to the Mediterranean diet is associated with lower abdominal adiposity in European men and women. J Nutr. 2009;139:1728–37.

Rosenheck R. Fast food consumption and increased caloric intake: a systematic review of a trajectory towards weight gain and obesity risk. Obes Rev. 2008;9:535–47.

Ruxton CH, Kirk TR, Belton NR, Holmes MA. Relationships between social class, nutrient intake and dietary patterns in Edinburgh schoolchildren. Int J Food Sci Nutr. 1996;47:341–9.

Saxena S, Ambler G, Cole TJ, Majeed A. Ethnic group differences in overweight and obese children and young people in England: cross sectional survey. Arch Dis Child. 2004;89:30–6.

Schaefer EJ, Augustin JL, Schaefer MM, Rasmussen H, Ordovas JM, Dallal GE, et al. Lack of efficacy of a food-frequency questionnaire in assessing dietary macronutrient intakes in subjects consuming diets of known composition. Am J Clin Nutr. 2000;71:746–51.

Shin KO, Oh SY, Park HS. Empirically derived major dietary patterns and their associations with overweight in Korean preschool children. Br J Nutr. 2007;98:416–21.

Silva-Sanigorski AM, Bell AC, Kremer P, Nichols M, Crellin M, Smith M, et al. Reducing obesity in early childhood: results from Romp & Chomp, an Australian community-wide intervention program. Am J Clin Nutr. 2010;91:831–40.

Skinner JD, Bounds W, Carruth BR, Morris M, Ziegler P. Predictors of children's body mass index: a longitudinal study of diet and growth in children aged 2–8 y. Int J Obes Relat Metab Disord. 2004;28:476–82.

Song MK, Rosenthal MJ, Song AM, Yang H, Ao Y, Yamaguchi DT. Raw vegetable food containing high cyclo (his-pro) improved insulin sensitivity and body weight control. Metabolism. 2005;54:1480–9.

Song WO, Chun OK, Kerver J, Cho S, Chung CE, Chung SJ. Ready-to-eat breakfast cereal consumption enhances milk and calcium intake in the US population. J Am Diet Assoc. 2006;106:1783–9.

Spieth LE, Harnish JD, Lenders CM, Raezer LB, Pereira MA, Hangen SJ, et al. A low-glycemic index diet in the treatment of pediatric obesity. Arch Pediatr Adolesc Med. 2000;154:947–51.

Stenvers DJ, Jonkers CF, Fliers E, Bisschop PH, Kalsbeek A. Nutrition and the circadian timing system. Prog Brain Res. 2012;199:359–76.

St-Jules DE, Watters CA, Novotny R. Estimation of fish intake in Asian and white female adolescents, and association with 2-year changes in body fatness and body fat distribution: the female adolescent maturation study. J Acad Nutr Diet. 2014;114:543–51.

St Onge MP, Goree LL, Gower B. High-milk supplementation with healthy diet counseling does not affect weight loss but ameliorates insulin action compared with low-milk supplementation in overweight children. J Nutr. 2009;139:933–8.

Stroebele N, de Castro JM. Television viewing is associated with an increase in meal frequency in humans. Appetite. 2004;42:111–3.

Sugimori H, Yoshida K, Izuno T, Miyakawa M, Suka M, Sekine M, et al. Analysis of factors that influence body mass index from ages 3 to 6 years: A study based on the Toyama cohort study. Pediatr Int. 2004;46:302–10.

Suling M, Hebestreit A, Peplies J, Bammann K, Nappo A, Eiben G, et al. IDEFICS consortium. Design and results of the pretest of the IDEFICS study. Int J Obes (Lond). 2011;35(Suppl 1): S30–44.

Szajewska H, Ruszczynski M. Systematic review demonstrating that breakfast consumption influences body weight outcomes in children and adolescents in Europe. Crit Rev Food Sci Nutr. 2010;50:113–9.

Taylor SJ, Viner R, Booy R, Head J, Tate H, Brentnall SL, et al. Ethnicity, socio-economic status, overweight and underweight in East London adolescents. Ethn Health. 2005;10:113–28.

Teegarden D. The influence of dairy product consumption on body composition. J Nutr. 2005;135:2749–52.

Tektonidis TG, Akesson A, Gigante B, Wolk A, Larsson SC. A Mediterranean diet and risk of myocardial infarction, heart failure and stroke: a population-based cohort study. Atherosclerosis. 2015;243:93–8.

Thompson FE, Subar AF. Chapter 1—Dietary assessment methodology. In: Coulston A, Boushey CJ, Ferruzzi MG, editors. Nutrition in the prevention and treatment of disease. 3rd ed. Cambridge: Academic Press; 2013. p. 5–46.

Tognon G, Hebestreit A, Lanfer A, Moreno LA, Pala V, Siani A, et al. IDEFICS consortium. Mediterranean diet, overweight and body composition in children from eight European countries: cross-sectional and prospective results from the IDEFICS study. Nutr Metab Cardiovasc Dis. 2014;24:205–13.

USDA. National nutrient database for standard reference. Beltsville, MD: USDA Agricultural Research Service, 2010.

Valdes J, Rodriguez-Artalejo F, Aguilar I., Jaen-Casquero MB, Royo-Bordonada MA. Frequency of family meals and childhood overweight: a systematic review. Pediatr Obes. 2013;8:e1–13.

van den Boom A, Serra-Majem L, Ribas L, Ngo J, Perez-Rodrigo C, Aranceta J, et al. The contribution of ready-to-eat cereals to daily nutrient intake and breakfast quality in a Mediterranean setting. J Am Coll Nutr. 2006;25:135–43.

Vergnaud AC, Norat T, Romaguera D, Mouw T, May AM, Travier N, et al. Meat consumption and prospective weight change in participants of the EPIC-PANACEA study. Am J Clin Nutr. 2010;92:398–407.

Villa I, Yngve A, Poortvliet E, Grjibovski A, Liiv K, Sjostrom M, et al. Dietary intake among under- , normal- and overweight 9- and 15-year-old Estonian and Swedish schoolchildren. Public Health Nutr. 2007;10:311–22.

Wang YC, Ludwig DS, Sonneville K, Gortmaker SL. Impact of change in sweetened caloric beverage consumption on energy intake among children and adolescents. Arch Pediatr Adolesc Med. 2009;163:336–43.

Wang Y, Wang L, Xue H, Qu W. A review of the growth of the fast food industry in China and its potential impact on obesity. Int J Environ Res Public Health. 2016;13:1112.

Wardle J, Carnell S, Cooke L. Parental control over feeding and children's fruit and vegetable intake: how are they related? J Am Diet Assoc. 2005;105:227–32.

Warren JM, Henry CJ, Simonite V. Low glycemic index breakfasts and reduced food intake in preadolescent children. Pediatrics. 2003;112:e414.

Weker H. Simple obesity in children. A study on the role of nutritional factors. Med Wieku Rozwoj. 2006;10:3–191.

Willett WC, Howe GR, Kushi LH. Adjustment for total energy intake in epidemiologic studies. Am J Clin Nutr. 1997;65:1220S–8S.

Wolford ST, Argoudelis CJ. Measurement of estrogens in cow's milk, human milk, and dairy products. J Dairy Sci. 1979;62:1458–63.

World Cancer Research Fund/American Institute for Cancer Research. Food, nutrition, physical activity, and the prevention of cancer: a global perspective. Washington DC: AICR; 2007.

You WP, Henneberg M. Type 1 diabetes prevalence increasing globally and regionally: the role of natural selection and life expectancy at birth. BMJ Open Diab Res Care. 2016;4(1):e000161.

Chapter 7
Accelerometry-Based Physical Activity Assessment for Children and Adolescents

Kenn Konstabel, Swati Chopra, Robert Ojiambo, Borja Muñiz-Pardos and Yannis Pitsiladis

Abstract Accurate assessment of physical activity (PA) is important to study the associations between PA and health outcomes, to evaluate the effectiveness of interventions and to derive public health recommendations. Despite limitations, accelerometry-based methods generate the best available measures for epidemiological research involving a large number of children and adults. In this chapter, we review the most important methodological issues pertaining to the use of accelerometers to assess the overall volume of PA. We stress the importance of recording and keeping the raw data whenever possible. We review the validation studies using accelerometry to determine energy expenditure and calibration studies

On behalf of the IDEFICS and I.Family consortia

K. Konstabel (✉)
National Institute for Health Development, Tallinn, Estonia
e-mail: kenn.konstabel@tai.ee

K. Konstabel
Institute of Psychology, University of Tartu, Tartu, Estonia

K. Konstabel
School of Natural Sciences and Health, Tallinn University, Tallinn, Estonia

S. Chopra
Leeds Institute of Rheumatic and Musculoskeletal Medicine,
University of Leeds, Leeds, UK

R. Ojiambo
Department of Medical Physiology, Moi University, Eldoret, Kenya

B. Muñiz-Pardos
GENUD Research Group, University of Zaragoza, Zaragoza, Spain

Y. Pitsiladis
Department of Movement, Human and Health Sciences, University of Rome
"Foro Italico", Rome, Italy

Y. Pitsiladis
Collaborating Centre of Sports Medicine, University of Brighton, Eastbourne, UK

© Springer Nature Switzerland AG 2019
K. Bammann et al. (eds.), *Instruments for Health Surveys in Children and Adolescents*, Springer Series on Epidemiology and Public Health,
https://doi.org/10.1007/978-3-319-98857-3_7

135

that attempt to derive thresholds ("cut-offs") for differentiating between activity intensity categories. Conceptual and measurement issues due to the use of different thresholds are reviewed, as well as the temporal resolution issues such as sampling rate and epoch length. Different wear time detection algorithms and inclusion criteria are reviewed as well as options in data reduction (deriving meaningful variables from accelerometer data). We present an R package automatising most of the steps in accelerometer data analysis. The chapter concludes with some insights into the future of accelerometry given the wearable revolution and logistical considerations in using accelerometers in large field studies.

7.1 Introduction

7.1.1 Physical Activity and Health

Physical activity (PA) can be defined as any bodily movement produced by skeletal muscles that result in energy expenditure (EE) (Caspersen et al. 1985). PA is related to all-cause mortality (Lee and Skerrett 2001); we therefore need objective methods of PA assessment to elucidate the dose–response relationship between PA and health outcomes. Evidence of the detrimental effects of a sedentary lifestyle on the health of children is constantly growing (Dencker and Anderson 2008). For example, an association between inactivity and childhood obesity is now generally accepted (Miller et al. 2004; Ekblom et al. 2004; Trost et al. 2001). On the one hand, obese children and adolescents are prone to significant short- and long-term health problems such as cardiovascular diseases, hyperlipidaemia, hypertension, glucose intolerance, type 2 diabetes, psychiatric disorders, and orthopaedic complications (Miller et al. 2004; Reilly et al. 2003) and have an increased risk of developing adult obesity (Whitaker et al. 1997; Mossberg 1989). On the other hand, increasing PA can counter the adverse effects of childhood obesity such as reducing visceral fat (Byrd-Williams et al. 2010). The effects of PA are not confined to the risks associated with obesity and overweight: the direct and indirect effects include bone health, muscular fitness, mood disorders, and cognitive ageing (Miles 2007; de Vet and Verkooijen 2018).

7.1.2 Physical Activity Guidelines

In view of alarming levels of sedentariness and physical inactivity, several PA guidelines and recommendations have been worked out. In the global recommendations compiled by the expert group appointed by the World Health Organization (WHO), low level of PA is mentioned as fourth leading risk factor of mortality (World Health Organization 2010), preceded by high blood pressure, tobacco use, and high blood glucose and followed by overweight and obesity. It is noteworthy that PA is often mentioned as an effective strategy of prevention regarding the other leading causes of mortality (e.g. hypertension: Whelton et al. 2002; overweight and obesity: Tremblay et al. 2005; Jakicic and Otto 2005; Ortega et al. 2007). The WHO guidelines recommend for children and young people:

(a) Accumulating at least 60 min daily moderate-to-vigorous physical activity (MVPA), whereas more than that amount would provide additional health benefit;
(b) Most of the activity should be aerobic, some of it should be of vigorous intensity, and bone- and muscle-strengthening activities should be done at least three times a week.

Several national guidelines [e.g. US (Barlow and Expert Committee 2007), UK (Bull and Expert working groups 2010), and Estonia (Pitsi ct al. 2017)] recommend reducing sedentary (sitting) time. For example, the American Academy of Pediatrics (Barlow and Expert Committee 2007) has recommended that television and video time should be restrained to a maximum of 2 h per day for the prevention of paediatric overweight and obesity and resultant comorbidities. There is emerging evidence that the health effects of sedentariness go beyond those of lack of PA (Zhou and Owen 2017).

The promotion of PA among children is important for its direct health effects but also because of its potential to instil lifelong behaviour patterns that, if maintained into adulthood, will result in a more active and physically fit adult population (Sallis and Patrick 1994; Twisk et al. 1997). This notion is dependent on the assumption that PA is tracked from childhood to adulthood; there are not many long-term tracking studies using objective methods (the short-term studies in children and adolescents have typically found moderate tracking, e.g. Rääsk et al. 2015a), whereas moderate to high stability of PA is found using parental and self-reports over several decades (Telama et al. 2014).

A second indirect effect of PA in childhood is the development of both physical fitness (Ortega et al. 2015) and fundamental movement skills (Lubans et al. 2010; Barnett et al. 2009) that are important on their own right, and also as enabling a wider choice of PA later in life.

7.1.3 Importance of Physical Activity Assessment

The current focus on accurate assessment of PA levels is essential for the determination of the dose–response relationship between PA and health outcomes (Wareham and Rennie 1998). For example, valid and reliable measures of PA are necessary for studies designed to (1) determine the association between PA and health outcomes; (2) document the frequency and distribution of PA in defined populations; (3) determine the level of PA required to influence specific health parameters; (4) identify the psychosocial and environmental factors that influence

PA behaviour; and (5) evaluate the effectiveness of health promotion programmes to increase habitual PA in individuals group or communities (Wareham and Rennie 1998; Trost 2007).

Questionnaires have been widely used in PA assessment due to their affordability and ease of administration. Depending on the type of the study, a questionnaire may be the only feasible option. The differences between questionnaires and objective methods are not confined to the former being less accurate—using questionnaires, one should consider that the information is based on self-perception and memory, and is always multidimensional, reflecting not only the behaviour of interest but also concerns like self-concept and self-presentation. Therefore:

(a) Questionnaire assessments of PA may be subject to misclassification, to a different degree in different respondents (Gorber and Tremblay 2016).
(b) Respondents may be particularly poor at estimating the volume or frequency of a behavioural category that is artificial from their point of view (e.g. light-intensity activity or, in general, any unstructured activity), but they may be quite reliable in estimating the frequency of personally meaningful behaviours or other relevant facts (e.g. the frequency of walking from home to school or the distance from school to home) (Rääsk et al. 2015a, 2017).
(c) Questionnaire assessments may not be sensitive to change or may change differently from the behavioural change; for example, Rääsk et al. (2015a) found a considerable decline in objective PA in adolescents over 2 years, but no change in self-reports and only a very small decline in parent reports.

Consequently, questionnaires can be highly useful in initial stages of research and in assessing certain types of questions, but their use is highly problematic when one intends to estimate quantitative relationships, for example dose–response relationships between PA and health outcomes, or the effect of an intervention. Caution must be exerted when treating questionnaire data as quantitative, even if they are expressed in terms of physical units such as minutes of MVPA. Potentially, questionnaires can complement accelerometry-based assessment in several ways, e.g. regarding the types of activities that the participant has performed.

PA is a complex and multidimensional phenomenon; in every study, one must make some choices as to which parameters to assess. From a public health point of view, one of the most important parameters is the total volume of PA. This can be expressed (a) as daily or weekly energy expenditure in physical units, (b) in arbitrary units, e.g. "counts" per minute (CPM), (c) in natural units, e.g. daily steps, (d) in units referring to time in intensity categories, e.g. daily minutes of MVPA. In addition to the MVPA, the importance of light activity is being emphasised in more and more studies (Powell et al. 2011; Levine 2004). More complex variables that can be of public health interest are breaks in sedentary activities (Healy et al. 2008; Bailey and Locke 2015) and "bouts" of either MVPA or light activity—that is, periods where a certain intensity level has persisted for at least a certain amount of time (Mark and Janssen 2009). These variables can be easily derived from accelerometer output and are directly related to PA recommendations.

Some more specific health-relevant aspects of PA may be more difficult to assess with accelerometers. For example, for the fundamental movement skills to develop in an optimal way, it is important that the child has a reasonable amount of practice at a range of different activities (e.g. throwing, balancing, jumping, running). These skills could be tested directly and assessed via self-report or proxy reports, but using just one sensor on the waist it is probably impossible to figure out how often the sensor bearer has engaged in the act of throwing something. The same logic applies to bone- and muscle-strengthening exercises, as well as balance exercises: at least, using only one sensor, it is probably impossible to tell whether these have been performed in recommended amounts. The motivation, enjoyment, or interest in PA may play a role in the lifelong continuity of PA behaviours, but are, again, difficult to assess with accelerometry-based devices. Depending on the research question, it may thus be of crucial importance to complement accelerometry-based data by assessments of fitness and skills, and/or self- or proxy reports of motivation, enjoyment, and context.

Not all aspects of PA that are relevant to any given health outcome are fully known. For example, research into the chronobiology of PA has only recently started, but there are data showing that a fragmented rhythm of daily PA is associated with lower cardiorespiratory fitness and higher metabolic risk (Garaulet et al. 2017). This example is one among the many showing that the public health relevance of the data collected in large-scale studies using accelerometry-based PA assessment is not limited to a few summary variables that are typically used. It is thus of crucial importance to find ways to keep the data in their original form, not just the summary variables.

The IDEFICS study is one of the largest European studies on childhood obesity and includes eleven countries and more than 16,000 children aged between 2 and 9.9 years (Bammann et al. 2006; Ahrens et al. 2011). One of the aims of the IDEFICS study was to investigate the primary factors leading to childhood obesity by assessing the lifestyle patterns of children within the European Union in order to develop suitable interventions aimed at countering the obesity epidemic. A number of novel interventions were utilised within the IDEFICS study in order to improve health awareness and encourage healthy eating and physical activity in children. The IDEFICS study is the first large-scale study to assess PA objectively (i.e. accelerometry) among preschool and primary school children (Ahrens et al. 2011).

The I.Family study continued the IDEFICS study with a focus on the familial, social, and physical environment to assess the determinants of eating behaviour and food choice and its impact on health outcomes (Ahrens et al. 2017).

7.2 Accelerometry-Based Activity Monitoring

An activity monitor must be able to detect motion, transform the motion information into some usable units, and store this information over a period of time. A simple mechanical pedometer (or passometer in earlier use) may contain a pendulum that would move back and forth with every step and some mechanism to make a gear wheel advance by one position with every movement of the pendulum, etc. Mechanical pedometers can detect steps with some accuracy but are, by definition, restricted by the concept of step (thus ignoring the intensity and speed dimensions); in addition, pedometers are not good at detecting slow-paced movement (Martin et al. 2012). Accelerometry-based monitoring provides a reasonable compromise between validity and feasibility (see the review by Esliger and Tremblay 2007). More affordable methods such as diaries and pedometers have lower validity; methods with higher validity such as direct observation, calorimetry, and doubly labelled water (DLW) tend to be costly and more burdensome to the participants. In comparing accelerometry with the latter methods with better validity, one must notice that accelerometry-based monitors offer an excellent temporal resolution (differently from DLW) and, at the same time, good ecological validity (participants can carry the equipment with them for weeks and, in principle, years, with no major interference for their daily life—differently from both observation and calorimetry).

The term **accelerometer** means, in strict sense, only the **sensor**, which is a crucial but not the only component of the activity monitor. Today, most of the activity monitors contain a capacitive "microelectromechanical systems" (MEMS) or a piezoelectric sensor (John and Freedson 2012). MEMS sensor is used, for example, in the devices used in the IDEFICS and I.Family studies: ActiGraph models GT1M and GT3X, ActiTrainer, as well as the 3DNX that was used in the IDEFICS validation study (Bammann et al. 2011; Ojiambo et al. 2012; Horner et al. 2011). A piezoelectric sensor is used, for example, in Actical, as well as older models from ActiGraph such as AM 7164 (John and Freedson 2012). As to our knowledge, there is yet no systematic comparison of the advantages and disadvantages of different sensor types in activity monitors. ActiGraph's decision to change the sensor type seems to have been motivated by cost efficiency and feasibility, whereas the claim is that the later and the earlier models yield comparable results (John and Freedson 2012). There are studies comparing devices with different sensors: for example, Fudge et al. (2007) have compared sensors of a different type (piezoelectric sensor in CSA 7164 vs. MEMS sensor in GT1M and GT3X), but these comparisons are confounded with differences in firmware.

Studies of technical variability support the notion that MEMS sensor used in GT3X is reliable in estimating PA in the frequencies that are common to most types of human daily activities (Santos-Lozano et al. 2012).

Bouten et al. (1997) have reviewed studies on human body acceleration and concluded that a sensor with amplitude range of about −6 to + 6 G and with frequency range of about 20–100 Hz would be sufficient if the sensor is placed at waist level. One cannot but notice that several older devices, including GT1X, fall short of this requirement; however, it is unclear whether this causes a serious bias in the estimates of daily activity volume.

The activity monitoring device must also contain a unit for **filtering** and pre-storage processing of the signal. The pre-processing may be done at the hardware level (as in ActiGraph AM 7164), in updatable firmware within the device (as in GT1M), or in the computer when downloading the data (as in GT3X+). Given the memory limitations in the earlier (pre-GT3X) models, storing the raw data over a period of several days was not possible, so the data must have been processed within the device and stored as values aggregated within an "**epoch**" (this term is used in the literature to denote the time interval of measurement; typical values of an epoch are between 1 and 60 s). Temporary malfunctioning at this level may result in implausible and impossible values (Rich et al. 2013) which must be corrected before analysis. Another set of issues is related to the band-pass filter included in ActiGraph firmware: the signal outside the range of 0.25–2.5 G is markedly attenuated by the software (John and Freedson 2012). This is likely to be the reason for the "plateau" seen in GT1M output when the device is worn while running: the output (counts per minute) rises linearly until a certain speed (9–10 km/h) and then either declines or continues to rise at a much gentler slope (Fudge et al. 2007). Other researchers (possibly using different versions of firmware) have even noticed a decrease in counts with increasing running speed; as a consequence, running at 18 km/h might look identical to running at 8 km/h in the data (John et al. 2010). Indeed, Chen et al. (2012) saw a plateau effect in post-filtered activity in GT3X and in the 60 s integrated data ("counts"), but not in the original pre-filtered data. Due to firmware features, thus, the ActiGraph monitors may underestimate the intensity of vigorous activity. This is, however, unlikely to influence the estimates of the duration of vigorous activity, and it is probably not very influential for estimating the total daily volume of PA, as running faster than 9 or 10 km/h is, regrettably, a rare and short-lived event for most participants in epidemiological studies. Nevertheless, as the reason for the band-pass filter is to exclude the movement frequencies unlikely to occur in humans, it remains to be determined whether a better trade-off can be achieved (i.e. better representation of high-speed running, but not at the expense of including more non-humanly possible movement).

The **memory** capacity of the ActiGraph devices has been constantly rising: from 64 kB in AM 7164 to 1 MB in GT1M to 512 MB (possibly more) in GT3X+. The recording time will depend on both memory and temporal resolution: choosing a shorter epoch in older models means that the memory is filled up faster.

Note that the recording capacity of the device also depends on the battery capacity. As the battery time tends to shorten with use, it is advisable to check the batteries regularly and charge them occasionally even when the devices are not in use (e.g. between the fieldwork periods).

The sensor, processing unit, memory, and the battery comprise the functional parts of an activity monitor. These are, however, not the only parts that can influence the results. The **casing** is important to protect the inner workings of the device from the external forces, but one should also consider the aesthetic component: participants are to carry this with them for at least several days. In large studies, the casing is often the first component to show the signs of wear. The **belt** to attach the device on waist has some important features to pay attention to: (1) ease of use (can it be used to attach the device firmly in an easy way?) and (2) washability.

Nowadays, on the one hand, there is consensus that **raw measurements** (in physical units) should be used whenever possible, (1) to minimise dependence on proprietary algorithms and filters, (2) to allow maximal comparability between different devices, and (3) to record data at maximal temporal resolution. On the other hand, a large number of studies have used older-generation devices where raw recordings are not available due to memory restrictions. Thus, ActiGraph counts have become a de facto standard of comparison. Some authors have argued for converting the counts back to physical units, but it is only possible to do it approximately (John and Freedson 2012)—so the comparability achieved with this step may be an illusion. The potential benefits that using raw data may once bring have so far remained largely just that: potential benefits. There is no convincing evidence, for example, that using high-resolution data would bring about a qualitative jump in the accuracy of estimation of daily energy expenditure or the gross volume of PA. It is likely that high-resolution data may allow better accuracy at activity recognition, but even this has its limits with a single sensor whose exact location regarding body parameters is not known. Applications with more sensors with more exact placement, however, are not likely to be feasible in large epidemiological studies.

For the time being, thus, while we recognise the need of recording and storing the data at maximum available resolution and in physical units, we restrict the following discussion to the "counts" output of ActiGraph devices. This is admittedly a temporary solution but is relevant as long as the older generation of activity monitors (not capable of recording at high resolution) or data thereof is used.

7.3 Practical and Methodological Issues in Accelerometry-Based PA Assessment

7.3.1 Issues in Choice of the Device

When the IDEFICS study started in 2006, the question of choosing an activity monitor was essentially that of a choice between brands: hypothetically, is ActiX better than ActiY? The decision to use ActiGraph's GT1M and ActiTrainer devices in the study was based on the widespread use of these monitors and lower costs compared to other devices in the same category. Since then, the focus has slowly but steadily moved towards establishing non-proprietary algorithms and metrics working on raw acceleration data (John and Freedson 2012; van Hees et al. 2013): with this approach, the brands are to be decomposed into functional units such as sensor, memory, and algorithms. From this perspective, a clear and simple recommendation is to select a device that allows recording and downloading raw data in physical units (see, e.g. van Hees et al. 2013; de Almeida et al. 2018; van Hees 2018 on the analysis of such data).

Using physical units and recording raw data are essential for interbrand comparability, for being able to separate sensor-related and algorithmic components of PA assessment and for being able to use any algorithms derived in future. Whether the raw data provide a higher level of precision is open to debate, and the conclusion will probably depend on which parameter of PA one intends to estimate.

Besides openness and validity, one also needs to pay attention to feasibility and affordability. When planning the IDEFICS study, there was a remarkable price difference between activity monitors with uniaxial and three-axial recording. We therefore investigated the question whether the other spatial axes besides vertical add anything worthwhile to the assessment of general volume of PA. In the validation study with doubly labelled water (Ojiambo et al. 2012), we compared two devices: GT1M (only longitudinal/vertical axis) and 3DNX (three axes: longitudinal, mediolateral, and anterior–posterior) and found that while all three axes were correlated with PA energy expenditure (PAEE), only vertical axis contributed unique predictive variance. In terms of variance explained, using the vertical axis alone was better than a combination of all three axes (vector length). The main reason for this result is probably that the movements along the vertical axis are the most laborious because they go half of the time, in exactly opposite direction to that of gravity. A study by Howe et al. (2009) reached the same conclusion using a different device (RT3): vector magnitude counts were no more predictive of EE than vertical counts (unfortunately, the other axes besides vertical were not analysed separately). In a recent study using GT3X, Chomistek et al. (2017) found the triaxial composite to have a higher correlation with DLW-derived daily and PA energy expenditure than the vertical counts alone. The difference was, however, small (unadjusted correlations between total EE and counts were 0.59 versus 0.55 for women, and 0.58 versus 0.54 for men). It is unfortunate that the raw files were not preserved in that study, so it is not possible to check whether the result depends on proprietary algorithms used to derive counts (e.g. the band-pass filter discussed above; cf. John and Freedson 2012) or would remain the same with open-source algorithms (e.g. van Hees 2018). The main conclusion of our DLW study, however, remains unaltered: the vertical axis counts are the most important in predicting daily EE, with the other axes adding, if anything, only a small fraction of variance. This should not be taken as a recommendation to use uniaxial sensors if there is a choice: on the contrary, more information is generally preferable to less. However, when one is interested in predicting the gross volume of PA, it should not be taken for granted that the "vector magnitude" (vector length) metric should be preferred to the use of vertical axis alone.

7.3.2 Validity and Calibration

In this section, we are mostly interested in methods to estimate the total volume of PA, as well as the time spent in different levels of intensity of activity. Consequently, two types of validation studies are relevant: (a) validating the accelerometer output against doubly labelled water and (b) studies of classifying activities into intensity categories, typically using indirect calorimetry as a criterion. The DLW enables EE to be accurately measured in free-living conditions, which makes it the method of choice in validating the total volume of PA.

The studies relating accelerometer output to DLW have been of variable quality (Plasqui et al. 2013) and have yielded varying results (Sardinha and Júdice 2017); the zero-order correlation of accelerometer output and energy expenditure is, at best, moderate. Below, we would like to point out two studies that have used ActiGraph devices and a similar age group to that of the IDEFICS study.

Butte et al. (2014) validated two complex multivariate prediction models (cross-sectional time series and multivariate adaptive regression splines, described in Zakeri et al. (2013) in more detail) including biometric variables, accelerometer counts, and heart rate (HR) as predictors and achieved good accuracy in prediction (root-mean-square error [RMSE] = 105 kcal/day); the accuracy was slightly lower without including HR (RMSE = 116 kcal/day). Due to the choice of modelling strategy, however, it is not easy to find out the independent contribution of accelerometer counts to the prediction. In addition, even though this strategy may optimise predictive accuracy, it is less optimal for understanding the functional relationships in question.

In the IDEFICS validation study (Ojiambo et al. 2012), we found, using multiple linear regressions, that body mass alone predicted 71% of the variance in daily energy expenditure (EE); vertical counts from an ActiGraph device (ActiTrainer, compatible with GT1M but capable of recording HR as well) added another 11 percentage points. The prediction formula was:

$$EE = 0.72196 + 0.15984 \times weight + 0.00332 \times CPM.$$

The RMSE for this model was 0.49 MJ/day (approximately 117 kcal), thus not very different from that found by Butte and colleagues using a more complex model (note, however, that this is a biased comparison as Butte's study included separate model development and testing steps).

The other device included in the study, 3DNX, was equally predictive of the EE: the model R^2 increased by 10 percentage points when vertical counts of 3DNX were added to body mass:

$$EE = 0.03109 + 0.16699 \times weight + 0.00856 \times CPM_{vertical},$$

where $CPM_{vertical}$ represents the vertical (longitudinal) axis counts of the 3DNX device. The other two axes, however, were not significant when added to the model and had, in fact, negative regression coefficients:

$$EE = 0.61127 + 0.16328 \times weight + 0.01662 \times CPM_{vertical}$$
$$- 0.00391 \times CPM_{anteroposterior} - 0.00593 \times CPM_{mediolateral}.$$

It is interesting to note that not only did the counts from anterioposterior and mediolateral axis not reach statistical significance in the model (the p-value for mediolateral axis was 0.066), but their corresponding regression coefficients were negative. It would be premature to offer a substantive interpretation to the sign of these coefficients, but it does seem to indicate that the lack of prediction was not due to insufficient statistical power.

We are far from claiming that our study represents the optimal strategy in predicting DLW from accelerometer output. On the contrary, the relationship between PA, body parameters, and EE is unlikely to be confined to linear main effects. Using allometric modelling as suggested by Carter et al. (2008) may be a better strategy from a substantive point of view, even if the predictive advantage is modest.

One should also note that the percentages of explained variance depend on both the variance in body parameters and the diversity of lifestyles in the population under study. For example, Ojiambo et al. (2013) studied a highly active group, children and adolescents in Kenya, and found that accelerometer counts (average counts per minute) explained about 12% of the variance in daily energy expenditure when added to the model after body weight. Interestingly, time spent in light-intensity activity contributed another 12%. Tentatively, this may mean that time spent in low-intensity activities is an independent predictor of EE, regardless of the intensity of these activities. To see this effect in data, however, one needs a population where there is a large variance in the amount of light-intensity activities: a large share of light PA in Ojiambo's study was likely to involve going to school and back; the distance between home and school varied from 0.8 to 13.4 km. As another example, Horner et al. (2013) studied a highly active military population (mean PAEE 6.4 MJ/day (SD = 2.3 MJ/day), which is even more than the 5.7 MJ/day (SD = 3.0 MJ/day) in Ojiambo's very highly active population, and found the largest share of total EE to be explained by body parameters, with accelerometer counts adding only 4%. Superficially, one might think that in a highly active population, the contribution of PA in EE should be higher. This seeming paradox is explained by the highly structured nature of military activities, offering little room for individual choice over the intensity or duration of an activity.

We have heretofore discussed validity as a problem of prediction of variance. In the research using DLW as a criterion, there is little data on validity in the absolute sense, including possible bias in estimating EE from a regression-based model like the ones described above. This would probably depend on not just the device being validated, but also the anthropometric parameters, as well the level and patterning of PA in the population under question. However, predicting the absolute value of EE is rarely a primary objective (among other reasons, because PA recommendations are not expressed in the units of EE); there is more reason to demand accuracy and lack of bias in the estimation of time spent in different categories of activity intensity. For example, to estimate whether a child conforms to the recommendation of at least 60-min daily MVPA, one would need an unbiased estimate of daily minutes of MVPA. To obtain such measures, one needs to calibrate the accelerometer output against some other measure. There are several ways of doing it, but the most common are (1) developing a regression formula relating accelerometer counts to EE and using this formula to find cut-points for successive intensity categories (e.g. Freedson et al. 2005; Treuth et al. 2004; Puyau et al. 2002; Mattocks et al. 2007; Pate et al. 2006) and (2) finding an optimal trade-off between sensitivity and specificity when using accelerometer counts to predict the intensity category of an activity (e.g. Sirard et al. 2005; Evenson et al. 2008; van Cauwenberghe et al. 2010). Butte et al. (2014) implemented a combination of these strategies by using EE via oxygen uptake as a criterion but sensitivity/specificity analysis via receiver operating characteristic (ROC) curves as an analytical approach. In some cases, there is a confusion about which criterion has been actually used. For example, Hislop et al. (2012) have cited the Evenson et al. (2008) study as being based on oxygen uptake (VO_2) as a criterion; in fact, $\dot{V}O_2$ was only used to describe the activities and calculating maximum $\dot{V}O_2$, but cut-points were developed based on pre-classified activities. One might thus say that $\dot{V}O_2$ was only indirectly used as validation criterion, as it was used to demonstrate the validity of classification of activity intensities, but it was not used in data analysis to develop cut-points.

Migueles et al. (2017) offer a comprehensive overview of ActiGraph cut-points for all age groups and metrics; a subset (restricted to vertical counts and younger age groups) is shown in Table 7.1. In studies comparing different sets of cut-points, there is no clear winner. The second strategy is specifically targeted for maximising accuracy and minimising bias; thus, it is not surprising that it has worked out best in a comparison using these criteria. Namely, Trost et al. (2011) have concluded that "*Of the five sets of cut points examined, only the EV cut points provided acceptable classification accuracy for all four levels of physical activity intensity*". With this in mind, the Evenson cut-points were applied in the IDEFICS study. It is interesting to compare it with two more recent calibration studies by Butte et al. (2014) and van Cauwenberghe et al. (2010). First of all, the cut-points differentiating between light and moderate activity are all at approximately 2200 counts per minute (CPM) (range 2120–2336 CPM, see Table 7.1), differing from each other by no more than 10%. This is roughly consistent with several other studies (Martinez-Gomez et al. 2011), even though some studies suggest a higher threshold of about 3000 CPM (Guinhouya et al. 2011). The thresholds for vigorous activity range from 3520 to 4450 CPM, the largest difference being thus about 20%. The picture is drastically different with the threshold between sedentary and light activity: 100 CPM (25 counts per 15 s) as estimated by Evenson et al. (2008), 240 CPM as estimated by Butte et al. (2014), and 1492 CPM (373 counts per 15 s) as estimated by van Cauwenberghe et al. (2010)—a 1500% difference between the lowest and the highest estimate. The latter cut-point is not uniquely high, being similar to that obtained by Sirard et al. (2005) in a calibration study with direct observation as criterion.

How can one reconcile this degree of divergence? One can first notice that some activities would certainly be misclassified by van Cauwenberghe et al.'s criterion: for example, slow walking would almost certainly produce less than 373 ActiGraph counts per 15 s: the average was 295 in Evenson et al.'s (2008) study for walking at 3.2 km/h, while the mean VO_2 was 12.7 ml/kg/min. However, the mean counts for sedentary play were 447.9, that is, more than for slow walking (265.3).

Table 7.1 Cut-points (lower thresholds for light, moderate, and vigorous intensity) for children, using ActiGraph vertical counts

First author, year	Activity monitor, activities	Method, prediction equation	Age (N)	Thresholds: LIG/ MOD/VIG (epoch)
Freedson et al. (2005)	CSA 7164 Walking and jogging on treadmill	METs = 2.757 + 0.0015 × CPM − 0.08957 × age − 0.000038 × CPM × age	6–17 (80)	101/2220/4136 (60)
Puyau et al. (2002)	CSA 7164 SED: Nintendo, arts, play LIG: aerobic warm-up, walk MOD: tae bo, play, walk 3.5 mph VIG: jog, jump rope, walk, skip, soccer	AEE = 0.0183 + 0.000010 × CPM	6–16 (26)	800/3200/8200 (60)
Treuth et al. (2004)	ActiGraph 7164 Rest, watch TV, play computer game, sweep floor, walk (2.5 mph, 3.5 mph), aerobics, bicycling, shoot baskets, stair walk, run	METs = 2.01 + 0.00171 × CP30 s = 2.01 + 0.000856 × CPM	14.1 ± 0.3 (74 girls)	101/3000/5200 (60)
Sirard et al. (2005)	ActiGraph 7164 SED: talk, play LIG: walk (3.2 ± 0.6) MOD: walk (4.3 ± 0.6) VIG: jog (6.9 ± 3.9)	ROC, direct observation	3–5 (16)	Age-specific: 3y: 302/ 615/1231 4y: 364/812/ 1235 5y: 399/891/ 1255 (15)
Pate et al. (2006)	ActiGraph 7164 Rest, walk/jog (2, 3, 4 mph)	VO$_2$ (ml/kg/min) = 10.0714 + 0.02366 × CP15 s[a]	3–6 (29)	../420/842 (15)
Mattocks et al. (2007)	ActiGraph 7164 Lie, sit, walk/jog (4.4 ± 0.7, 5.8 ± 0.8, 9.2 ± 1.5), hopscotch	EE (kJ/kg/min) = −0.933 + 0.000098 × CPM + 0.091 × age + 0.0422 × sex (m = 0, f = 1)	12.4 ± 0.2 (163)	101[b]/2306 [3 METs]/ 3581 [4 METs]/6130 (60)

(continued)

Table 7.1 (continued)

First author, year	Activity monitor, activities	Method, prediction equation	Age (N)	Thresholds: LIG/ MOD/VIG (epoch)
Evenson et al. (2008)	ActiGraph#AM7164-2.2 SED: sit, watch DVD, colour books LIG: walk (2 mph) MOD: stair climbing, walk (3 mph), dribble basketball Vigorous: basketball, jumping jacks, run (4 mph)	ROC, direct observation (activity intensities validated by VO_2)	5–8 (33)	26/574/1003 (15) >100/2296/4012 (60[b])
van Cauwenberghe et al. (2010)	ActiGraph GT1M SED: sit/stand on floor listening to a story, draw sitting on the floor, play LIG: walk (3.2; 4.0), play MOD: walk (4.8; 5.6; self-paced), play VIG: walk/jog (6.4; 7.2; 8.0), play	ROC, direct observation	5.8 ± 0.4 (18)	373/585/881 (15) 1492/2340/3524 (60)
Butte et al. (2014)	ActiGraph GT3X+ Watch TV, colouring, play video games, play with toys, dance, aerobics, run in place, nap, free activities	VO_2 (room respiration calorimetry), smoothing splines, ROC	4.5 ± 0.8 (50)	240/2120/4450 (60)

Notes CPM = counts per minute; CP15s = counts per 15 s; CP30s = counts per 30 s

Activities are categorised into SED (sedentary), LIG (light), MOD (moderate), and VIG (vigorous) if this classification is given in the original paper

Age is reported as range (min–max) or mean ± SD. Activity monitors are cited as reported in the original papers

Intensity categories are usually defined as <1.5 METs for sedentary, 1.5–3 for light, 3–6 for moderate, and >6 for vigorous intensity (Trost et al. 2001). There are different definitions of 1 MET, two of the most common being EE at resting state, and 3.5 ml O_2/kg/min (approximately 1 kcal/kg/h). Pate et al. (2006) used a different criterion (see note below); Mattocks et al. (2007) developed cut-points for both 3 METs (usual threshold for moderate activity) and 4 METs (their preferred threshold). Puyau et al. (2002) reported their criteria in kcal/kg/min as 0.015, 0.05, and 0.1, corresponding to 0.9, 3, and 6 kcal/kg/h. The first threshold may be an error or a typographical error, as 0.025 would correspond to the usual threshold of 1.5 METs

[a]20 and 30 ml/kg/min used as criteria for moderate and vigorous level, based on visual inspection of VO_2 data points

[b]From review by Trost et al. (2001)

The relationship between counts (acceleration measured at waist level) and energy expenditure is thus dependent on activity type, particularly at a low-intensity spectrum. Sedentary free play may involve frequent upper-body movements that cause acceleration at the site of the sensor but do not involve displacement of the whole-body mass like in walking. Maintaining a single threshold for all activities may thus result in misclassifying some of the sedentary activities (e.g. active play) as light or, alternatively, misclassifying some of the light activities (e.g. slow walking) as sedentary. To avoid both of these sins at the same time, one might consider an algorithm similar to Crouter and Bassett's (2008) or Crouter et al.'s (2012) branched regression approach—applying different formulae depending on the coefficient of variation (CV) of the counts or using different thresholds depending on the position of the body, which can be estimated by the "inclinometer" function included in some more recent devices such as GT3X. However, the accuracy of classification based on CV or inclinometer is far from perfect, which introduces an additional source of error.

In addition, one should take into account that the threshold estimates depend on the design of the study. In Evenson et al.'s (2008) study, for instance, there was a noticeable gap between sedentary and light activities: the average output from the accelerometer was 6.6 counts per 15 s for the highest averaging sedentary activity, whereas the average was 294.7 for the lowest averaging light activity (walking at 3.2 km/h). If this middle range were filled with sedentary and light activities of various grades of intensity, the discrimination would become a more difficult task, and the estimated threshold might shift up or down, depending on how the tasks are selected. Using measured EE values instead of task indicators (as in Butte et al. 2014) may be a partial solution to this problem.

In conclusion, cut-points are not arbitrary criteria, but neither do they represent the absolute truth. Because the relationship between EE and accelerometer output differs across activities, the statistically optimal set of thresholds could be derived in a calibration study with a representative sample of activities. The representative activities would, however, be different across individuals.

Some authors discourage the use of cut-points, arguing that average acceleration (preferably measured in physical units) per time unit is a better summary of the data set and a better predictor of EE than time in intensity categories. This is only partly justified as the estimates of time in intensity categories contain at least two sources of error that are not present when using average acceleration: (1) uncertainty of the threshold estimates and (2) ignoring the differences of intensity within categories; i.e. light activity at 1.51 MET (metabolic equivalent of task) is treated as equal to light activity at 2.99 MET, whereas the first is almost sedentary and the second is almost moderate. These difficulties may be alleviated by converting counts to EE units (METs, calories, or joules) using some of the approximate formulae in the literature or using MET·minutes or count·minutes instead of simple minutes as a statistic. One would need, however, additional calibration studies (or reanalyses of existing studies) to do this in the optimal way, as most of the calibration formulae are based on linear equations, and some have implausible implications. For example, Treuth formula (Treuth et al. 2004) for predicting METs from counts has

2.1 as intercept and a positive slope for counts: that is, the result can never be less than 2.1 METs. In other words, the formula can never predict sedentariness (MET < 1.5), even for 0 counts. In addition, it is possible that the optimal cut-points may depend on the anthropometric parameters such as height or weight.

It is thus clear that using cut-points for activity intensity categories does not only allow a finer description of activity: it also introduces additional sources of error to the estimates. Selecting the best threshold is not always possible as we do not yet have complete information; as a minimum precaution, it is therefore important to recognise that the choice of thresholds may make a difference with huge clinical and biological implications (Pate et al. 2006; Vanhelst et al. 2014a). However, it is an oversimplification to consider using cut-points an ad hoc solution to the imperfections in our data collection procedures that we will eventually get rid of. Indexing of PA as time in intensity categories has a number of shortcomings from a measurement theoretical point of view; however, such summaries are meaningful from a physiological and practical point of view, e.g. when justifying health recommendations or planning interventions. More fine-grained summaries may be useful for more specialised purposes, but one needs to take into account that finer distinctions tend to be less reliable.

Finally, it is a common practice to adjust cut-points when using a different epoch from that of the calibration study. For example, a calibration study found that 25 counts per 15 s can be used to differentiate light activities from sedentariness; using 60 s epoch, the threshold would thus be 100 CPM. This is a potential source of error: the optimal cut-point would probably be slightly different if 60 s epoch was used in the calibration study. There are, however, no studies making this direct comparison; meanwhile, one may conjecture that the difference is likely to be small. It is important, however, to use the exact, unrounded multipliers when adjusting the cut-points. For example, the methods section of one study (Gabriel et al. 2010) contained this sentence: *"For classification of 10 s epochs, NHANES threshold values were multiplied by a factor of 0.17 (i.e., 10 s/60 s)"*. The value 0.17 is 2% higher than the true value (1/6); hopefully, the authors had used the true value instead of the rounded value, but this is not clear from the text. For comparing studies using different sets of cut-offs and if original raw data are not available, one can use equating based on linear models (e.g. Brazendale et al. 2016).

7.3.3   Accelerometer Placement

Following the general principle that more data are better than less, one should try using as many sensors as possible; in addition, according to the law of diminishing returns, each additional sensor is likely to give less extra information than the previous one. The possibilities are limited by budget, logistics, and burden on participants; all these considerations typically lead to using a single sensor in moderate to large cohort studies.

If a single sensor is used, it should ideally be placed as close to the mass centre of the body as possible (Rosenberger et al. 2013), which means approximately at the hip level. Wearing the device at the back would probably minimise the distance from the mass centre, but placement at left or right side may be more convenient, and the difference in distance is not large. The hip location, being close to the centre of gravity of the body, correlates well with EE associated with movement against gravitational resistance which is a major component of EE as corroborated by the studies referred above, where the vertical axis was the best predictive of EE (Ojiambo et al. 2012; Howe et al. 2009; Chomistek et al. 2017). The right side of the body may be preferred for convenience as most people are right-handed (Corder et al. 2008). Ward et al. (2005) reported that it made very little difference if the accelerometer was worn on the right or left side.

At high ambulatory speeds (>9 km/h), ankle placement may supersede hip (Kyröläinen et al. 2001). This is partly due to biomechanical shifts in the transition from walking to running leading to altered joint kinematics. This is, however, a secondary consideration when assessing children's overall volume of PA, which only infrequently includes such speeds. Ankle placement may be useful for capturing fast running and biking, and it also probably captures sedentary fidgeting. Thus, it would be most useful in combination with another sensor at the hip level and perhaps as a way of detecting the posture. Moreover, considering the "plateau" effect in ActiGraph devices (and possibly other devices using band-pass filter), one would recommend using either raw signal or other devices when fidelity in capturing locomotion at high speeds is important.

Wrist placement can be more convenient than hip: typically, watches are worn on wrist. As a corollary, this means that if the device does not include a watch, it should be worn on the watch-less hand, which is usually the right hand; so, placement on non-dominant wrist, which seems to be preferable (Sirichana et al. 2017), may be inconvenient for right-handed watch-wearers. Other researchers (Dieu et al. 2017) have found little difference between dominant and non-dominant hand, but there is evidence (Sirichana et al. 2017) that the difference is there for low-intensity activities.

With both wrist and hip placement, one must consider that the correlation between acceleration and EE may be different for different activities. As a thought experiment, imagine giving a pedometer to three persons. Person A is instructed to collect 1000 steps in walking (wearing the device at waist), whereas person B's task is to hold the device in hand and collect the same number of "steps" while sitting. Person C is instructed to walk while holding the device in his right hand and to raise the hand up above his head with every second step while lowering it at the next step. Which one of them used the most energy? Who covered more distance, A or C?

Now imagine that for yet another person, D, the pedometer is hidden inside a 5 kg dumb-bell; otherwise, he is instructed to walk and move hand in synchrony with person C. He will expend considerably more energy in this process, but chances are that the final step counts will be identical.

On theoretical grounds, one would say that for capturing the overall volume of PA, the wrist placement is suboptimal because in addition to the energy costly counter-gravity movements of the whole body it reflects the less energy costly hand-only movements. These components cannot be disentangled without additional information. Accordingly, several studies have found considerably higher correlations between oxygen uptake and hip-placed sensor as compared to wrist sensor (Rosenberger et al. 2013; Swartz et al. 2000). In one study, however, similar correlations were found (Phillips et al. 2013; $r = 0.90$ versus 0.97); this result may be partly explained by a small number of activities included in the study and a different metric that was used (average within-individual r's, which do not adequately reflect the predictability of EE from counts *without* individual calibration). It thus seems likely that both sites can be used to estimate the overall volume of PA, but site-specific calibration has to be undertaken. For instance, Shiroma et al. (2016) have found that ActiGraph GT3X counts from wrist are up to 5 times higher than for hip, and their variance is higher.

Other sites that could be worth considering include chest (wearing the device in the form of neck pendant, Zhang et al. 2016), shoe (Lin et al. 2016), and ear (Manohar et al. 2009). Several multiple sensor systems have been used, e.g. Wockets (Rosenberger et al. 2013). Studies using multiple sensors have brought about only a modest increase in the predictability of EE from accelerometer data: for example, in one study (Montoye et al. 2016), predictions based on three sites (wrist, thigh, ankle) had slightly higher correlations with EE than the hip accelerometer ($r = 0.79$ versus 0.72). This is in concordance with the view that counter-gravity movements of the whole body (best captured by a vertical sensor placed near the mass centre of the body) are the major component of EE.

In the second decade of the twenty-first century, it would be difficult not to notice that many people are, most of the time, carrying a cell phone containing an accelerometer sensor. Besides their primary application of rotating the screen orientation when necessary, these sensors are used in PA applications and have been used in research. For example, Manohar et al. (2011) have successfully used iPhone (fixed at back) in PA assessment. In addition to being a success, this study illustrates two difficulties with using cell phone sensors: (1) for reliable PA assessment, the placement of the sensor has to be known (or devised); (2) people use a large number of different devices with considerable variability in accelerometer sensors.

In conclusion, for measuring the overall activity level, the best site for the sensor is as close to the mass centre of the body as possible; hip is the most often used site; other sites (e.g. back at waist level) may be as informative, but each site needs specific calibration. Other sites add little information that would be directly relevant to EE but can be highly useful for activity recognition. In this regard, only crude distinctions, e.g. distinguishing bipedal locomotion (walking, jogging, and running), from other activities might be possible with a single sensor at hip.

7.3.4 Temporal Resolution, Epochs, and Bouts

The question of temporal resolution consists of at least four subquestions: sampling rate of the sensor, sampling rate of the recording, sampling rate used in the analysis, and, finally, minimal length of an episode that one considers to be meaningful or important. These questions are interrelated.

The **sampling rate of the sensors** is typically in the range of about 20 Hz to about 100 Hz in the commercially available activity monitors. This is probably enough to register the volume of everyday activities (Chen et al. 2012); however, if one is interested in the question of intensity of the load to weight-bearing bones (which ultimately has an impact on bone density), then one may need much higher frequencies, up to 1000 Hz (Kitamura et al. 2009).

Not all of the activity monitors allow storing the original unprocessed measurements. In these cases, the pre-processed and integrated signal is stored, using arbitrary units (counts) and in pre-specified time units (epochs). The length of the epoch depends on the memory capacity of the device and the desired period of observation and, to a lesser extent, on the battery capacity. Within these limits, it is always advisable to select the lowest possible **epoch length for recording**. Some monitors (such as the newer ActiGraph devices) offer the possibility to download raw data and, at the same time, a pre-processed file with counts using an epoch set by the user. The most useful option is to do both and set the lowest possible epoch value for the file with counts. First, processing the raw data files is time consuming and still more complicated than processing the count data files. One might thus want to do the preliminary or even all of the analyses using the count data. Even in this case, however, it is important to keep the raw measurements (e.g. the .gt3x files in the case of GT3X) as this is the only way to ensure independence from proprietary algorithms. Second, even if one has decided to use, say, 60 s epoch in the analysis, these data can be easily derived from a 1 s epoch file, whereas it is (at least, for the time being) more tedious to derive it from the raw data. In the absence of raw data, it is not possible to go back from a longer epoch (say, 60 s) to a shorter (say, 1 s) one. That is, one can always aggregate if one has the unaggregated data, but, in the absence of time machine, it is not possible to disaggregate the data that are already aggregated. There is a further consideration in choosing the epoch: for comparability with other studies, it is sensible to use epochs that are submultiples of both 60 and 15 (i.e. 1 and 5) as these can be reintegrated to the most commonly used epochs.

If the previous questions have been successfully solved, one has a choice regarding the **epoch to use in further analyses**. This choice affects some of the summary variables derived from the data (e.g. wear time; time in intensity categories) but not others (e.g. average counts per minute; total counts). There is no simple answer to the question of an optimal epoch, but one should think of biological relevance. For example, consider a single 30 ms (ms) long period of vigorous activity in the middle of 10 min of sedentariness. Does this data point reflect the activity of the organism? In other words, can one say that during a 10-min period, the organism was otherwise sedentary, but vigorously active for 30 ms? This would probably not make sense. But what about 100 ms? 500 ms? 1 s? It seems reasonable to assume that within a few seconds one can do something vigorous, for instance jump, or lift a heavy dumb-bell; it is, however, difficult to imagine any activity that is much faster. Thus, an analytical epoch much lower than "a few seconds" does probably not make sense.

There are a number of studies showing that the choice of epoch has an impact on the estimates of time in intensity categories (Ojiambo et al. 2011; Edwardson and Gorely 2010; McClain et al. 2008). Gabriel et al. (2010) have shown that MVPA estimates had a comparable correlation with self-reported MVPA at 10 and 60 s epochs, but the correlations with meaningful outcome variables (e.g. body weight, body mass index (BMI), fat, and lean mass) were stronger at 60 s epoch. The generalisability of these results is unknown, but in any case this should not be taken as an argument for *recording* at a higher (60 s) epoch. Rather, one should make a difference between an analytical epoch and the minimum required length of PA episodes to be relevant to health. The latter issue also comes under the name of "bouts". Gabriel et al.'s (2010) results could mean that the MVPA episodes with shorter duration than 1 min are irrelevant for health. However, integrating the data into longer epochs is not an optimal solution to this question; rather, one should make a difference between very short episodes (<60 s), and not so short (≥ 60 s) episodes, and compare their respective contributions to the prediction. This is a potential complement to Mark and Janssen's (2009) result that short (5–9 min) and medium-to-long (≥ 10 min) bouts of MVPA are incrementally protective of overweight. In future studies, it is recommendable to keep the effects of epoch and bouts analytically separate and analyse different lengths of bouts while keeping the lowest possible epoch.

7.3.5   Wear Time Detection

Wear time detection is of crucial importance if the device cannot be worn continuously for the whole period of observation: for example, in the IDEFICS study, the participants were instructed to remove the accelerometer at night and for certain activities (e.g. taking a shower). With waterproof devices worn on wrist, it is feasible to have an uninterrupted period of observation, but this gives rise to another problem: distinguishing sleep time from wake time.

It has been argued that wear time validation can be considerably more exact using raw data as compared to time-integrated counts: high-resolution data are sensitive to the very small movements which almost invariably occur when the device is worn but can be "integrated out" when the count units are calculated. To our knowledge, no direct comparison between wear time validation methods used in raw and time-integrated data has been made so far. Van Hees et al. (2011) describe a wear time detection algorithm that can be used with wrist-worn accelerometer using raw data. Zhou et al. (2015) describe a method to improve the accuracy of this method by combining it with data from an integrated sensor of body temperature.

In time-integrated data, there are three commonly used algorithms:

(1) Consecutive zeroes method: Janssen et al. (2015) compared different versions of this rule and found ≥ 20 min to be the best criterion.
(2) Troiano et al. (2008): Non-wear was defined by an interval of at least 60 consecutive minutes of zero activity intensity counts, with allowance for 1–2 min of counts between 0 and 100.
(3) Choi et al. (2011a) method: "*1-min time intervals with consecutive zero counts for at least 90 min time window (w1), allowing a short time interval with nonzero counts lasting up to 2 min (allowance interval) if no counts are detected during both the 30 min (window 2) of upstream and downstream from that interval; any nonzero counts except the allowed short interval are considered as wearing*".

Choi et al. (2012) have compared the last two methods and found the latter to be more accurate, and both perform better at vector length metric than on vertical counts.

The choice of a wear time validation algorithm is most influential on the estimates of sedentary time; the other parameters estimated from data (time in intensity categories; average acceleration or counts per time unit) are only influenced if expressed as proportions of wear time.

Another occasionally used method for detecting non-wear time is using diaries (e.g. Ottevaere et al. 2011); this method shares many problems with other self-report methods but could provide useful information if high compliance is ensured and if concordant with the recorded activity data. Our experience in the IDEFICS study is that activity diary is the component with the poorest compliance; one cannot be sure whether all non-wear events are recorded; in addition, the degree of retrospectiveness of the diaries is unknown (i.e. whether the times were recorded right after the event, or in the evening, or reconstructed right before returning the diary to the survey centre). These are among the reasons why algorithmic methods are preferred in most studies. However, there are occasions where significant PA occurs, but the activity monitors cannot be worn for technical, convenience-related, or aesthetic reasons: for example, swimming, dance competitions, or different contact sports. In these cases, using activity diaries to impute missing data can be a viable strategy to avoid underestimating the true PA levels (de Meester et al. 2011).

In estimating the amount of time that needs to be observed, the calendar day is most often used as a unit. This is one of the natural units by which human activities are organised (in addition to weeks, months, and years), but from a data analytical point of view the period between 00:00 and 24:00 is no different from any other 24-h period. This means, in principle, that incomplete days could be used in analyses if the missing time could be imputed from another day. However, this would make it more difficult to analyse, for example, the effects of weekdays, so keeping day as a natural unit of analysis has some obvious advantages.

There is a lot of discussion in the literature about (a) the **valid day** issue: the number of hours of wearing time in a day that is needed in order to keep that day in the analyses and (b) the issue of **minimum number of valid days** required to consider the recording representative of a participant's usual levels of PA.

There is no universal answer to these questions: it depends on the organisation of daily activities in the population under study. In a hypothetical population where there are consistent individual differences in activity levels but no within-individual differences between hours in a day or days in a year, 1 h of recording would be sufficient to characterise any individual's level of activity. In real populations, however, these premises do not hold: individuals' activity levels fluctuate, and days and hours differ widely from each other. For an empirically based answer on minimum recording time, one would thus need to observe a population for a considerable period (say, a few years) to get a truly representative estimate of all kinds of different fluctuations in PA that may occur and their regularity or irregularity (e.g. seasonal variation may be different depending on the weather in a particular year; so at least a few years of observation are needed for a true picture of seasonal variation). If this becomes too difficult for participants, one could sample random hours, days, or weeks from a year. Based on this data set, one could derive a sampling algorithm to minimise the necessary recording time to get a credible estimate of a person's yearly activity. To our knowledge, such a study has not yet been carried out, but it is not unrealistic given today's technical capabilities.

In (temporary) lack of long-term studies, shorter ones have been used to predict the reliability of data, presuming that the future resembles the past. For example, Trost et al. (2000) studied youth in different age groups and found, using Spearman–Brown prophecy formula, that to achieve a reliability (measured as intraclass correlation, ICC) of 0.90, one would need to observe 11 days in first to third-graders, but 20 days in tenth to twelfth graders. In contrast, Vanhelst et al. (2014b), using a slightly different method, found that any combination of a weekday and a weekend day was sufficient to explain >90% of the variance in PA in obese youth (aged 7–18 years). Ojiambo et al. (2011) found 1-day ICCs of 0.32, 0.33, and 0.35 of average counts per minute, sedentary time, and MVPA, respectively, which in combination with the Spearman–Brown formula predicted that about 5 days would be needed to achieve a reliability of 0.7, 7 to 9 days for an ICC of 0.8, and 17–19 days for an ICC of 0.9. Such studies can, however, only serve as a rough guide, for several reasons.

(1) Intraclass correlations are based on random effects models and assume interchangeability of observations (Shrout and Fleiss 1979). However, consecutive days are not independent of each other, which means one would need a longer study to estimate the level of autocorrelation, and they are not randomly selected. Randomly selected 3 days from a year might give us an unbiased estimate of a person's yearly activity, but in a typical study these would be three consecutive days, which is highly improbable to happen by chance (the probability is about 2.07×10^{-8}).

(2) Under specific conditions, ICCs may underestimate the true reliability (Hallgren 2012); the amount to which this happens in PA studies is unknown—to ask this question, one should first make sure that the assumption of interchangeability holds.

(3) With the exception of the Vanhelst et al. (2014b) study, the difference between weekdays and weekends is often ignored, and a general recommendation regarding the number of days is given.

(4) ICC, as typically applied in PA studies, considers only one source of reliable variance ("true" levels of PA that are different between individuals) whereas there are many (e.g. there is an interaction between time of the day and person: some people are more active in the morning and some in the afternoon). This situation could be more adequately modelled by generalisability theory (Brennan 2001) or similar methods.

(5) Using the day as the unit of analysis seems natural but is not without problems. A single day of measurement seems likely to reflect, to a certain degree, the habitual activity of people, but its reliability cannot be computed using ICC without subdividing it, say, by hours. Dividing a day by hours, however, is not a full solution because (a) it is an arbitrary division which needs to be justified against alternatives such as half-hours or "academic hours" (45 min); (b) in this case, one would need to consider additional components of variance—time of day and person by time-of-day interaction, e.g. in the generalisability theory framework (Brennan 2001); and (c) more fine-grained divisions mean more units of observation from each person, possibly leading to higher estimates of reliability of the composite; however, reliability estimates should not depend on the arbitrary selection of unit of analysis.

(6) Most severely, the ICC as ratio of the between-individual variance to the total variance is a group-based and sample-dependent measure of reliability. In other words, according to this model, the accuracy of a single measurement occasion depends on how different the other people are from the person being measured. A larger ICC could be achieved by increasing the between-individual variance of the sample, for example including a few more sedentary individuals and competing athletes. To find a small ICC, it suffices to find a highly homogenous sample. This is counter-intuitive: a seeming change in reliability of a measurement has occurred without anything having been changed in the measurement itself. It would thus be desirable to develop a way to assess the accuracy of PA measures that would not depend on individual differences.

Against this background, one cannot fully rely on the ICC-based estimates as a guide. This information should be complemented by common sense, former studies, and knowledge of the target population. In addition, the desired level of reliability is not fixed: higher reliability is needed for individual diagnosis and in smaller samples. In population-based studies, one has to simultaneously manage two risks: (a) poor representativeness of individual measurements due to a too short period of measurement and (b) poor representativeness of the sample due to low compliance in PA measurements. Because protocol adherence tends to decrease with days of wear (Trost 2007; Corder et al. 2008), a compromise between feasibility and accuracy is necessary.

Seasonality of PA is a question that may need more attention: for example, Rääsk et al. (2015b) found a correlation of 0.19 between minutes of MVPA and time of measurement (indexed as absolute difference in days between winter solstice and the first day of accelerometry). This is a small correlation, but it results in a considerable mean difference when measurements from different seasons are compared. There are other studies of seasonality of PA (e.g. Kolle et al. 2009), but a consensus has not yet found of how and to which extent the seasonality must be taken into account.

It is common knowledge that people's PA differs by time of day, and there are usually differences between weekdays and weekends. From this, the minimum requirement for PA recording is one full weekday and one full weekend day. Recoding more weekdays and, if possible, a whole week, is desirable to capture the between-day differences that are likely to occur; longer periods are even better but may reduce compliance. Repeating the assessment at a different time of the year would probably do more for representativeness than prolonging an assessment by the same number of days.

In the IDEFICS study, the initial decision was to record at least 3 days of activity for each child, including one weekend day, whereas it strived for a recording time of 1 week in the I.Family study. This decision was based on the number of activity monitors available in each centre, the time available for fieldwork and the time needed to set up the devices including downloading the data, charging the batteries, and setting the device up for next recording. In some centres, more devices were available, and longer recording times were thus possible. For deriving reference values for the whole sample (Konstabel et al. 2014), it was decided to use the inclusion criterion of at least one weekend day and one weekday (with at least 8 h of wear time)—this way, 7684 children could be included (only 5047 when two weekdays were required instead of one—that is, the sample size would have been about 35% less).

Ideally, the recording period should cover a whole week or all different days of the week. In many studies, this is not possible to achieve, given common difficulties such as the number of available devices, the study period, or the desired sample size. A simple way to compactly present PA variables in these cases is to use a weighing scheme that is proportional to the number of weekdays and weekend days in a week: either a weighted sum $(5 \times WD + 2 \times WE)$ or a weighted average $(5 \times WD + 2 \times WE)/7$, where WD is the average value in weekdays and WE is the average value in weekend days (Konstabel et al. 2014; Ortega et al. 2013). Note that the result applies to the typical week, not to the average week: for that purpose, one should consider holidays, school breaks, vacations, illness days, and the like; the corrected proportion of non-business days could be used, but one cannot assume that all non-business days are like typical weekend days—consequently, this additional correction could do more harm than good.

7.3.6 Aspects of Data Reduction

Ideally, participants in a study comply with the study protocol. In the IDEFICS study, this meant putting on the accelerometer the first thing in the morning and taking it off every night right before going to sleep; removing it only for taking shower and swimming (or other events which may do harm to the device); and recording all non-wear events in the activity diary. However, protocols are not completely observed and there will be differences in wear time for unknown reasons. Several ways to correct or adjust for these differences have been used, the simplest of them being controlling for wear time (either for number of valid days or average daily wear time; Ortega et al. 2013) or expressing time in activity intensity categories as percentage of wear time (Rääsk et al. 2015a). We have also used a hybrid method: to find adjusted MVPA, the daily MVPA was first expressed as a fraction of wear time and then multiplied by average wear time in minutes (Konstabel et al. 2014). The rationale for this was that the outcome in minutes is easier to communicate and understand than a fraction, especially if that fraction is, unfortunately, close to zero. Additionally, wear times were different across sexes and age groups, thus adjusting provided a simple way of factoring wear time out of the group comparisons. This form of "adjusted minutes" (of, say, MVPA) would, however, presume that the activity at non-wear times is, on the average, as intensive as the activity at the time when the device was worn. There are two complementary ways to minimise the impact of such assumptions: (a) trying to achieve good compliance and (b) imputing the periods of missing data either using closest-in-time activity form the same day or another day from the same individual or using activity diaries. In some special cases, one could consider using group averages from the same period in imputing. Conceptually, this might make sense in groups sharing a common daily schedule of activities, e.g. the military (Horner et al. 2013) or, possibly, students at school time.

Minutes in activity categories are useful summary statistics for ease of communication and understandability. They have, however, a disadvantage of ignoring the within-category differences: activities at 1.51 MET and 2.99 MET are, for example, treated equally as light, even though there is an almost twofold difference in intensity. For some purposes (e.g. public health recommendations—and, consequently, studies validating such recommendations), ignoring the within-category variance is probably inevitable, or if one believes that the error becomes too large, the solution might be to create an additional category. However, there are questions (e.g. the relative contribution of activities at different intensity levels to the energy balance) where ignoring the within-category differences is simply not possible. For these purposes, one could decompose the total daily counts into intensity categories. Using formulae from the literature (Alhassan et al. 2012), one can transform these decomposed counts into EE units (METs or kcal or kcal/kg) or EE-per-time units (e.g. MET·minutes). For example, Rääsk et al. (2015a) have found longitudinal decreases in both light activity and MVPA in a study of adolescent boys. In addition, Konstabel et al. (2017) showed that in terms of EE, the decreases in light activity mattered more.

7.4   Software for Data Analysis

At the time when data collection in the IDEFICS study was finished, the standard way to analyse GT1M data was a combination of manual pre-processing in spreadsheet software (e.g. deleting manually the long sequences of counts where the participant either appears not to be wearing the device or has written in the activity diary that the device was not being worn), then using the macros or spreadsheet functions to compute summary statistics and then copying these summary statistics into another table for final analysis. In small samples, this does not result in too extensive workload and may even lead to important insights into the data, as everything is checked by the human eye. For a large epidemiological study, this method is obviously unpractical and could lead to human errors. There were also a number of software programs available, such as MAHUffe, MeterPlus, and Kinesoft, which allowed some laborious steps of pre-processing to be automatised. We needed, however, a fully customisable system which would be well integrated with a good statistical platform. Therefore, we decided to write a program using the software R (Ihaka and Gentleman 1996; R Core Team 2017). To date, this has evolved into an R add-on package "accelerate" (Konstabel 2018; for access see also Sect. 7.7) which provides a comprehensive set of functions to process the ActiGraph (7164, GT1M, and GT3X count data) and 3DNX data. The previous versions of the package have been used in analysing data from several projects (e.g. Rääsk et al. 2017; Garaulet et al. 2017; Ortega et al. 2013).

7.4.1   Design Choices

R was chosen as a platform because of its widespread use, integration of a statistical environment with programmability, availability of a large number of statistical and data analysis methods as add-on packages, integration with literate programming tools, and extensibility. The main goals of the package are comprehensiveness and ease of use which means inclusion of all commonly used methods and tasks in a simple workflow. The package was designed to be modular and easily extensible. Each subtask is programmed as a separate function; the user can change each part separately without the need of changing the whole program (e.g. new functions can be added for new data file formats or new analytical methods). For extensibility and robustness, the number of dependencies was kept at minimum. Finally, as accelerometer data files can be quite large, sparing use of memory had to be kept in mind. For example, data files are processed sequentially rather than loading them all into the memory and, instead of storing a timestamp with each data point, the timestamp is reconstructed when necessary, given the start time and time interval between the observations ("epoch").

7.4.2   Reading in and Pre-processing the Data

The first layer in the `accelerate` package is functions to read in the data files in various formats. There are three separate functions to read in plain text file formats from ActiGraph: `read.actigraph.dat` (for "dat" files), `read.actigraph.csv` (for "csv" files), and `read.csa` (for "dat" files from older models such as CSA 7164). These plain text formats store date and time information in local formats (e.g. 02/06/2018, 06.02.2018, and 2018-02-06 all refer to the same date, 6 February 2018); the functions thus contain algorithms to automatically try to interpret such information in a meaningful way (e.g. taking into account that downloading the data is a later event than initialising the device and that there are no more than 12 months in a year). Alternatively, one can set the date format to be used in an extra argument named `dateformat`. The newer "agd" file format used by ActiGraph, as well as the 3DNX device (read in respectively by `read.agd` and `read.3dnx`), stores dates in unambiguous format, so reading in is more straightforward. Finally, the `read.actigraph` function accepts any of the ActiGraph file formats (except for the older CSA format) and chooses the appropriate function to use based on file extension (e.g. "agd" files are redirected to `read.agd`).

All the reading-in functions accept a `get.id` argument which refers to a function to derive an identification number (ID) of the participant based on the file name or any information within the file. Two such functions are provided, `getID` which uses all digits in the file name as an ID and `getNAME` which deletes the file extension and any digits and uses the rest as an ID. An appropriate function should be chosen or written based on the conventions of the study.

The data are stored as a list of two components, X, a data frame containing the data, and HD, a vector containing all other relevant information such as start date/time of recording, the epoch, serial number of the device, ID code of the participant, file name.

By default, the reading-in functions do some pre-processing, such as filtering out the faulty data (e.g. negative counts) and detecting the wear and non-wear times (the latter are replaced by missing data codes). This behaviour is controlled by two arguments, `.filter`, and `preprocess`; to suppress all pre-processing, one can set both of these to `identity`.

Two algorithms of wear time detection are available: the `delete.zeros` function implementing the "consecutive zeros" algorithm (detecting the periods with at least N minutes of consecutive zeros, where N is, by default, 20) and the `wmChoi` function implementing the algorithm proposed by Choi and colleagues (2011a) adapted with slight changes from the PhysicalActivity package (Choi et al. 2011b).

For sequential processing of many files, the package includes a function `process.folder` that can be adapted to various tasks that involve applying similar rules to every file. This mechanism is used in `read.actigraph.folder` which reads in, pre-processes, and summarises all ActiGraph files in a folder (reintegrating every file to a common epoch to avoid treating files with different epochs in the same way), producing a data frame where each day is represented by a row and participants are identified by different values in the ID column. The mechanism can be easily adapted to different sets of rules and different tasks, such as producing a feedback sheet to every participant and possibly sending it via e-mail. The function takes care of errors when reading in or summarising the files: instead of quitting and giving an error message, the messages are recorded and saved for later inspection. By default, `process.folder` does timing in all cases, so it is possible to estimate how much time each operation might take, even retrospectively.

For example, to read in and summarise all over 2000 Hungarian files from the IDEFICS baseline survey (T_0), the following code was used:

```
> HT0 <- read.actigraph.folder("Hungary_T0")
```

This can take some time, so for estimating when the processing will be complete one might try the argument `LIST` to read in just a few files first:

```
> HT0 <- read.actigraph.folder("Hungary_T0", LIST = 1:5)
> attr(HT0, "timing")
```

7.4.3   Summarising the Data

Suppose we have read in a file using ...

```
> x <- read.actigraph("sampledata/1036.dat")
```

We can now summarise the data by some time unit. Usually, this would be days, but in some cases shorter periods such as hours or half-hours can be useful. The code uses R's built-in function `cut.POSIXt` to divide the time sequence, so specifications like "30 min" or "hours" or "2 days" are all valid. Thus, the first line in the following code segment summarises x by days and the other one by 30 min segments:

```
> summary(x, "DSTday") # the default
> summary(x, "30 min") # each row summarises a 30 min period
```

One could use just "days" in the first line, but "DSTday" takes care of the daylight saving time; due to this, in many countries, one day in a year will only have 23 h, while another has as many as 25.

The summary outputs a data frame with some information about each time period in the file. First, the file name, subject's ID, epoch, model, and serial number of the device are included; these data are, obviously, identical for all rows based on the same file. The next three variables can be different for each row in the summary: `Period` (the start of the time period, as a date/time variable with class), `Length` (nominal length of the period, including non-wear time), and `POSIXctWkdy` (day of the week, coded as integers from 0 to 6, starting from Sunday). The following variables depend on what has been recorded in the data file and the functions one chooses using the argument STATS to summary. The CNTSTATS function outputs some of the most common statistics used for counts: valid time (val.time), total counts (tot.-counts), average counts per minute (avg.cpm), and time in intensity categories. One or more sets of cut-points can be specified using the cutoffs argument; both minutes in intensity category and the corresponding proportion of valid time are computed. The CNTSTATS2 function uses the cut-points in a slightly different way. In addition to minutes in each intensity category, it outputs the sum of counts in each intensity category, which can be converted to quasi EE units (Konstabel et al. 2017), as discussed in Sect. 7.3.6. If the file contains information on steps or heart rate, this can be analysed using STEPSTATS and HRSTATS. Finally, HRSTATS2 combines count and heart rate data to find median heart rate in each category of activity intensity (an analysis by Ojiambo et al. 2012).

As an example, the following line will compute the count and step statistics by each day in category *x*, using Evenson cut-points; the results will be expressed in a compact way; i.e. errors in the data file (e.g. negative counts) are not included in the table, and time in intensity categories is expressed only as minutes (instead of minutes and a fraction of valid time):

```
>  summary(x,  STATS = c(CNTSTATS,  STEPSTATS),  cutoffs =
Cutoffs.Evenson, short = TRUE)
```

The data can be plotted using the generic plot function. The plot.acc method will plot counts as lines, using time as the *x*-axis. Figure 7.1 is produced by the following code:

```
> plot(x, cutoffs = Cutoffs.Evenson) # Figure 7.1
```

Another way to visualise the daily PA profile is to partition the time periods into activity categories in the order of increasing intensity (see Fig. 7.2). This can be done with aciPlot:

```
> aciPlot(x, select = Wkdy %in% 5) # Figure 7.2
```

Finally, the function summarize is intended to summarise the data at the next level with one row per participant. This can be applied to a summary of a single file [such as the output summary(x)] or of a number of files (such as the output of read.actigraph.folder). The two main arguments to summarize are: condition (an expression using variables in the output of summary, such as val.time > 8*60) and no.days (number of valid time periods—typically days—that a participant must have in order to be included). Another version, summarize2, treats weekdays and weekend days differently: the reqdays argument can be set as a named vector, such as c(wd = 5, we = 2) to require at least five valid weekdays and two weekend days for a participant's data to be included.

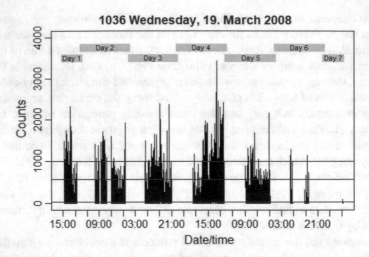

Fig. 7.1 A single participant's activity across 6 days (red lines correspond to Evenson cut-points)

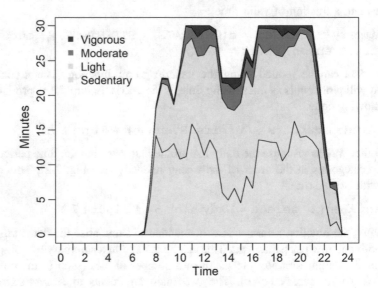

Fig. 7.2 Activity profile in a single day ("Day 4" in Fig. 7.1) by 30-min segments

7.5 Future Perspectives in Accelerometry

Accelerometry is among the best ways to measure PA, but it has inherent limitations: for example, static efforts and weight carrying seem unlikely to be captured, especially with a single sensor. In addition, the relationship between movement and EE may be different in different types of activity (e.g. biking as compared to running). There seem to be two ways forward for more accurate prediction of EE. First, while portable $\dot{V}O_2$ systems do already exist, they are not convenient for carrying along during several days of ordinary life. The advancement of technology may provide even better solutions that, if not affordable for large-scale testing, could provide a breakthrough in calibrating and validating the accelerometry-based monitors. Secondly, activity recognition algorithms could be developed based on either the advancements of Crouter and Bassett's (2008) two-regression model, multiple accelerometer sensors or a combination of different sensors. While the "black box" modelling strategy (e.g. using artificial neural networks) is guaranteed to give a result, joining the efforts of biomechanics and metabolic physiology is more likely to advance our substantive understanding of the nature of PA energy expenditure at different activities.

As many contemporary devices allow downloading the raw data, and software for analysing such data is becoming easily accessible (van Hees 2018), using raw data should be considered especially in the cases where counts-based methods of analysis are known to be suboptimal as, e.g. in wear time detection as well as at the low and high end of the intensity spectrum. Combining different sensors (e.g. temperature or light sensors) could be an alternative way of wear time detection.

There is a large number of sensors that can be used in combination with accelerometry and probably an even larger field of unexplored or underexplored possibilities. For example, altimeters (pressure sensors) could be used to classify inclined locomotion (e.g. walking upstairs) to enhance the accuracy in EE estimation (Yang and Hsu 2010).

For understanding and intervening on PA, it has to be treated as a meaningful human activity rather than just physical movement. For that purpose, linking the accelerometer data with information on mood and behaviour (e.g. diaries, experience sampling, or electronically activated recording), physiological reactions, and context [e.g. geographical location from geographic information systems (GIS)] is crucial. GIS, in particular, offers a large array of possibilities to relate PA to what is changeable in the environment (Buck et al. 2015a, b).

7.6 Assessing Physical Activity in the Field

Besides technology and algorithms, the data quality also depends on human factors and fieldwork logistics. The first, crucial, task is to make sure that the person who wore a device is **identifiable**. In the IDEFICS study, this was done in slightly different ways in different survey centres, depending on the local conditions. In one participating country, for example, it was necessary to label the devices with child's name. This was especially important in the younger, kindergarten-aged group, who, in the workdays, had organised nap time from approximately 1 pm to 3 pm. Typically, the teacher would collect the devices before the nap and distribute them again after it; this would not be possible without the labels. In school-aged children, in contrast, the labelling was more of a precaution, as the devices were typically not removed during the day. Nevertheless, the labels were occasionally lost, and the devices were uncoupled from the participants for other reasons. For example, it happened that several siblings from the same family were wearing the activity monitors at the same time, or classmates inadvertently (or perhaps advertently) swapped their devices. In such cases, if the swapping happened on the first day or right before returning the devices, the data could be used, in case the bearers of the devices were identified by parents' or teachers' reports, comparing activity diaries with the recorded data or other information. In a few cases, the device was returned but was not worn or contained mostly missing data because the child either could not or forgot to wear it or was ill at the time. If logistically possible, the child was then offered a new opportunity, and the latter file was used in analyses.

There are some reports on **reactivity** on wearing accelerometers (Dössegger et al. 2014), that is, higher than usual activity on the first day of measurement, which thereafter returns to the presumably usual level. The IDEFICS study was not planned for assessing reactivity. For example, the first day of wearing was not chosen at random but determined based on logistics and device availability; however, indirect assessment of reactivity might be possible. We did try to minimise reactivity by emphasising in the instructions that the participants should continue with their usual activities. The problem is, of course, that the reactivity might not always be intentional or even conscious: by being given an activity monitor, participants are inevitably reminded about physical activity, and this may be enough to prompt an increase in activity. In addition, reactivity due to the personnel at schools or kindergartens may have a longer lasting effect and be even more difficult to control.

The **motivation** and **compliance** of the participants are an important factor in data quality. Feedback on PA has potential to increase motivation; quick and fully automatic ways of creating feedback were not available to us at the baseline survey of the IDEFICS study, but by the end of the study period we had developed a rudimentary script, which is included in a simplified form in the `accelerate` package (`do.feedback`). However, providing feedback (as well as other ways of boosting interest in PA assessment) could increase reactivity. One might also want to consider the potentially adverse effect of negative feedback. Thus, the "too little PA" message should be framed in a positive and encouraging way.

There are logistic issues that may do harm to motivation even if the participant is otherwise interested in PA assessment. One of these is the fear of losing or damaging the device. There is a trade-off involved in eliminating this fear completely because for obvious reasons we do not want the participants to lose or damage the devices. Another issue is that of aesthetics and hygiene. First, the devices tend to look less and less new with every user, up to a point when one must do something about it; second, in study logistics, one must plan sufficient time for washing and drying the belts sufficiently often.

When downloading the data, it is useful to regularly **check** the files, for example, making a plot similar to Fig. 7.1. If the data do not look like human activity, one should investigate the reason. The malfunctioning hardware may need to be repaired or removed from use; temporary problems at download time are unlikely but can be repaired by downloading the data anew (which is impossible if the device is already set up to record new data); incompatibilities with new versions of firmware may be resolved by using other (newer or older) versions of download software; finally, during the IDEFICS study, several data files with firmware-related problems were successfully repaired in collaboration with the device manufacturer. It is useful to become aware of these problems as early as possible; thus, having a look at the files right after downloading is probably a good idea.

7.7 Provision of Instruments and Standard Operating Procedures to Third Parties

All standard operating procedures (SOPs) described in this chapter are provided by the General Survey Manuals that can be accessed on the following website: www. leibniz-bips.de/ifhs after registration. The R package "accelerate" can also be downloaded from this website.

Each third partner using the SOPs provided in this chapter is kindly requested to cite this chapter as follows:

Konstabel K, Chopra S, Ojiambo R, Muñiz-Pardos B, Pitsiladis Y, on behalf of the IDEFICS and I.Family consortia. Accelerometry-based physical activity assessment for children and adolescents. In: Bammann K, Lissner L, Pigeot I, Ahrens W, editors. Instruments for health surveys in children and adolescents. Cham: Springer Nature Switzerland; 2019. pp. 135–173.

Acknowledgements The development of instruments, the baseline data collection, and the first follow-up work as part of the IDEFICS study (www.idefics.eu) were financially supported by the European Commission within the Sixth RTD Framework Programme Contract No. 016181 (FOOD). The most recent follow-up including the development of new instruments and the adaptation of previously used instruments was conducted in the framework of the I.Family study (www.ifamilystudy.eu) which was funded by the European Commission within the Seventh RTD Framework Programme Contract No. 266044 (KBBE 2010–14).

We thank all families for participating in the extensive examinations of the IDEFICS and I. Family studies. We are also grateful for the support from school boards, headmasters, and communities.

References

Ahrens W, Bammann K, Siani A, Buchecker K, De Henauw S, Iacoviello L, et al. IDEFICS consortium. The IDEFICS cohort: design, characteristics and participation in the baseline survey. Int J Obes (Lond). 2011;35(Suppl 1):S3–15.

Ahrens W, Siani A, Adan R, De Henauw S, Eiben G, Gwozdz W, et al. I. Family consortium. Cohort profile: the transition from childhood to adolescence in European children—how I. Family extends the IDEFICS cohort. Int J Epidemiol. 2017;46(5):1394–5j.

Alhassan S, Lyden K, Howe C, Kozey Keadle S, Nwaokelemeh O, Freedson PS. Accuracy of accelerometer regression models in predicting energy expenditure and METs in children and youth. Pediatr Exerc Sci. 2012;24(4):519–36.

Bailey DP, Locke CD. Breaking up prolonged sitting with light-intensity walking improves postprandial glycemia, but breaking up sitting with standing does not. J Sci Med Sport. 2015;18:294–8.

Bammann K, Sioen I, Huybrechts I, Casajús J, Vicente-Rodríguez G, Cuthill R, et al. IDEFICS consortium. The IDEFICS validation study on field methods for assessing physical activity and body composition in children: design and data collection. Int J Obes (Lond). 2011;35(Suppl 1): S79–87.

Bammann K, Peplies J, Sjöström M, Lissner L, De Henauw S, Galli C, et al. IDEFICS consortium. Assessment of diet, physical activity and biological, social and environmental factors in a multi-centre European project on diet- and lifestyle-related disorders in children (IDEFICS). J Pub Health. 2006;14(5):279–89.

Barlow SE, Expert Committee. Expert committee recommendations regarding the prevention, assessment, and treatment of child and adolescent overweight and obesity: summary report. Pediatrics. 2007;120(Suppl 4):S164–92.

Barnett LM, van Beurden E, Morgan PJ, Brooks LO, Beard JR. Childhood motor skill proficiency as a predictor of adolescent physical activity. J Adoles Health. 2009;44(3):252–9.

Bouten CV, Koekkoek KT, Verduin M, Kodde R, Janssen JD. A triaxial accelerometer and portable data processing unit for the assessment of daily physical activity. IEEE Trans Biomed Eng. 1997;44(3):136–47.

Brazendale K, Beets MW, Bornstein DB, Moore JB, Pate RR, Weaver RG, et al. Equating accelerometer estimates among youth: the Rosetta Stone 2. J Sci Med Sport. 2016;19(3):242–9.

Brennan RL. Generalizability theory. New York: Springer; 2001.

Buck C, Kneib T, Tkaczick T, Konstabel K, Pigeot I. Assessing opportunities for physical activity in the built environment of children: interrelation between kernel density and neighborhood scale. Int J Health Geogr. 2015a;22:14–35.

Buck C, Tkaczick T, Pitsiladis Y, De Bourdehaudhuij I, Reisch L, Ahrens W, et al. Objective measures of the built environment and physical activity in children: from walkability to moveability. J Urban Health. 2015b;92(1):24–38.

Bull FC, Expert working groups. Physical activity guidelines in the U.K.: review and recommendations. School of Sport, Exercise and Health Sciences, Loughborough University. 2010. https://www.gov.uk/government/uploads/system/uploads/attachment_data/file/213743/dh_128255.pdf. Accessed 8 Feb 2018.

Butte NF, Wong WW, Lee JS, Adolph AL, Puyau MR, Zakeri IF. Prediction of energy expenditure and physical activity in preschoolers. Med Sci Sports Exerc. 2014;46(6):1216–26.

Byrd-Williams CE, Belcher BR, Spruijt-Metz D, Davis JN, Ventura EE, Kelly L, et al. Increased physical activity and reduced adiposity in overweight Hispanic adolescents. Med Sci Sports Exerc. 2010;42:478–84.

Carter J, Wilkinson D, Blacker S, Rayson M, Bilzon J, Izard R, et al. An investigation of a novel three-dimensional activity monitor to predict free-living energy expenditure. J Sports Sci. 2008;26(6):553–61.

Caspersen CJ, Powell KE, Chistenson GM. Physical activity, exercise, and physical fitness: definitions and distinctions for health-related research. Public Health Rep. 1985;100:126–31.

Chen KY, Janz KF, Zhu W, Brychta RJ. Redefining the roles of sensors in objective physical activity monitoring. Med Sci Sports Exerc. 2012;44:S13–23.

Choi L, Liu Z, Matthews CE, Buchowski MS. Validation of accelerometer wear and nonwear time classification algorithm. Med Sci Sports Exerc. 2011a;43(2):357–64.

Choi L, Liu Z, Matthews CE, Buchowski MS. Physical activity: process physical activity accelerometer data. R package version 0.1–1. 2011b. https://CRAN.R-project.org/package=PhysicalActivity. Accessed 3 May 2018.

Choi L, Ward SC, Schnelle JF, Buchowski MS. Assessment of wear/nonwear time classification algorithms for triaxial accelerometer. Med Sci Sports Exerc. 2012;44(10):2009–16.

Chomistek AK, Yuan C, Matthews CE, Troiano RP, Bowles HR, Rood J, et al. Physical activity assessment with the ActiGraph GT3X and doubly labeled water. Med Sci Sports Exerc. 2017;49(9):1935–44.

Corder K, Ekelund U, Steele RM, Wareham NJ, Søren Brage S. Assessment of physical activity in adolescents. J Appl Physiol. 2008;105:977–87.

Crouter SE, Bassett DR Jr. A new 2-regression model for the Actical accelerometer. Br J Sports Med. 2008;42(3):217–24.

Crouter SE, Horton M, Bassett DR. Use of a 2-regression model for estimating energy expenditure in children. Med Sci Sports Exerc. 2012;44(6):1177–85.

de Almeida Mendes M, da Silva ICM, Ramires VV, Reichert FF, Martins RC, Tomasi E. Calibration of raw accelerometer data to measure physical activity: a systematic review. Gait Posture. 2018;61:98–110.

de Meester F, De Bourdeaudhuij I, Deforche B, Ottevaere C, Cardon G. Measuring physical activity using accelerometry in 13–15-year-old adolescents: the importance of including non-wear activities. Public Health Nutr. 2011;14(12):2124–33.

de Vet E, Verkooijen KT. Self-control and physical activity. Disentangling the pathways to health. In: de Ridder D, Adriaanse M, Fujita K, editors. The Routledge international handbook of self-control in health and well-being. London: Routledge; 2018. p. 276–87.

Dencker M, Andersen LB. Health-related aspects of objectively measured daily PA in children. J Sports Med. 2008;28:133–44.

Dieu O, Mikulovic J, Fardy PS, Bui-Xuan G, Béghin L, Vanhelst J. Physical activity using wrist-worn accelerometers: comparison of dominant and non-dominant wrist. Clin Physiol Funct Imaging. 2017;37(5):525–9.

Dössegger A, Ruch N, Jimmy G, Braun-Fahrländer C, Mäder U, Hänggi J, et al. Reactivity to accelerometer measurement of children and adolescents. Med Sci Sports Exerc. 2014;46 (6):1140–6.

Edwardson CL, Gorely T. Epoch length and its effect on physical activity intensity. Med Sci Sports Exerc. 2010;42(5):928–34.

Ekblom O, Oddsson K, Ekblom B. Prevalence and regional differences in overweight in 2001 and trends in BMI distribution in Swedish children from 1987 to 2001. Scan J Public Health. 2004;32:257–63.

Esliger DW, Tremblay MS. Physical activity and inactivity profiling: the next generation. Appl Physiol Nutr Metab. 2007;32:195–207.

Evenson KR, Cattellier D, Gill K, Ondrak K, McMurray RG. Calibration of two objective measures of physical activity for children. J Sports Sci. 2008;26:1557–65.

Freedson P, Pober D, Janz KF. Calibration of accelerometer output for children. Med Sci Sports Exerc. 2005;37:523–30.

Fudge BW, Wilson J, Easton C, Irwin L, Clark J, Haddow O, et al. Estimation of oxygen uptake during fast running using accelerometry and heart rate. Med Sci Sports Exerc. 2007;39:192–8.

Gabriel KP, McClain JJ, Schmid KK, Storti KL, High RR, Underwood DA, et al. Issues in accelerometer methodology: the role of epoch length on estimates of physical activity and relationships with health outcomes in overweight, post-menopausal women. Int J Beh Nutr Phy Activ. 2010;7:53.

Garaulet M, Martinez-Nicolas A, Ruiz JR, Konstabel K, Labayen I, González-Gross M, et al. HELENA study group. Fragmentation of daily rhythms associates with obesity and cardiorespiratory fitness in adolescents: the HELENA study. Clin Nutr. 2017;36(6):1558–66.

Gorber SC, Tremblay MS. Self-report and direct measures of health: bias and implications. In: Shephard RJ, Tudor-Locke C, editors. The objective monitoring of physical activity: contributions of accelerometry to epidemiology, exercise science and rehabilitation. New York: Springer; 2016. p. 369–76.

Guinhouya BC, Hubert H, Zitouni D. Need for unbiased computation of the moderate-intensity physical activity of youth in epidemiologic studies. Am J Prev Med. 2011;41(1):e1–2.

Hallgren KA. Computing inter-rater reliability for observational data: an overview and tutorial. Tutor Quant Methods Psychol. 2012;8(1):23–34.

Healy GN, Dunstan DW, Salmon J, Cerin E, Shaw JE, Zimmet PZ, et al. Breaks in sedentary time —beneficial associations with metabolic risk. Diabetes Care. 2008;31:661–6.

Hislop JF, Bulley C, Mercer TH, Reilly JJ. Comparison of accelerometry cut points for physical activity and sedentary behavior in preschool children: a validation study. Pediatr Exerc Sci. 2012;24(4):563–76.

Horner F, Bilzon JL, Rayson M, Blacker S, Richmond V, Carter J, et al. Development of an accelerometer-based multivariate model to predict free-living energy expenditure in a large military cohort. J Sports Sci. 2013;31(4):354–60.

Horner FE, Rayson MP, Bilzon JLJ. Reliability and validity of the 3DNX accelerometer during mechanical and human treadmill exercise testing. Int J Obes (Lond). 2011;35(Suppl 1):S88–97.

Howe CA, Staudenmayer JW, Freedson PS. Accelerometer prediction of energy expenditure: vector magnitude versus vertical axis. Med Sci Sports Exerc. 2009;41(12):2199–206.

Ihaka R, Gentleman R. R: A language for data analysis and graphics. J Comput Graph Stat. 1996;5:299–314.

Jakicic JM, Otto DA. Physical activity considerations for the treatment and prevention of obesity. Am J Clin Nutr. 2005;82(Suppl 1):226S–9S.

Janssen X, Basterfield L, Parkinson KN, Pearce MS, Reilly JK, Adamson AJ, et al. Gateshead millennium study core team. Objective measurement of sedentary behavior: impact of non-wear time rules on changes in sedentary time. BMC Public Health. 2015;23:504.

John D, Freedson P. Actigraph and actical physical activity monitors: a peek under the hood. Med Sci Sports Exerc. 2012;44:S86–9.

John D, Tyo B, Bassett DR. Comparison of four ActiGraph accelerometers during walking and running. Med Sci Sports Exerc. 2010;42(2):368–74.

Kitamura K, Nemoto T, Sato N, Chen W. Development of a new accelerometer-based physical activity-monitoring system using a high-frequency sampling rate. Biol Sci Space. 2009;23: 77–83.

Kolle E, Steene-Johannessen J, Andersen LB, Anderssen SA. Seasonal variation in objectively assessed physical activity among children and adolescents in Norway: a cross-sectional study. Int J Behav Nutr Phys Act. 2009;6:36.

Konstabel K, Mäestu J, Rääsk T, Lätt E, Jürimäe J. Decline in light-intensity activity is a major component of the longitudinal decline in physical activity in adolescent boys. Acta Paediatr. 2017;106(Suppl 470):24.

Konstabel K, Veidebaum T, Verbestel V, Moreno LA, Bammann K, Tornaritis M, et al. IDEFICS consortium. Objectively measured physical activity in European children: the IDEFICS study. Int J Obes (Lond). 2014;38(Suppl 2):S135–43.

Konstabel K. accelerate: an R package for accelerometry data analysis version 1.0.1. 2018. https:// osf.io/s42a3/.

Kyröläinen H, Belli A, Komi PV. Biomechanical factors affecting running economy. Med Sci Sports Exerc. 2001;33:1330–7.

Lee IM, Skerrett PJ. Physical activity and all-cause mortality: what is the dose-response relation? Med Sci Sports Exerc. 2001;33:459–71.

Levine JA. Non-exercise activity thermogenesis (NEAT). Nutr Rev. 2004;62:S82–97.

Lin SY, Lai YC, Hsia CC, Su PF, Chang CH. Validation of energy expenditure prediction modelling using real-time shoe-based motion detectors. IEEE Trans Biomed Eng. 2016;64:2152–62.

Lubans DR, Morgan PJ, Cliff DP, Barnett LM, Okely AD. Fundamental movement skills in children and adolescents. Review of associated health benefits. Sports Med. 2010;40 (12):1019–35.

Manohar C, McCrady S, Pavlidis IT, Levine JA. An accelerometer-based earpiece to monitor and quantify physical activity. J Phys Act Health. 2009;6(6):781–9.

Manohar CU, McCrady SK, Fujiki Y, Pavlidis IT, Levine JA. Evaluation of the accuracy of a triaxial accelerometer embedded into a cell phone platform for measuring physical activity. J Obes Weight Loss Ther. 2011;1(106):3309.

Mark AE, Janssen I. Influence of bouts of physical activity on overweight in youth. Am J Prev Med. 2009;36(5):416–21.

Martin JB, Krč KM, Mitchell EA, Eng JJ, Noble JW. Pedometer accuracy in slow walking older adults. Int J Ther Rehabil. 2012;19(7):387–93.

Martinez-Gomez D, Ruiz JR, Ortega FB. Author response. Am J Prev Med. 2011;41(1):e2–3.

Mattocks C, Leary S, Ness A, Deere K, Saunders J, Tilling K, et al. Calibration of an accelerometer during free-living activities in children. Int J Pediatr Obes. 2007;2:218–26.

McClain JJ, Abraham TL, Brusseau TA Jr, Tudor-Locke C. Epoch length and accelerometer outputs in children: comparison to direct observation. Med Sci Sports Exerc. 2008;40 (12):2080–7.

Migueles JH, Cadenas-Sanchez C, Ekelund U, Delisle Nyström C, Mora-Gonzalez J, Löf M, et al. Accelerometer data collection and processing criteria to assess physical activity and other outcomes: a systematic review and practical considerations. Sports Med. 2017;47(9):1821–45.

Miles L. Physical activity and health. Nutr Bull. 2007;32:314–63.

Miller J, Rosenbloom A, Silverstein J. Childhood obesity. J Clin Endocrinol Metab. 2004;89:4211–8.

Montoye AHK, Dong B, Biswas S, Pfeiffer KA. Validation of a wireless accelerometer network for energy expenditure measurement. J Sports Sci. 2016;34(21):2130–9.

Mossberg H. 40-year follow-up of overweight children. Lancet. 1989;26:491–3.

Ojiambo R, Cuthill R, Budd H, Konstabel K, Casajus JA, Gonzalez-Agüero A, et al. IDEFICS consortium. Impact of methodological decisions on accelerometer outcome variables in young children. Int J Obes (Lond). 2011;35(Suppl 1):S98–103.

Ojiambo R, Gibson AR, Konstabel K, Lieberman DE, Speakman JR, Reilly JJ, et al. Free-living physical activity and energy expenditure of rural children and adolescents in the Nandi region of Kenya. Ann Hum Biol. 2013;40(4):318–23.

Ojiambo RM, Konstabel K, Veidebaum T, Reilly JJ, Verbestel V, Casajús JA, et al. IDEFICS consortium. Validity of hip-mounted uniaxial accelerometry with heart-rate monitoring versus triaxial accelerometry in the assessment of free-living energy expenditure in young children: the IDEFICS validation study. J Appl Physiol. 2012;113(10):1530–6.

Ortega FB, Cadenas-Sánchez C, Sánchez-Delgado G, Mora-González J, Martínez-Téllez B, Artero EG, et al. Systematic review and proposal of a field-based physical fitness-test battery in preschool children: the PREFIT battery. Sports Med. 2015;45(4):533–55.

Ortega FB, Konstabel K, Pasquali E, Ruiz JR, Hurtig-Wennlöf A, Mäestu J, et al. Objectively measured physical activity and sedentary time during childhood, adolescence and young adulthood: a cohort study. PLoS ONE. 2013;8(4):e60871.

Ortega FB, Ruiz JR, Sjöström M. Physical activity, overweight and central adiposity in Swedish children and adolescents: the European Adolescents Heart Study. Int J Behav Nutr Phys Act. 2007;4:61.

Ottevaere C, Huybrechts I, De Meester F, De Bourdeaudhuij I, Cuenca-Garcia M, De Henauw S. The use of accelerometry in adolescents and its implementation with non-wear time activity diaries in free-living conditions. J Sports Sci. 2011;29(1):103–13.

Pate RR, Almeida MJ, McIver KL, Pfeiffer KA, Dowda M. Validation and calibration of an accelerometer in preschool children. Obes (Silver Spring). 2006;14(11):2000–6.

Phillips LRS, Parfitt G, Rowlands AV. Calibration of the GENEA accelerometer for assessment of physical activity intensity in children. J Sci Med Sport. 2013;16:124–8.

Pitsi T, Zilmer M, Vaask S, Ehala-Aleksejev K, Kuu S, Löhmus K, et al. Eesti toitumis- ja liikumissoovitused 2015 (Estonian guidelines on nutrition and physical activity). Tallinn: Tervise Arengu Instituut. 2017. https://intra.tai.ee//images/prints/documents/149019033869_eesti%20toitumis-%20ja%20liikumissoovitused.pdf. Assessed 2 Feb 2018.

Plasqui G, Bonomi AG, Westerterp KR. Daily physical activity assessment with accelerometers: new insights and validation studies. Obes Rev. 2013;14(6):451–62.

Powell KE, Paluch AE, Blair SN. Physical activity for health: What kind? How much? How intense? On top of what? Annu Rev Public Health. 2011;32:349–65.

Puyau MR, Adolph AL, Vohra FA, Butte NF. Validation and calibration of physical activity monitors in children. Obes Res. 2002;10(3):150–7.

R Core Team. R. A language and environment for statistical computing. Vienna, Austria: R Foundation for Statistical Computing. 2017. https://www.R-project.org/. Accessed 3 May 2018.

Rääsk T, Konstabel K, Mäestu J, Lätt E, Jürimäe T, Jürimäe J. Tracking of physical activity in pubertal boys with different BMI over two-year period. J Sports Sci. 2015a;33:1649–57.

Rääsk T, Lätt E, Jürimäe T, Mäestu J, Jürimäe J, Konstabel K. Association of subjective ratings to objectively assessed physical activity in pubertal boys with differing BMI. Percept Mot Skills. 2015b;121(1):245–59.

Rääsk T, Mäestu J, Lätt E, Jürimäe J, Jürimäe T, Vainik U, et al. Comparison of IPAQ-SF and two other physical activity questionnaires with accelerometer in adolescent boys. PLoS ONE. 2017;12(1):e0169527.

Reilly JJ, Methven E, McDowell Z. Health consequences of obesity. Arch Dis Child. 2003;88:748–52.

Rich C, Geraci M, Griffiths L, Sera F, Dezateux C, Cortina-Borja M. Quality control methods in accelerometer data processing. PLoS ONE. 2013;8(6):e67206.

Rosenberger ME, Haskell WL, Albinali F, Mota S, Nawyn J, Intille S. Estimating activity and sedentary behavior from an accelerometer on the hip or wrist. Med Sci Sports Exerc. 2013;45 (5):964–75.

Sallis JF, Patrick K. Physical activity guidelines for adolescents: consensus statement. Pediatric Exerc Sci. 1994;6:302–14.

Santos-Lozano A, Marín PJ, Torres-Luque G, Ruiz JR, Lucía A, Garatachea N. Technical variability of the GT3X accelerometer. Med Eng Phys. 2012;34(6):787–90.

Sardinha LB, Júdice PB. Usefulness of motion sensors to estimate energy expenditure in children and adults: a narrative review of studies using DLW. Eur J Clin Nutr. 2017;71(8):1026.

Shiroma EJ, Schepps MA, Harezlak J, Chen KY, Matthews CE, Koster A, et al. Daily physical activity patterns from hip- and wrist-worn accelerometers. Physiol Meas. 2016;37(10):1852–61.

Shrout PE, Fleiss JL. Intraclass correlations: uses in assessing rater reliability. Psychol Bull. 1979;86(2):420–8.

Sirard JR, Trost SG, Pfeiffer KA, Dowda M, Pate RR. Calibration and evaluation of an objective measure of physical activity in preschool children. J Phys Act Health. 2005;2(3):345–57.

Sirichana W, Dolezal BA, Neufeld EV, Wang X, Cooper CB. Wrist-worn triaxial accelerometry predicts the energy expenditure of non-vigorous daily physical activities. J Sci Med Sport. 2017;20:761–5.

Swartz AM, Strath SJ, Bassett WI, O'Brien DR, King GA, Anisworth BE. Estimation of energy expenditure using CSA accelerometers at hip ad wrist sites. Med Sci Sports Exerc. 2000;32: S450–6.

Telama R, Yang X, Leskinen E, Kankaanpää A, Hirvensalo M, Tammelin T, et al. Tracking of physical activity from early childhood through youth into adulthood. Med Sci Sports Exerc. 2014;46(5):955–62.

Tremblay MS, Barnes JD, Copeland JL, Esliger DW. Conquering childhood inactivity: is the answer in the past? Med Sci Sports Exerc. 2005;37:1187–94.

Treuth MS, Schmitz K, Catellier DJ, McMurray RG, Murray DM, Almeida MJ, et al. Defining accelerometer thresholds for activity intensities in adolescent girls. Med Sci Sports Exerc. 2004;36(7):1259–66.

Troiano RP, Berrigan D, Dodd KW, Mâsse LC, Tilert T, McDowell M. Physical activity in the United States measured by accelerometer. Med Sci Sports Exerc. 2008;40(1):181–8.

Trost S, Kerr L, Ward D, Pate R. Physical activity and determinants of physical activity in obese and non-obese children. Int J Obes Relat Metabol Disord. 2001;25:822–9.

Trost SG, Pate RR, Freedson PS, Sallis JF, Taylor WC. Using objective physical activity measures with youth: how many days of monitoring are needed? Med Sci Sports Exerc. 2000;30(2):426–31.

Trost SG, Loprinzi PD, Moore R, Pfeiffer KA. Comparison of accelerometer cut-points for predicting activity intensity in youth. Med Sci Sports Exerc. 2011;43:1360–8.

Trost SG. State of the art reviews: measurement of physical activity in children and adolescents. Am J Lifestyle Med. 2007;1:299–314.

Twisk J, Mellenbergh G, van Mechelen W. Tracking of biological and lifestyle cardiovascular risk factors over a 14-year period. Am J Epidemiol. 1997;145:888–95.

van Cauwenberghe EV, Labarque V, Trost SG, De Bourdeaudhuij I, Cardon G. Calibration and comparison of accelerometer cut points in preschool children. Int J Pediatr Obes. 2010;6(2–2): e582–9.

van Hees VT, Gorzelniak L, Dean León EC, Eder M, Pias M, Taherian S, et al. Separating movement and gravity components in an acceleration signal and implications for the assessment of human daily physical activity. PLoS ONE. 2013;8(4):e61691.

van Hees VT, Renström F, Wright A, Gradmark A, Catt M, Chen KY, et al. Estimation of daily energy expenditure in pregnant and non-pregnant women using a wrist-worn tri-axial accelerometer. PLoS ONE. 2011;6(7):e22922.

van Hees VT. GGIR: raw accelerometer data analysis. R package version 1.5–16. 2018. https://CRAN.R-project.org/package=GGIR. Accessed 2 May 2018.

Vanhelst J, Béghin L, Salleron J, Ruiz JR, Ortega FB, Ottevaere C, et al. Impact of the choice of threshold on physical activity patterns in free living conditions among adolescents measured using a uniaxial accelerometer: the HELENA study. J Sports Sci. 2014a;32(2):110–5.

Vanhelst J, Fardy PS, Duhamel A, Béghin L. How many days of accelerometer monitoring predict weekly physical activity behaviour in obese youth? Clin Physiol Funct Imaging. 2014b;34 (5):384–8.

Ward DS, Evenson KR, Vaughn A, Rodgers AB, Troiano RP. Accelerometer use in physical activity: Best practices and research recommendations. Med Sci Sports Exerc. 2005;37 (11):582–8.

Wareham N, Rennie K. The assessment of physical activity in individuals and populations: why try to be more precise about how physical activity is assessed? Int J Obes (Lond). 1998;22: S30–8.

Whelton PK, He J, Appel LJ, Cutler JA, Havas S, Kotchen TA, et al. National high blood pressure education program coordinating committee. Primary prevention of hypertension: clinical and public health advisory from the national high blood pressure education program. JAMA. 2002;288(15):1882–8.

Whitaker R, Wright J, Pepe M, Seidel K, Dietz W. Predicting obesity in young adulthood from childhood and parental obesity. N Engl J Med. 1997;337:869–73.

World Health Organization. Global recommendations on physical activity for health. 2010. http://www.who.int/dietphysicalactivity/publications/9789241599979/en/. Accessed 2 May 2018.

Yang CC, Hsu YL. A review of accelerometry-based wearable motion detectors for physical activity monitoring. Sensors. 2010;10(8):7772–88.

Zakeri IF, Adolph AL, Puyau MR, Vohra FA, Butte NF. Cross-sectional time series and multivariate adaptive regression splines models using accelerometry and heart rate predict energy expenditure of preschoolers. J Nutr. 2013;143(1):114–22.

Zhang JH, Macfarlane DJ, Sobko T. Feasibility of a chest-worn accelerometer for physical activity measurement. J Sci Med Sport. 2016;19(12):1015–9.

Zhou SM, Hill RA, Morgan K, Stratton G, Gravenor MB, Bijlsma G, et al. Classification of accelerometer wear and non-wear events in seconds for monitoring free-living physical activity. BMJ Open. 2015;5(5):e007447.

Zhou W, Owen N. Sedentary behavior and health concepts, assessments, and interventions. Champaign, IL: Human Kinetics; 2017.

Chapter 8
Pre- and Postnatal Factors Obtained from Health Records

Wolfgang Ahrens, Fabio Lauria, Annarita Formisano,
Luis A. Moreno and Iris Pigeot

Abstract Collection of secondary data on an individual level, e.g. from official sources, may complement primary data from questionnaires and examinations in epidemiological field studies. Retrieval of individual-level secondary data thus represents an important step to constitute a comprehensive epidemiological database: secondary health data potentially represent an added value for the inference of causal relationships because they provide information without recall bias. In the IDEFICS/I.Family studies, health records of routine child visits reaching back to birth as well as medical records for the prenatal period were collected. Several studies suggest that both intra-uterine and early infancy growth may influence the development of overweight during childhood, adolescence and even adulthood (Poston 2012). The IDEFICS/I.Family studies were conducted in different cultural

On behalf of the IDEFICS and I.Family consortia

W. Ahrens (✉) · I. Pigeot
Leibniz Institute for Prevention Research and Epidemiology—BIPS,
Bremen, Germany
e-mail: ahrens@leibniz-bips.de

W. Ahrens · I. Pigeot
Faculty of Mathematics and Computer Science, University of Bremen,
Bremen, Germany

F. Lauria · A. Formisano
Unit of Epidemiology and Population Genetics, Institute of Food Sciences,
National Research Council, Avellino, Italy

L. A. Moreno
Facultad de Ciencias de la Salud, Growth, Exercise, NUtrition and Development
(GENUD) Research Group, Universidad de Zaragoza, Zaragoza, Spain

© Springer Nature Switzerland AG 2019
K. Bammann et al. (eds.), *Instruments for Health Surveys in Children
and Adolescents*, Springer Series on Epidemiology and Public Health,
https://doi.org/10.1007/978-3-319-98857-3_8

settings using a standardised protocol that sometimes needed adaptation to local characteristics. The latter was the case for the documentation of routine child visits and maternity cards that varied across countries with regard to data sources and the type of information recorded. This chapter summarises the methodology of retrieval and harmonisation of secondary health data in the IDEFICS/I.Family studies and describes the differences and similarities of these records across countries.

8.1 Introduction

In the framework of both studies, medical records related to the child and the mother were collected to assess pre- and postnatal factors that are related to the environment (including intra-uterine environment) in which a child grows up. Early growth is a period of life during which, according to available scientific evidence, the predisposition to certain pathologic conditions is programmed (Wells et al. 2007; Singhal 2017; Matthews et al. 2017). This is, for instance, the case for overweight and obesity and for several metabolic disorders (Poston 2012).

Epidemiological studies investigating the association between early life factors and adult health are often based on parental (maternal) recall (Terry et al. 2009). Actually, most published results on early life factors of the IDEFICS study were based on perinatal data collected by questionnaire focusing on birth weight (Sparano et al. 2013; Van den Bussche et al. 2012), gestational weight gain (Dello Russo et al. 2013; Bammann et al. 2014) or gestational hypertension (Pohlabeln et al. 2017). However, collecting information in this way could also represent a limitation for statistical analysis because of the possible bias due to the impaired reliability of maternal recall. Several studies (Buka et al. 2004; Rice et al. 2007; Tehranifar et al. 2009) investigated this issue and found that the validity of maternal recall may depend upon several factors. The most important determinant of accuracy of the recall is the type of parameter: for example, almost all findings are consistent for a high accuracy of maternal recall for breastfeeding (Cupul-Uicab et al. 2009) and birth weight (Catov et al. 2006; Rice et al. 2007; Tehranifar et al. 2009), while reliability was lower when recalling birth length (Dubois and Girard 2007). In the IDEFICS study, maternal reports on pregnancy and birth were highly reproducible, but parental recall of early infant nutrition was weaker (Herrmann et al. 2011). Additional factors that may influence the reliability of maternal recall include educational level, socioeconomic level, parity, time lag of the recalled event and weight status of the child (Rice et al. 2007; Elliott et al. 2010).

Secondary health data may be more accurate and valid than self-reports. Their collection can be more cost-effective than lengthy interviews and may reduce participant burden. Associations may only become apparent if they are assessed using objective records because true associations can be masked by non-differential misclassification of self-reported data. Routine records of child growth are particularly valuable for the analysis of growth dynamics requiring several repeated measurements in the same individual. We therefore used objective records to investigate growth trajectories in the IDEFICS/I.Family studies (Reeske et al. 2013; Börnhorst et al. 2016a, b, 2017). Objective health records may also allow for validation of self-reports.

In the following, we will distinguish between prenatal and postnatal factors. Prenatal factors refer to the intra-uterine environment during pregnancy. Postnatal factors refer to data collected starting from the delivery. The length of the postnatal period may vary depending on the type of characteristics under investigation.

8.2   Prenatal Factors

Health records on prenatal factors usually refer to both the mother and the child. All conditions that shape the intra-uterine environment in which the foetus grows up and that influence the level of exposure of the child to potential risk factors are of interest. These may not only occur during pregnancy but also during the time before conception. Information referring to the health status of the mother before the beginning of her pregnancy may become available through the physician or may be obtained from health records while data on routine visits during pregnancy are often recorded on maternity cards.

In the IDEFICS/I.Family studies, records on prenatal factors had to be retrieved from various sources. In some countries, part of this information was kept in birth (Sweden, Estonia) or hospital registries (Belgium). In Hungary, a central electronic medical registry was introduced only after the IDEFICS study. However, in most countries linkage of registry data with study data is strictly regulated. In Sweden, for instance, data from the maternal birth registry (e.g. maternal age, weight, height, smoking) or the social registry (e.g. family disposable income, parental education, foreign background) may not leave the country, but manually retrieved archival data (on growth in weight and height) were not subject to the restrictions.

Filled in by a physician or a nurse and kept by the mother, maternity cards/booklets include the prenatal factors summarised in Table 8.1. In many countries (Germany, Italy, Cyprus, Spain), information about prenatal factors was only personally kept by the mother. In Germany, maternity cards were available for almost all participants while the corresponding data had to be retrieved from hospital records in Belgium.

Access to registries facilitates the collection of the respective data in large population samples while, in case that these records are to be kept by mothers, data may get lost. In the latter case, bias may occur because mothers who take more care of health-related problems regarding themselves and/or their children may more often retain the respective documents. For instance, records of routine child visits were provided for only 7% of participating children in Cyprus but for 83% in Germany (see Table 8.2).

Box 8.1 shows the type of records, either related to the mother and the foetus, and the gestational phase which they refer to. During pregnancy, several data regarding the health status of the mother and the child, potentially useful to assess prenatal exposure, are collected, either at the first visit (only) or at various time

Table 8.1 Sources and accessibility of pre- and postnatal health records in the countries participating in the IDEFICS/I.Family studies

	Belgium	Cyprus	Estonia	Germany	Hungary	Italy	Spain	Sweden
Child prenatal factors								
Echo-estimated infant body size indices	–	–	MC	MC	–	Medical records	–	CHR
Child postnatal factors								
Child birth weight and height	CHB	CHB	Med BirthReg	CHB	CHB	CHB	CHB	NatReg
Gestational age at delivery	CHB	CHB	Med BirthReg	CHB	CHB	CHB	CHB	NatReg
Type of feeding (breast, formula, mixed)	CHB	–	–	MC (BF at 6–8 week)	–	CHB	CHB	CHR, NatReg
Duration of breastfeeding	CHB	–	–	–	–	CHB	CHB	CHR, NatReg
Age at weaning/complementary feeding introduction	CHB	–	–	–	–	CHB	CHB	CHR, NatReg
Type of complementary feeding foods	CHB	–	–	–	–	–	CHB	CHR, NatReg
Weight, height and head circumference at age 1, 6, 12, 24 mo.	CHB	CHB	CHB	CHB	CHB	CHB	CHB	CHR
Maternal factors								
Placental weight	Hospital records	–	–	Hospital records	–	Hospital records	Hospital records	NatReg
Number of foetuses gestated	Hospital records	–	Med BirthReg	MC	MC	Medical records	Hospital records	NatReg
Pre- and post-pregnancy maternal weight and height	Hospital records	–	MC	MC	MC	Medical records	Medical records	NatReg

BF Breastfeeding; *CHB* Child health booklet/card; *CHR* Child health record; *MC* Maternity card/booklet; *Med BirthReg* Medical birth registry; *NatReg* National registry

Table 8.2 Number of children with available records on prenatal factors and routine child visits in the IDEFICS/I.Family cohort

	Belgium		Cyprus		Estonia		Germany		Hungary		Italy		Spain		Sweden		All	
	n	%	n	%	n	%	n	%	n	%	n	%	n	%	n	%	n	%
Prenatal factors, e.g. abortions, stillbirths, previous severe diseases, pre-pregnancy weight	0	0	0	0	2042	95.0	1554	70.3	133	4.1	0	0	0	0	0	0	3729	19.9
Prenatal care, e.g. SBP, DBP, glucose, protein, weight at antenatal visit	0	0	0	0	0	0	1542	69.7	97	3.0	0	0	0	0	0	0	1639	8.7
Postnatal/ neonatal factors, e.g. Apgar score, method of delivery, gestational week, weight/height at birth	566	23.6	231	7.8	2042	95.0	1854	83.9	547	16.5	603	24.7	363	23.6	0	0	6206	33.0
Child examination, e.g. head circumference, height, weight	531	22.2	198	6.7	0	0	1829	82.7	513	15.8	488	20.0	349	22.6	0	0	3908	20.8
All participants	2396	100.0	2970	100.0	2150	100.0	2211	100.0	3244	100.0	2440	100.0	1541	100.0	1831	100.0	18783	100.0

Due to data protection regulations, Swedish data are only provided upon request on a case-by-case basis points during pregnancy (Box 8.1). Data about personal history of hypertension or diabetes (as well as of other pre-existing pathologic conditions) may be obtained from medical records. Such information is important since, for instance, pre-pregnancy diabetes is associated with the development of obesity in offspring (Philipps et al. 2011). Pre-pregnancy body weight and height are usually recorded at the first physical examination where pre-pregnancy body weight is often based on self-reports and thus has limited validity. However, pre-pregnancy body weight is needed to assess the adequacy of gestational weight gain according to current guidelines (Rasmussen and Yaktine 2009).

Box 8.1 Pre-/postnatal factors from records of routine child visits and pregnancy logs in the countries participating in the IDEFICS/I.Family studies

Factors related to the mother
Pre-pregnancy period
Diagnosis of hypertension
Diagnosis of diabetes
Body weight
Blood pressure
Antenatal visits (at the beginning of pregnancy)
Last menstruation and calculated date of delivery
Number of foetuses gestated
Antenatal visits (at various time points)
Blood cell count
Urine analysis
Proteinuria
Glycosuria
Blood glucose
Blood pressure
Antenatal visits (at the end of pregnancy)
Weight gain during pregnancy
Duration of gestation
Type of delivery
Factors related to the child
Antenatal visits (at various time points)
Total length of the foetus
Length of bone segments
Echo-estimated foetal body weight
Postnatal visits (at various time points)
Height and body weight
Head circumference
Breastfeeding (type and duration)
Age and type of weaning

In the IDEFICS/I.Family studies, health records on the date of the last menstruation and the calculated date of delivery were compared with mothers' recall and/or with other records, e.g. on weeks of gestation. The duration of gestation needs to be assessed accurately because it may influence the metabolic programming of the offspring (Tamashiro and Moran 2010). The number of foetuses in the corresponding pregnancy needs to be known because it influences the composition of the intra-uterine environment in which a child grows up.

During pregnancy, mothers usually undergo several clinical laboratory checks and ultrasonographic examinations: in most cases, these data may be found in medical records and only rarely in central registries. Laboratory parameters may provide information about the metabolic profile of the mother and the occurrence of concomitant diseases, such as urinary tract infections or proteinuria that may have long-term consequences on child health. The ultrasonographic examination of the child's intra-uterine development is usually repeated at different times during pregnancy. Recorded anthropometric indices usually include estimated foetal weight, foetal length, length of specific bone segments as well as head and abdominal circumferences. These parameters were available from central registries in Sweden. Ultrasonographic estimates of the anthropometric indices in the foetus were available also in Estonia from national registries but access required specific authorisations. In Italy, medical records of ultrasonographic examinations were generally kept by the mothers themselves. In the remaining countries, no records from the ultrasonographic examinations during pregnancy were available. Thus, the number of children for whom ultrasonographic estimates of foetal anthropometric indices were available in the IDEFICS/I.Family cohort was small. Due to these methodological problems, the association between foetal anthropometric indices and the development of overweight and obesity has been scarcely investigated; thus, even if restricted to a small sample, the IDEFICS/I.Family cohort may provide new insights into this largely unexplored issue.

Duration (number of weeks) of gestation, weight gain during pregnancy and type of delivery are the most important records collected at the end of the gestation (Table 8.1). Preterm birth is associated with a high risk of abnormal brain function as well as with long-term metabolic consequences (Saigal and Doyle 2008). Gestational weight gain was the object of some recently published studies that suggest excess weight gain of the mother during pregnancy increases the risk of obesity in offspring independently of birth weight (Schack-Nielsen et al. 2010; Mamun et al. 2014).

Type of delivery, caesarean or spontaneous, is mostly correctly recalled by the mother. However, this information is usually recorded together with other parameters of interest that are less well recalled, such as the Apgar score or the occurrence of specific medical problems during delivery. Having information about the type of delivery is of interest as it was observed that during the first three months of life, the diversity and colonisation pattern of the infant gut microbiota depends on the mode of delivery (Rutayisire et al. 2016).

Birth weight and height may belong to the most important prenatal factors that reflect the growth of the foetus during gestation. Bland–Altman plots of the

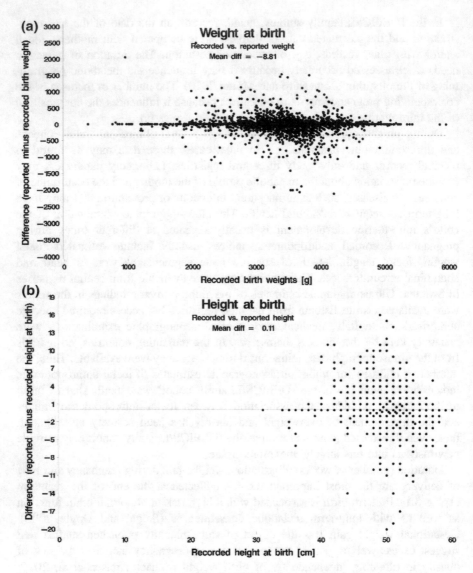

Fig. 8.1 Agreement between maternal recall of birth weight (**a**) and birth height (**b**) and routine health records

IDEFICS study showed a high concordance between birth weight from official records and recalled birth weight (Fig. 8.1a), while it was lower for birth length (Fig. 8.1b). Our data support previous studies showing that maternal recall of birth weight is usually quite accurate (Catov et al. 2006; Rice et al. 2007). However, this accuracy declines the longer the period of the recall and the higher the number of pregnancies of the mother (Rice et al. 2007; Elliott et al. 2010). The relevance of birth weight as a determinant of the future development of the child is well known.

High birth weight is an independent predictor of obesity during infancy, adolescence and adulthood (Yu et al. 2011). There is also evidence that birth weight is associated with metabolic disorders and cardiovascular risk (Harder et al. 2009). Both, children with low birth weight (Boney et al. 2005; Druet and Ong 2008) and macrosomic infants (Das et al. 2009; Evagelidou et al. 2006; Gillman et al. 2003), are at higher risk of developing insulin resistance and abnormalities in lipid profile as well as overweight and obesity.

8.3 Postnatal Factors

The sources and the types of postnatal medical records available in the countries participating in the IDEFICS/I.Family studies are summarised in Table 8.1. In Sweden, postnatal data on weight and height trajectories were accessible through child health care and school health archives, after obtaining a special permission. In Estonia, national registries are incomplete regarding postnatal factors; information from the child health card was not accessible.

In the other European countries where health records were collected for the IDEFICS/I.Family studies, a "child health booklet" (CHB) was the main source of postnatal data on the children's development. CHBs are completed by a paediatrician or a nurse and are usually kept by the parents. Therefore, parents were asked to provide their child's CHB for abstraction or photocopying at the examination in the survey centre.

CHBs cover the medical history of the child from the delivery up to preschool age, school age or adolescence—depending on the country—with routine visits at time points that differed across countries. CHBs provide information about anthropometric indices at various ages. The most common anthropometric indices recorded in CHBs are body weight, height and head circumference. In some countries, child body weight is manually plotted on growth charts in the CHB which may introduce a writing/reading error that adds to the (technical) measurement error (Fig. 8.2). The age and time intervals at which such information is collected differ by country. In general, body weight, height and head circumference were recorded at ages 6 months, 1 year and 2 years. In some countries, more time points are available: every month up to the first year and at six-month intervals up to preschool age. These data allow to estimate the growth trajectory of a child, e.g. to investigate its association with overweight during childhood. In particular, the period of life during which the so-called adiposity rebound occurs can be determined. The adiposity rebound, i.e. the increase in body mass index at roughly 5–7 years of age that follows its physiological reduction, is considered an independent determinant of adiposity in children. It was observed that early occurrence and magnitude of this adiposity rebound were both positively associated with the risk of developing overweight or obesity during childhood (Taylor et al. 2005; Chivers et al. 2010). However, our own data revealed that the adiposity rebound cannot be assessed in children with higher than average BMI growth of body mass index (BMI) (Börnhorst et al. 2017).

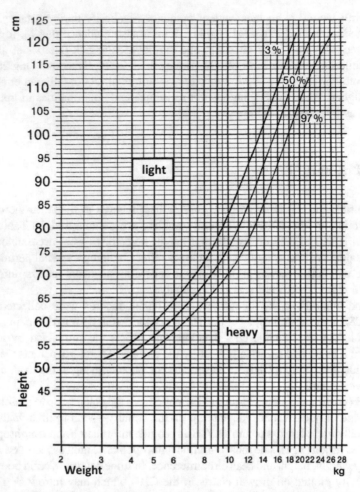

Fig. 8.2 Growth chart used to record body height against body weight at routine child visits in Germany (*Source* Scan of the respective page in the so-called Yellow Booklet in Germany, where the check-ups for children up to six years, referred to as U1, U2, U3, etc., are recorded)

CHBs also provided useful information on infant nutrition, another potential determinant of the subsequent development of overweight and obesity. In particular, breastfeeding, complementary feeding and weaning were retrieved from this source. However, CHB content differed in this regard across the countries participating in the IDEFICS/I.Family studies. Information on breastfeeding, complementary feeding and weaning was recorded in CHBs in Belgium, Italy and Spain. In Germany, this information was available from maternity cards. An overview of the variables compiled in the common dataset is given in Table 8.2.

The abstraction of data on complementary feeding and weaning turned out to be more complex, because it included either quantitative (i.e. age of complementary feeding introduction) or qualitative (type of foods) information. Age of complementary feeding was available for almost all participants while records on qualitative aspects of weaning showed greater heterogeneity across countries. Especially the type of foods used for complementary feeding and the sequence of introduction of new foods were only available in a subgroup.

8.4   Conclusions

The IDEFICS/I.Family studies take advantage of the opportunity to combine secondary health records of pre- and postnatal factors possibly influencing the future development of overweight and obesity, with a complete set of primary data collected in a large cohort of children from eight European countries. By amalgamation of primary and secondary data, the observation period was extended by several years to investigate growth trajectories in a life course perspective (Börnhorst et al. 2016a, b, 2017). The need for harmonisation of these records—because of country differences—and the sometimes-limited availability of health records—due to lack of compliance by parents or the restricted access to registries—resulted in some loss of information. The resulting reduction in sample size may, however, be counterbalanced by the higher accuracy of health records as compared to self-reports.

Data from the pre- and postnatal periods of life constituted the largest part of secondary data collected during the IDEFICS/I.Family study. Further, secondary data collected during both studies included demographic and economic indices as well as data from geographic information systems (GISs) of the study regions (Buck et al. 2015). National or local statistics were available from all participating countries, thus allowing for a satisfactory portrait of the environment(s) in which the target population(s) lived.

Summarising, it turned out to be quite time-consuming to collect health records from parents or from other sources. In some countries, these records were only provided by a small number of parents. This may have led to some bias, in particular to selection bias. Based on our experience in two large international population-based studies, we strongly encourage the implementation of birth registries according to common standards all over Europe and to use this important source of information for health monitoring and research.

8.5   Provision of Instruments and Standard Operating Procedures to Third Parties

The General Survey Manuals that provide among other all standard operating procedures can be accessed on the following website: www.leibniz-bips.de/ifhs after registration.

Each third partner using the information on health records provided in this chapter is kindly requested to cite this chapter as follows:

Ahrens W, Lauria F, Formisano A, Moreno LA, Pigeot I, on behalf of the IDEFICS and I.Family consortia. Pre- and postnatal factors obtained from health records. In: Bammann K, Lissner L, Pigeot I, Ahrens W, editors. Instruments for health surveys in children and adolescents. Cham: Springer Nature Switzerland; 2019. p. 175–188.

Acknowledgements This chapter is based on a draft that was created by Gianvincenzo Barba from the Institute of Food Sciences, National Research Council (Avellino, Italy). Gianni unexpectedly passed away before this chapter was completed. He played a prominent part in the harmonisation of data from routine child visits and maternity cards across the countries collecting data for the IDEFICS/I.Family cohort. We are grateful for his valuable contributions.

The development of instruments, the baseline data collection and the first follow-up work as part of the IDEFICS study (www.idefics.eu) were financially supported by the European Commission within the Sixth RTD Framework Programme Contract No. 016,181 (FOOD). The most recent follow-up including the development of new instruments and the adaptation of previously used instruments was conducted in the framework of the I.Family study (www.ifamilystudy.eu) which was funded by the European Commission within the Seventh RTD Framework Programme Contract No. 266044 (KBBE 2010–14).

We thank all families for participating in the extensive examinations of the IDEFICS and I. Family studies. We are also grateful for the support from school boards, headmasters and communities.

References

Bammann K, Peplies J, De Henauw S, Hunsberger M, Molnar D, Moreno LA, et al. IDEFICS consortium. Early life course risk factors for childhood obesity: the IDEFICS case-control study. PLoS ONE. 2014;9(2):e86914.

Boney CM, Verma A, Tucker R, Vohr BR. Metabolic syndrome in childhood: association with birth weight, maternal obesity, and gestational diabetes mellitus. Pediatrics. 2005;115:e290–6.

Börnhorst C, Tilling K, Russo P, Kourides Y, Michels N, Molnár D, et al. IDEFICS consortium. Associations between early body mass index trajectories and later metabolic risk factors in European children: the IDEFICS study. Eur J Epidemiol. 2016a;31(5):513–25.

Börnhorst C, Siani A, Russo P, Kourides Y, Sion I, Molnár D, et al. Early life factors and inter-country heterogeneity in BMI growth trajectories of European children: the IDEFICS study. PLoS ONE. 2016b;11(2):e0149268.

Börnhorst C, Siani A, Tornaritis M, Molnár D, Lissner L, Regber S, et al. IDEFICS and I. Family consortia. Potential selection effects when estimating associations between the infancy peak or adiposity rebound and later body mass index in children. Int J Obes (Lond). 2017; 41(4):518–26.

Buck C, Tkaczick T, Pitsiladis Y, De Bourdeaudhuij I, Reisch L, Ahrens W, et al. Objective measures of the built environment and physical activity in children: from walkability to moveability. J Urban Health. 2015;92(1):24–38.

Buka SL, Goldstein JM, Spartos E, Tsuang MT. The retrospective measurement of prenatal and perinatal events: accuracy of maternal recall. Schizophr Res. 2004;71:417–26.

Catov JM, Newman AB, Kelsey SF, Roberts JM, Sutton-Tyrrell KC, Garcia M, et al. Accuracy and reliability of maternal recall of infant birth weight among older women. Ann Epidemiol. 2006;16:429–31.

Chivers P, Hands B, Parker H, Bulsara M, Beilin LJ, Kendall GE, et al. Body mass index, adiposity rebound and early feeding in a longitudinal cohort (Raine Study). Int J Obes (Lond). 2010;34:1169–76.

Cupul-Uicab LA, Gladen BC, Hernández-Avila M, Longnecker MP. Reliability of reported breastfeeding duration among reproductive-aged women from Mexico. Matern Child Nutr. 2009;5:125–37.

Das S, Irigoyen M, Patterson MB, Salvador A, Schutzman DL. Neonatal outcomes of macrosomic births in diabetic and non-diabetic women. Arch Dis Child Fetal Neonatal Ed. 2009;94: F419–22.

Dello Russo M, Ahrens W, De Vriendt T, Mårild S, Molnár D, Moreno LA, et al. IDEFICS consortium. Gestational weight gain and adiposity, fat distribution, metabolic profile, and blood pressure in offspring: the IDEFICS project. Int J Obes (Lond). 2013;37(7):914–9.

Druet C, Ong KK. Early childhood predictors of adult body composition. Best Pract Res Clin Endocrinol Metab. 2008;22:489–502.

Dubois L, Girad M. Accuracy of maternal reports of pre-schoolers' weights and heights as estimates of BMI values. Int J Epidemiol. 2007;36:132–8.

Elliott JP, Desch C, Istwan NB, Rhea D, Collins AM, Stanziano GJ. The reliability of patient-reported pregnancy outcome data. Popul Health Manage. 2010;13:27–32.

Evagelidou EN, Kiortsis DN, Bairaktari ET, Giapros VI, Cholevas VK, Tzallas CS, et al. Lipid profile, glucose homeostasis, blood pressure, and obesity-anthropometric markers in macrosomic offspring of nondiabetic mothers. Diabetes Care. 2006;29(6):1197–201.

Gillman MW, Rifas-Shiman S, Berkey CS, Field AE, Colditz GA. Maternal gestational diabetes, birth weight, and adolescent obesity. Pediatrics. 2003;111:e221–6.

Harder T, Roepke K, Diller N, Stechling Y, Dudenhausen JW, Plagemann A. Birth weight, early weight gain, and subsequent risk of type 1 diabetes: systematic review and meta-analysis. Am J Epidemiol. 2009;169:1428–36.

Herrmann D, Suling M, Reisch L, Siani A, De Bourdeaudhuij I, Maes L, et al. IDEFICS consortium. Repeatability of maternal report on prenatal, perinatal and early postnatal factors: findings from the IDEFICS parental questionnaire. Int J Obes (Lond). 2011;35(Suppl 1): S52–60.

Mamun AA, Mannan M, Doi SA. Gestational weight gain in relation to offspring obesity over the life course: a systematic review and bias-adjusted meta-analysis. Obes Rev. 2014;15 (4):338–47.

Matthews EK, Wei J, Cunningham SA. Relationship between prenatal growth, postnatal growth and childhood obesity: a review. Eur J Clin Nutr. 2017;71(8):919–30.

Philipps LH, Santhakumaran S, Gale C, Prior E, Logan KM, Hyde MJ, et al. The diabetic pregnancy and offspring BMI in childhood: a systematic review and meta-analysis. Diabetologia. 2011;54:1957–66.

Pohlabeln H, Rach S, De Henauw S, Eiben G, Gwozdz W, Hadjigeorgiou C, et al. IDEFICS consortium. Further evidence for the role of pregnancy-induced hypertension and other early life influences in the development of ADHD: results from the IDEFICS study. Eur Child Adolesc Psychiatry. 2017;26(8):957–67.

Poston L. Maternal obesity, gestational weight gain and diet as determinants of offspring long term health. Best Pract Res Clin Endocrinol Metab. 2012;26:627–39.

Rasmussen KM, Yaktine AL, editors. Institute of Medicine (US) and National Research Council (US) Committee to reexamine IOM pregnancy weight guidelines. Weight gain during pregnancy: reexamining the guidelines. Washington, DC: National Academies Press; 2009.

Reeske A, Spallek J, Bammann K, Eiben G, De Henauw S, Kourides Y, et al. Migrant background and weight gain in early infancy: results from the German study sample of the IDEFICS study. PLoS ONE. 2013;8(4):e60648.

Rice F, Lewis A, Harold G, van den Bree M, Boivin J, Hay DF, et al. Agreement between maternal report and antenatal records for a range of pre and peri-natal factors: the influence of maternal and child characteristics. Early Hum Dev. 2007;83:497–504.

Rutayisire E, Huang K, Liu Y, Tao F. The mode of delivery affects the diversity and colonization pattern of the gut microbiota during the first year of infants' life: a systematic review. BMC Gastroenterol. 2016;16(1):86.

Saigal S, Doyle LW. An overview of mortality and sequelae of preterm birth from infancy to adulthood. Lancet. 2008;371:261–9.

Schack-Nielsen L, Michaelsen KF, Gamborg M, Mortensen EL, Sørensen TI. Gestational weight gain in relation to offspring body mass index and obesity from infancy through adulthood. Int J Obes (Lond). 2010;34:67–74.

Singhal A. Long-term adverse effects of early growth acceleration or catch-up growth. Ann Nutr Metab. 2017;70(3):236–40.

Sparano S, Ahrens W, De Henauw S, Mårild S, Molnár D, Moreno LA, et al. Being macrosomic at birth is an independent predictor of overweight in children: results from the IDEFICS study. Matern Child Health J. 2013;17(8):1373–81.

Tamashiro KL, Moran TH. Perinatal environment and its influences on metabolic programming of offspring. Physiol Behav. 2010;100:560–6.

Taylor RW, Grant AM, Goulding A, Williams SM. Early adiposity rebound: review of papers linking this to subsequent obesity in children and adults. Curr Opin Clin Nutr Metab Care. 2005;8:607–12.

Tehranifar P, Liao Y, Flom JD, Terry MB. Validity of self-reported birth weight by adult women: sociodemographic influences and implications for life-course studies. Am J Epidemiol. 2009;170:910–7.

Terry MB, Flom J, Tehranifar P, Susser E. The role of birth cohorts in studies of adult health: the New York women's birth cohort. Paediatr Perinat Epidemiol. 2009;23:431–45.

Van den Bussche K, Michels N, Gracia-Marco L, Herrmann D, Eiben G, De Henauw S, et al. Influence of birth weight on calcaneal bone stiffness in Belgian preadolescent children. Calcif Tissue Int. 2012;91:267–75.

Wells JC, Chomtho S, Fewtrell MS. Programming of body composition by early growth and nutrition. Proc Nutr Soc. 2007;66:423–34.

Yu ZB, Han SP, Zhu GZ, Zhu C, Wang XJ, Cao XG, et al. Birth weight and subsequent risk of obesity: a systematic review and meta-analysis. Obes Rev. 2011;12(7):525–42.

Chapter 9
Core Questionnaires

Karin Bammann, Lucia A. Reisch, Hermann Pohlabeln,
Garrath Williams and Maike Wolters

Abstract This chapter sets out the core questionnaires used in the IDEFICS and I.
Family studies. Since the IDEFICS study looked at younger children, it used a
single questionnaire which was filled out by the parents. This focussed mainly on
the child but also included some questions about the family, such as socioeconomic
status. The I.Family study looked at the whole family, including children who were
now old enough to answer questions on their own behalf. It therefore used a wider
range of questionnaires, which this chapter outlines.

On behalf of the IDEFICS and I.Family consortia.

K. Bammann (✉)
Working Group Epidemiology of Demographic Change,
Institute for Public Health and Nursing Research (IPP),
University of Bremen, Bremen, Germany
e-mail: bammann@uni-bremen.de

L. A. Reisch
Department of Management, Society and Communication,
Copenhagen Business School, Frederiksberg, Denmark

H. Pohlabeln · M. Wolters
Leibniz Institute for Prevention Research and Epidemiology—BIPS,
Bremen, Germany

G. Williams
Department of Politics, Philosophy and Religion, Lancaster University,
Lancaster, UK

© Springer Nature Switzerland AG 2019   189
K. Bammann et al. (eds.), *Instruments for Health Surveys in Children
and Adolescents*, Springer Series on Epidemiology and Public Health,
https://doi.org/10.1007/978-3-319-98857-3_9

9.1   Introduction

Beyond dietary factors, genetics, environment and lifestyle, a wide range of behavioural, psychological and social factors play a role in children's healthy development—sometimes plausibly as direct determinants, and in other cases as mediating factors (Hruby and Hu 2015; Mazarello Paes et al. 2015; Fatima et al. 2015; Aranceta-Bartrina and Pérez-Rodrigo 2016). The IDEFICS study aimed to gain a wide range of relevant data, while I.Family took this a step further in seeking information about other family members. In this chapter, we set out the relevant instruments and briefly highlight some analyses that have made use of the data generated. Since I.Family involved a range of questionnaires, we first provide a summary list (Tables 9.1 and 9.2, for access see Sect. 9.5).

Table 9.1 Questionnaire used in the IDEFICS study (baseline and follow-up surveys)

Questionnaire	Target group	Assessment method	Length
Parental questionnaire	Children 2–11 years	Self-administered paper-pencil (parents)	70 questions

Table 9.2 Questionnaires used in I.Family

Questionnaire	Target group	Assessment method	Length
Children's questionnaire	Children 2–11 years	Self-administered paper-pencil (parents)	59 questions
Teen questionnaire	Adolescents ≥ 12 years	Self-administered via iPad	78 questions (Sweden: 80 questions because 2 questions on moist snuff use were included)
Maturation stage questionnaire	Children and adolescents ≥ 8 years	Self-administered paper-pencil	2 questions (boys); 3 questions (girls)
Parent's questionnaire	Parents	Self-administered paper-pencil	52 questions (Sweden: 56 questions, because 4 questions on moist snuff use were included)
Pregnancy and early childhood interview	Biological mother	Interview paper-pencil or computer-assisted, face-to-face or telephone; self-administered for specific questions (smoking, alcohol)	For IDEFICS children: 1 question For each sibling/half-sibling: 14 questions
Family questionnaire	Parents	Self-administered paper-pencil or telephone	20 questions

9.2 IDEFICS Parental Questionnaire

The IDEFICS parental questionnaire was a self-administered paper questionnaire. Since the majority of targeted children were in the age of 4–7 (sampled in preschools/kindergartens and classes of the first two grades of primary school) it was designed to be filled in by the children's parents or legal guardians.

The questionnaire was organised into several sections (see Table 9.3) on different topics, spanning from rather simple-to-answer factual questions on facts (general information on day care and (pre)school situation) as a general warm-up to the questionnaire to more difficult questions that are harder to answer and that required some thinking either regarding in terms of recall (pregnancy and childhood) or the necessity for judgment (appraising family lifestyle), or both (health and well-being, leisure time activities, children's spending). The questionnaire closed with sociodemographics and household income. A repeatability study showed that

Table 9.3 Content of IDEFICS parental questionnaire

Section	Length	Content	Source questionnaires
General information	9 questions	Formal relation of the questionnaire respondent to the child (1 question), age and self-reported height and weight of both parents/guardians, date of birth and sex of the child (5 questions), household composition (3 questions)	–
Day care, preschool and school	9 questions	Use of day care services (3 questions), attendance of kindergarten or (pre)school, consumption of kindergarten, or (pre)school meals, money to buy food, distance (3 questions) and mode of transport to kindergarten or (pre)school (3 questions)	–
Pregnancy and childhood	11 questions	Maternal age, alcohol consumption and smoking during pregnancy, gestational weight gain, gestational age, C-section, birth weight and length, health problems during first 4 postnatal weeks (8 questions), early infant feeding (3 questions)	–

(continued)

Table 9.3 (continued)

Section	Length	Content	Source questionnaires
Family lifestyle	4 questions	Parenting style, family life, size of social network, parental attitudes to responsibilities and policies regarding children's lifestyle	Abridged version of the API (Jackson et al. 1998; Cullen et al. 2001) Abridged version of the FKS (Schneewind 1988)
Health and well-being	10 questions	Health locus of control, subjective health of the child (2 questions), parental beliefs regarding weight status and eating of the child (2 questions), health-related quality of life (4 questions), stressful life events, child strengths and difficulties (2 questions)	Abridged version of MHLOC questionnaire (Wallston et al. 1978; Wallston 2005) Abridged version of the CFQ (Birch et al. 2001) KINDL questionnaire (Ravens-Sieberer and Bullinger 1998) Extended and adapted Social Readjustment Rating Scale (Holmes and Rahe 1967) Strengths and Difficulties Questionnaire (Goodman 1997)
Leisure time activities and consumer behaviour	14 questions	Outdoor playtime (4 questions), child member in a sports club, sports abilities (2 questions), media use, media socialisation and competence (3 questions), exposure to TV advertising, parental attitudes towards food advertising (5 questions)	Outdoor playtime checklist (Burdette et al. 2004) Abridged AFAC questionnaire (Diehl and Daum 1995)
Children's spending	6 questions	Children's buying power and independent spending (3 questions), family food buying practices, pester power (3 questions)	–
Sociodemographics	7 questions	Migrant status (2 questions), level of parental education (2 questions), parental occupational status and position, household net income (3 questions)	Country-specific answer categories suitable for coding in ISCED (UNESCO 2006) and ESeC (Harrison and Rose 2006), see also Bammann et al. (2013)

API = Authoritative Parenting Index; FKS = Familienklimaskalen; MHLOC = Multidimensional Health Locus of Control; CFQ = Child Feeding Questionnaire; AFAC = Attitudes Toward TV Food Advertising Aimed at Children; ISCED = International Standard Classification of Education; ESeC = European Socioeconomic Classification the information on pre- and perinatal factors had very high repeatability, whereas information on early infant nutrition scored lower (Herrmann et al. 2011).

To keep the questionnaires at a reasonable length, these questions were separated from questions on children's diet (see Chap. 6 of this book). Even then, pretest findings from the survey centres prompted a shortening of the questionnaire, including the removal of some items from previously published questionnaires, since parents complained about its length (Suling et al. 2011).

The questionnaire was developed in English, translated to the different national languages and most prevalent migrant languages (Russian, Turkish, Arabic) and back-translated to English by a separate person to detect translation problems. All available language versions had to be present at the survey centres. Help was offered to parents who were not able to fill in the questionnaire themselves. The questionnaire data were used in multiple ways to analyse different research questions, mostly in combination with other data sources from the IDEFICS study (Hunsberger et al. 2012, 2016; Lissner et al. 2012; Vanaelst et al. 2012a, b; Bammann et al. 2013, 2014; Fernandez-Alvira et al. 2013, 2015; Gwozdz et al. 2013, 2015; Reeske et al. 2013; Regber et al. 2013; Formisano et al. 2014; Foraita et al. 2015; Börnhorst et al. 2016; Iguacel et al. 2016).

9.3 I.Family Questionnaires

The I.Family project used a wider range of questionnaires, for two reasons. First in line with the name of the project, I.Family sought more detailed information on the family as a whole, including other siblings and on parents themselves. Second, many of the IDEFICS children had reached adolescence and were therefore able to answer questions on their own behalf.

With regard to the second aspect, a *teen questionnaire* was designed to be completed by participants from the age of 12 years. For younger children (aged <12 years), a *children's questionnaire* was used. This questionnaire was filled in by parents for IDEFICS children who had not yet reached the age of 12, as well as for siblings under 12 years old. Parents were asked to complete the I.Family *parent's questionnaire* on their views, behaviour and lifestyle. Additionally, one or both parents filled in a *family questionnaire*, addressing general questions regarding family rules, behaviour and socioeconomic status.

Wider parts of the I.Family questionnaires were adapted from the IDEFICS parental questionnaire. Also, the IDEFICS eating habits questionnaire (IDEFICS EHQ, see Chap. 6 "Dietary Behaviour in Children, Adolescents and Families: the Eating Habits Questionnaire (EHQ)" of this book), which was a separate questionnaire in the IDEFICS study, was integrated into the children's, teen and parent's questionnaires.

9.3.1   Questionnaires Referring to Children and Adolescents

9.3.1.1   I.Family Children's Questionnaire

Like the IDEFICS parental questionnaire, the I.Family children's questionnaire was completed by the parents, giving information about their children below the age of 12 years. It largely overlapped with the IDEFICS version, but also introduced some new questions also accounting for the older age range of the children (Table 9.4).

Table 9.4 Content of I.Family children's questionnaire

Section	Length	Content	Source questionnaires
General information (child)	2 questions	Birth date (1 question) and sex (1 question) of child	IDEFICS parental questionnaire
General information (parents)	4 questions	Formal relation to the child, age and sex of the questionnaire respondent (3 questions), situation of filling in the questionnaire (1 question)	IDEFICS parental questionnaire (extended answer categories for formal relation to the child)
Child's well-being	5 questions	Emotional and social well-being, self-esteem (4 questions), stressful life events (1 question)	Modified IDEFICS parental questionnaire
Child's spending	3 questions	Weekly available money, restrictions to spend money, things bought by the child (3 questions)	IDEFICS parental questionnaire (extended answer categories)
Media consumption and media use	7 questions	Media use per day by type of media (3 questions), media located in child's bedroom (1 question) Child's media use on the past day (2 questions), using computer and other media the same time (1 question)	IDEFICS parental questionnaire (extended media device list) Generation M^2 questions (Rideout et al. 2010)
Physical activity on way to kindergarten/ school	7 questions	Attendance of kindergarten or (pre)school, distance and mode of transport to kindergarten or (pre)school (3 questions) Time spent for transport (total and active) and activity intensity (4 questions)	Modified IDEFICS parental questionnaire MoMo-AFB (Jekauc et al. 2013)
Physical activity at school	2 questions	Physical education and school breaks (2 questions)	Questions taken from PATREC study (Sprengeler et al. 2017)

(continued)

Table 9.4 (continued)

Section	Length	Content	Source questionnaires
Physical activity in leisure time	5 questions	Playing outdoors on weekdays/-ends and activity intensity (2 questions), sports club membership, time spent in sports club, activity intensity and type of sport (3 questions)	IDEFICS parental questionnaire combined with MoMo-AFB for activity intensity (Jekauc et al. 2013)
Sleeping habits	11 questions	Sleep duration on weekdays (3 questions) and weekends (3 questions), other sleeping habits and sleep quality, bedroom light and noise (5 questions)	PSQI (Buysse et al. 1989)
Diet	13 questions	See Chap. 6 of this book for details	Modified IDEFICS EHQ, see Chap. 6 of this book for details

MoMo-AFB = Motorik-Modul Aktivitätsfragebogen; PSQI = Pittsburgh Sleep Quality Index

9.3.1.2 I.Family Teen Questionnaire (Age 12 and over)

The age range of the I.Family children who had already participated in the IDEFICS study was 5–17 years. Children age 12 or over were asked to fill in a specific teen questionnaire. This included the questions listed above in Table 9.4. It also included some aspects of health behaviour and lifestyle relevant to adolescents (Table 9.5). Smoking behaviour and alcohol consumption were evaluated using questions from The European School Survey Project on Alcohol and Other Drugs (ESPAD) (ESPAD 2011). For alcohol consumption, the questions covered the number of times alcoholic beverages had been consumed (over lifetime, during the last 12 months and during the last 30 days), the frequency and kind of beverages, frequency of binge drinking and self-assessment of intoxication from drinking alcohol. Regarding smoking, the number of occasions of having smoked cigarettes over lifetime, the quantity of cigarettes smoked during the last 30 days and the initiating age of smoking were assessed. For the Swedish survey only, questions on the use of moist snuff were added.

Questions on eating disorders, body image and impulsiveness were also added for this group, since adolescents are concerned about body weight and body image. These concerns can lead to dieting attempts as well as extreme distress, right up to severe eating disorders such as anorexia or bulimia nervosa. Adolescents from the age of 12 years were asked for dieting history and frequency as well as for the presence, frequency and severity of binge eating (Slof-Op 't Landt et al. 2009). Additionally, statements on body image were evaluated based on the eating disorder diagnostic scale (Stice et al. 2000). In this context, emotion-driven

Table 9.5 Content of the I.Family teen questionnaire

Section	Length	Content	Source questionnaires
General information	2 questions	Birth date and sex (2 questions)	IDEFICS parental questionnaire
Well-being	7 questions	Emotional and social well-being, self-esteem (6 questions), stressful life events (1 question)	Modified IDEFICS parental questionnaire extended by school-specific domains from KIDSCREEN (Ravens-Sieberer et al. 2005)
Family life and rules	9 questions	Perceived home atmosphere, activities with parents, parental knowledge of whereabouts (3 questions) Parental rules for staying out at evenings (2 questions) Parental rules for media use (1 question) Weekly amount of available money, buying restrictions and things usually bought (3 questions)	Modified from Latendresse et al. (2009) Modified from Pearson et al. (2010) Modified Generation M^2 questions (Rideout et al. 2010) IDEFICS parental questionnaire (extended answer categories)
Media consumption and media use	7 questions	Media use by type of media per day (3 questions), media located in the bedroom (1 question) Media use on the past day, using other media while using a computer (3 questions)	IDEFICS parental questionnaire (extended media device list) Generation M^2 questions (Rideout et al. 2010)
Physical activity on the way to school	6 questions	Distance and mode of transport to school (2 questions) Time spent for transport (total and active) and activity intensity (4 questions),	Modified IDEFICS parental questionnaire MoMo-AFB (Jekauc et al. 2013)
Physical activity at school	2 questions	Physical education and school breaks (2 questions)	Questions taken from PATREC study (Sprengeler et al. 2017)
Physical activity in leisure time	5 questions	Playing outdoors on weekdays/-ends and activity intensity (2 questions), sports club membership, time spent in sports club, activity intensity and type of sport (3 questions)	IDEFICS parental questionnaire combined with MoMo-AFB for activity intensity (Jekauc et al. 2013)
Body image	6 questions	Dieting (2 questions) and binge eating (3 questions) Perception of body weight (1 question)	Modified from Slof-Op 't Landt et al. (2009) Abridged and modified EDDS (Stice et al. 2000)

(continued)

Table 9.5 (continued)

Section	Length	Content	Source questionnaires
Impulsiveness	1 question	Impulsive behaviour (1 question)	Abridged version of the UPPS-P (Whiteside et al. 2005)
Sleeping habits	13 questions	Sleep duration on school days and on weekends/vacation (6 questions), other sleeping habits and sleep quality, bedroom light and noise (7 questions)	PSQI (Buysse et al. 1989)
Smoking	3 questions	Occasions of having smoked, frequency of smoking (2 questions), starting age of smoking (1 question) For Sweden: 2 additional questions on moist snuff use	Abridged ESPAD questionnaire (ESPAD 2013)
Alcohol consumption	5 questions	Occasions of alcoholic beverages use (2 questions), consumption of more than five drinks per occasion and level of drunkenness/ intoxication (3 questions)	Abridged ESPAD questionnaire (ESPAD 2013)
School marks	2 questions	Report marks in maths and national language (1 question), type of school attended (1 question)	Modified ESPAD questions (ESPAD 2013)
Diet	12 questions	See Chap. 6 of this book for details	Modified IDEFICS EHQ, see Chap. 6 of this book for details

MoMo-AFB = Motorik-Modul Aktivitätsfragebogen; EDDS = Eating Disorder Diagnostic Scale; UPPS-P = Urgency, Premeditation (lack of), Perseverance (lack of), Sensation Seeking, Positive Urgency; PSQI = Pittsburgh Sleep Quality Index; ESPAD – The European School Survey Project on Alcohol and Other Drugs

impulsiveness also plays an important role. This was assessed using the subscale negative urgency of the UPPS (Urgency, Premeditation (lack of), Perseverance (lack of), Sensation Seeking) impulsive behaviour scale (Whiteside et al. 2005).

School performance was also assessed. The report marks at the end of the last term in mathematics and the national language spoken in the respective country were asked. Since some systems do not give marks, it was also possible to tick "I do not (yet) get marks at school". As grading systems differ depending on the type of school even within one country, the type of school the participant was currently attending was also assessed. If the child was on holidays and was to attend a new school afterwards, they were asked to tick the last type of school attended.

Adolescents were particularly assured that their answers would be treated in strict confidence and would not be shared with their parents or anybody else outside the research team.

Because of their affinity for new media, the teen questionnaire was deployed as self-administered questionnaire to be completed via iPad. Participants sometimes complained about the length of the questionnaire, especially if all examinations and tests were conducted during only one visit to the survey centre.

9.3.1.3   I.Family Maturation Stage Questionnaire

Maturation (or pubertal) stage has an important relation to clinical, metabolic and psychological health outcomes. Children from the age of 8 years were asked by the medical study personnel to self-assess their pubertal development based on the Tanner stages including age of their first menstruation for girls and voice mutation for boys (Marshall and Tanner 1970). As children and adolescents may be embarrassed by these questions, the questionnaire was handed over to them and they completed it without being observed or disturbed. Afterwards, the completed questionnaire was folded and put into a box by the child (Table 9.6). In Italy, the illustrations of Tanner stages were perceived as embarrassing, and they were not used during the survey. Therefore, only information on age at first menstruation and on voice mutation is available for Italian participants.

9.3.2   Questionnaires Addressed to Parents

Apart from questionnaires about their children under the age of 12, parents were asked to complete questionnaires about themselves and about the family as a whole. We refer to these as the I.Family parent's questionnaire and the family questionnaire, respectively.

Table 9.6 Content of I.Family maturation stage questionnaire

Section	Length	Content	Source questionnaires
Boys: voice mutation	1 question	Stage of voice mutation	Modified from Carskadon and Acebo (1993)
Boys: pubic hair growth	1 question	Stage of pubic hair growth	Modified from Marshall and Tanner (1970) and illustrations from Morris and Udry (1980)
Girls: first menstruation	2 questions	First menstruation and age at first menstruation	Modified from Carskadon and Acebo (1993)
Girls: breast growth	1 question	Stage of breast growth	Modified from Marshall and Tanner (1969) and illustrations from Morris and Udry (1980)

9.3.2.1   I.Family Parent's Questionnaire

Table 9.7 gives an overview of the different behaviours and lifestyle that parents were asked about in the I.Family parent's questionnaire. Except for questions on well-being and media consumption which were only included in the children's and teen questionnaires, the topics are broadly similar to those adolescents were asked about.

Table 9.7 Content of I.Family parent's questionnaire

Section	Length	Content	Source questionnaires
General information	4 questions	Birth date, sex, formal relation to IDEFICS child of the questionnaire respondent (3 questions) and situation of filling in the questionnaire (1 question)	IDEFICS parental questionnaire (extended answer categories for formal relation to the child)
Family life and rules	2 questions	Parental attitudes to responsibilities and policies regarding children's lifestyle (1 question) Parental knowledge of whereabouts, encouragement of autonomy (1 question)	IDEFICS parental questionnaire (abridged) Modified from Latendresse et al. (2009)
Physical activity on the way to work	6 questions	Distance and mode of transport to work (2 questions) Time spent for transport (total and active) and activity intensity (4 questions),	Modified IDEFICS parental questionnaire MoMo-AFB (Jekauc et al. 2013)
Physical activity in leisure time	3 questions	Sports club membership, time spent in sports club and type of sport (3 questions)	IDEFICS parental questionnaire
Physical activity in the last 7 days	4 questions	Moderate and vigorous activity (2 questions), walking, sedentary time (2 questions)	Abridged IPAQ (IPAQ 2002)
Body image	6 questions	Dieting (2 questions) and binge eating (3 questions) Perception of body weight (1 question)	Modified from Slof-Op 't Landt et al. (2009) Abridged and modified EDDS (Stice et al. 2000)
Impulsiveness	1 question	Impulsive behaviour (1 question)	Abridged version of the UPPS-P (Whiteside et al. 2005)
Sleeping habits	12 questions	Sleep duration on working days and days off (6 questions), other sleeping habits and sleep quality, bedroom light and noise (6 questions)	PSQI (Buysse et al. 1989)

(continued)

Table 9.7 (continued)

Section	Length	Content	Source questionnaires
Smoking	4 questions	Smoking behaviour, start of smoking (2 questions), smoking frequency/habits (1 question), for Sweden: 4 additional questions on moist snuff use Smoking after waking up (1 question)	Modified from Latza et al. (2005) Heavy Smoking Index (Heatherton et al. 1989)
Alcohol	3 questions	Frequency of alcoholic beverage use (1 question), amount of drinks per occasion, frequency of drinking more than 5 drinks per day (2 questions)	Modified from WHO (2000)
Diet	9 questions	See Chap. 6 of this book for details	Modified IDEFICS EHQ, see Chap. 6 of this book for details

MoMo-AFB = Motorik-Modul Aktivitätsfragebogen; IPAQ = International Physical Activity Questionnaire; EDDS = Eating Disorder Diagnostic Scale; UPPS-P = Urgency, Premeditation (lack of), Perseverance (lack of), Sensation Seeking, Positive Urgency; PSQI = Pittsburgh Sleep Quality Index

Questions on adults' smoking behaviour were based on the German smoking standard assessment (Latza et al. 2005) comprising current smoking status, smoking amount, starting age of regular smoking and past smoking behaviour. Additionally, a question from the Heavy Smoking Index on smoking soon after waking up was added (Heatherton et al. 1989).

Regarding alcohol consumption, the suggested questions of the World Health Organization (2000) were used. These ask for the number of occasions drinking any alcoholic beverages and the usual amount of drinks on those days where alcoholic beverages have been consumed over the past year. The third question referred to the frequency of binge drinking in the past year defined as five or more drinks on one occasion.

Questions on eating disorders, body image and impulsiveness were the same as in the teen questionnaire.

9.3.2.2   I.Family Family Questionnaire

The I.Family family questionnaire was completed by one or both parents together and consisted of questions on family life and rules as well as on TV food advertisements, family meals and the parents' socioeconomic status (Table 9.8).

Table 9.8 Content of I.Family family questionnaire

Section	Length	Content	Source questionnaires
General information	4 questions	Birth date, sex and formal relation to IDEFICS child of the questionnaire respondent (3 questions) and situation of filling in the questionnaire (1 question)	IDEFICS parental questionnaire (extended answer categories for formal relation to the child)
Family life and rules	3 questions	Perceived home atmosphere, activities with parents (2 questions) Parental rules for media use (1 question)	Modified from Latendresse et al. (2009) Modified Generation M^2 questions (Rideout et al. 2010)
TV food advertisement	2 questions	Parental attitudes towards food advertising and discussion of contents with the child (2 questions)	IDEFICS parental questionnaire
Meals in the family	6 questions	See Chap. 6 of this book for details	Modified IDEFICS EHQ (see Chap. 6 of this book)
Socio-demographic information	7 questions	Parental education (4 questions), parental occupational status (2 questions), household income (1 question)	IDEFICS parental questionnaire (extended answer categories for occupational status)

9.3.2.3   I.Family Pregnancy and Early Childhood Questionnaire

In the IDEFICS study, information on pregnancy and early childhood, e.g. birth weight of child, risk factors like gestational weight gain, alcohol consumption and smoking during pregnancy, was collected from the biological mother in the parental questionnaire. In I.Family, this information was assessed for newly included siblings by a separate questionnaire, the pregnancy and early childhood questionnaire which consists of the same questions which were asked in the IDEFICS study plus an additional question on prepregnancy maternal weight (Table 9.9; see also Chap. 8 of this book). For the IDEFICS children in I.Family, only the latter question was asked, since the other information was already present from the IDEFICS study.

Table 9.9 Content of I.Family pregnancy and early childhood questionnaire

Section	Length	Content	Source questionnaires
General information	2 questions	Birth date (1 question) and sex (1 question)	IDEFICS parental questionnaire
Pregnancy	9 questions	Country of child's birth (1 question), alcohol consumption and smoking in pregnancy (2 questions), weight gain during pregnancy (1 question), preterm birth (2 questions), caesarean sect. (1 question), child's weight and height at birth (2 questions)	IDEFICS parental questionnaire and added question on prepregnancy body weight
Early childhood	4 questions	Health in the first four weeks after birth, breastfeeding/type of feeding (2 questions), age at introduction of specific foods, household's diet (2 questions)	IDEFICS parental questionnaire

9.4   Practical Experiences Gained

The study protocol of the IDEFICS study allowed participants to take part in the study without completing the questionnaires. Nevertheless, the proportion of completed questionnaires was very high in all participating countries (see Table 9.10). Also in I.Family, the proportion of completed questionnaires was high for children and teens. The participation of at least one parent was sought but not mandatory and in some countries parents were not willing to take part. Lower participation of parents particularly occurred in Belgium and Spain because of limited funding. Parents mostly completed the questionnaires at home. Usually, children, teens and parents were examined in the survey centre. However, in exceptional cases, if parents had very little time and were not able to come to the survey centre, a completed parent's questionnaire and self-reported height and weight were accepted for participation of a parent. As the completion of the teen questionnaire had to be done on the iPad in the survey centre, the required time for questionnaires and examinations was high and teens usually had to visit the survey centre.

In general, item response for completed questionnaires was very good (see Table 9.11). Exceptions were rare and not surprising, e.g. for household income (item response 85.8%, ranging from 56.5% in Cyprus to 95.5% in Sweden). In few cases, low item responses were matched by reservations expressed by the research

Table 9.10 Proportion of completed questionnaires in percentage

	Belgium	Cyprus	Estonia	Germany	Hungary	Italy	Spain	Sweden	All
IDEFICS parental questionnaire T_0	99.0	97.2	100	100	100	100	98.5	99.9	99.3
IDEFICS parental questionnaire T_1	100	97.2	97.7	98.0	87.7	100	97.1	92.6	96.2
I.Family children's or teen questionnaire	80.8	94.1	97.9	97.4	99.8	99.8	92.9	93.0	96.1
I.Family parent's questionnaire (at least one)	52.8	68.9	73.0	82.0	90.0	98.6	64.0	90.6	79.9
I.Family parent's questionnaire (each parent completed one)	9.4	38.0	28.6	32.5	51.1	30.4	31.0	17.8	32.7
I.Family family questionnaire	53.6	78.6	92.0	81.8	90.6	93.5	91.0	92.3	86.3

teams as, e.g. self-assessment of Tanner stage in Italy. Equally, concerns of questionnaire length expressed by the research team particularly in Cyprus were reflected by low item response especially for questions which consist of longer item lists as, e.g. parenting style.

9.5 Provision of Instruments and Standard Operating Procedures to Third Parties

All instruments described in this chapter including the General Survey Manuals that provide among other all standard operating procedures can be accessed on the following Web site: www.leibniz-bips.de/ifhs after registration.

Each third partner using the instruments provided in this chapter is kindly requested to cite this chapter as follows:

Bammann K, Reisch LA, Pohlabeln H, Williams G, Wolters M, on behalf of the IDEFICS and I.Family consortia. Core questionnaires. In: Bammann K, Lissner L, Pigeot I, Ahrens W, editors. Instruments for health surveys in children and adolescents. Cham: Springer Nature Switzerland; 2019. p. 189–207.

Table 9.11 Item response on selected variables in % (T_0, except where stated otherwise)

	Belgium	Cyprus	Estonia	Germany	Hungary	Italy	Spain	Sweden	All
Birth weight	96.8	83.8	94.7	94.9	96.5	97.8	95.2	94.5	94.1
Tanner stage (T_3): development of pubic hair (boys) or breast (girls)	94.4	83.6	92.7	81.3	94.1	n/a	84.0	84.1	73.1
Tanner stage (T_3): development of voice (boys) and menarche (girls)	93.8	89.0	97.0	82.5	95.2	97.2	83.6	91.1	91.5
Dietary habits: Food frequency (T_3)	82.0	84.1	93.3	93.7	99.6	98.7	92.0	92.3	91.9
Physical activity: Outdoor playtime	91.5	77.4	92.5	87.8	95.8	88.9	94.8	94.2	90.0
Household income	86.0	56.6	94.1	89.2	93.3	86.8	91.2	95.5	85.8
Parental education	97.6	85.1	96.7	96.1	97.7	99.2	98.1	97.2	95.7
Parenting style	96.7	62.0	94.7	96.1	94.6	94.6	96.4	97.2	90.7

n/a = not applicable

Acknowledgements The development of instruments, the baseline data collection and the first follow-up work as part of the IDEFICS study (www.idefics.eu) were financially supported by the European Commission within the Sixth RTD Framework Programme Contract No. 016181 (FOOD). The most recent follow-up including the development of new instruments and the adaptation of previously used instruments was conducted in the framework of the I.Family study (www.ifamilystudy.eu) which was funded by the European Commission within the Seventh RTD Framework Programme Contract No. 266044 (KBBE 2010-14).

We thank all families for participating in the extensive examinations of the IDEFICS and I.Family studies. We are also grateful for the support from school boards, headmasters and communities.

References

Aranceta-Bartrina J, Pérez-Rodrigo C. Determinants of childhood obesity: ANIBES study. Nutr Hosp. 2016;33(Suppl 4):339.

Bammann K, Gwozdz W, Lanfer A, Barba G, De Henauw S, Eiben G, et al. IDEFICS consortium. Socioeconomic factors and childhood overweight in Europe: results from the multi-centre IDEFICS study. Pediatr Obes. 2013;8(1):1–12.

Bammann K, Peplies J, De Henauw S, Hunsberger M, Molnar D, Moreno LA, et al. IDEFICS consortium. Early life course risk factors for childhood obesity: the IDEFICS case-control study. PLoS ONE. 2014;9(2):e86914.

Birch LL, Fisher JO, Grimm-Thomas K, Markey CN, Sawyer R, Johnson SL. Confirmatory factor analysis of the Child Feeding Questionnaire: a measure of parental attitudes, beliefs and practices about child feeding and obesity proneness. Appetite. 2001;36(3):201–10.

Börnhorst C, Siani A, Russo P, Kourides Y, Sion I, Molnar D, et al. Early life factors and inter-country heterogeneity in BMI growth trajectories of European children: the IDEFICS study. PLoS ONE. 2016;11(2):e0149268.

Burdette HL, Whitaker RC, Daniels SR. Parental report of outdoor playtime as a measure of physical activity in preschool-aged children. Arch Pediatr Adolesc Med. 2004;158(4):353–7.

Buysse DJ, Reynolds CF, Monk TH, Berman SR, Kupfer DJ. The Pittsburgh sleep quality index: a new instrument for psychiatric practice and research. Psychiatry Res. 1989;28:193–213.

Carskadon MA, Acebo C. A self-administered rating scale for pubertal development. J Adolesc Health. 1993;14(3):190–5.

Cullen KW, Baranowski T, Rittenberry L, Cosart C, Hebert D, de Moor C. Child-reported family and peer influences on fruit, juice and vegetable consumption: reliability and validity of measures. Health Educ Res. 2001;16(2):187–200.

Diehl JM, Daum I. Television food commercials aimed at children and parents. In: Curzon ME, Diehl JM, Ghraf R, Lentze MJ, editors. Carbohydrates in infant nutrition and dental health. Munich, Germany: Urban and Vogel; 1995. p. 169–83.

ESPAD. Questionnaire on substance use. Student questionnaire. Stockholm, Sweden: The European School Survey Project on Alcohol and Other Drugs (ESPAD); 2011.

ESPAD. A supplement to the 2011 ESPAD report. Appendix IV. Student questionnaire. Stockholm, Sweden: The European School Survey Project on Alcohol and Other Drugs (ESPAD); 2013.

Fatima Y, Doi SA, Mamun AA. Longitudinal impact of sleep on overweight and obesity in children and adolescents: a systematic review and bias-adjusted meta-analysis. Obes Rev. 2015;16(2):137–49.

Fernandez-Alvira JM, Börnhorst C, Bammann K, Gwozdz W, Krogh V, Hebestreit A, et al. Prospective associations between socio-economic status and dietary patterns in European children: the Identification and prevention of Dietary- and lifestyle-induced health EFfects In Children and infantS (IDEFICS) study. Br J Nutr. 2015;113(3):517–25.

Fernandez-Alvira JM, Mouratidou T, Bammann K, Hebestreit A, Barba G, Sieri S, et al. Parental education and frequency of food consumption in European children: the IDEFICS study. Public Health Nutr. 2013;16(3):487–98.

Foraita R, Günther F, Gwozdz W, Reisch LA, Russo P, Lauria F, et al. IDEFICS consortium. Does the FTO gene interact with the socioeconomic status on the obesity development among young European children? Results from the IDEFICS study. Int J Obes (Lond). 2015;39(1):1–6.

Formisano A, Hunsberger M, Bammann K, Vanaelst B, Molnar D, Moreno LA, et al. Family structure and childhood obesity: results of the IDEFICS project. Public Health Nutr. 2014;17 (10):2307–15.

Goodman R. The strengths and difficulties questionnaire: a research note. J Child Psychol Psychiatry. 1997;38(5):581–6.

Gwozdz W, Sousa-Poza A, Reisch LA, Ahrens W, Eiben G, Fernandéz-Alvira JM, et al. Maternal employment and childhood obesity—a European perspective. J Health Econ. 2013;32(4):728–42.

Gwozdz W, Sousa-Poza A, Reisch LA, Bammann K, Eiben G, Kourides Y, et al. Peer effects on obesity in a sample of European children. Econ Hum Biol. 2015;18:139–52.

Harrison E, Rose D. The European Socioeconomic Classification (ESeC). User guide. Colchester: University of Essex; 2006.

Heatherton TF, Kozlowski LT, Frecker RC, Rickert W, Robinson J. Measuring the heaviness of smoking: using self-reported time to the first cigarette of the day and number of cigarettes smoked per day. Br J Addic. 1989;84(7):791–9.

Herrmann D, Suling M, Reisch L, Siani A, De Bourdeaudhuij I, Maes L, et al. IDEFICS consortium. Repeatability of maternal report on prenatal, perinatal and early postnatal factors: findings from the IDEFICS parental questionnaire. Int J Obes (Lond). 2011;35(Suppl 1):S52–60.

Holmes TH, Rahe RH. The social readjustment rating scale. J Psychosom Res. 1967;11(2):213–8.

Hruby A, Hu FB. The epidemiology of obesity: a big picture. Pharmacoeconomics. 2015;33 (7):673–89.

Hunsberger M, Formisano A, Reisch LA, Bammann K, Moreno L, De Henauw S, et al. Overweight in singletons compared to children with siblings: the IDEFICS study. Nutr Diab. 2012;2:e35.

Hunsberger M, Lehtinen-Jacks S, Mehlig K, Gwozdz W, Russo P, Michels N, et al. IDEFICS consortium. Bidirectional associations between psychosocial well-being and body mass index in European children: longitudinal findings from the IDEFICS study. BMC Public Health. 2016;16:949.

Iguacel I, Fernandez-Alvira JM, Bammann K, De Clercq B, Eiben G, Gwozdz W, et al. IDEFICS consortium. Associations between social vulnerabilities and dietary patterns in European children: the Identification and prevention of Dietary- and lifestyle-induced health EFfects In Children and infantS (IDEFICS) study. Br J Nutr. 2016;116(7):1288–97.

IPAQ. International Physical Activity Questionnaire. Short last 7 days self-administered format. For use with young and middle-aged adults (15–69 years). www.ipaq.ki.se. 2002. Accessed 15 Mar 2018.

Jackson C, Henriksen L, Foshee VA. The authoritative parenting index: predicting health risk behaviors among children and adolescents. Health Educ Behav. 1998;25(3):319–37.

Jekauc D, Wagner MO, Khalert D, Woll K. Reliabilität und Vailidität des MoMo-Aktivitätsfragebogens für Jugendliche (MoMo-AFB). Diagnostica. 2013;59:100–11.

Latendresse SJ, Rose RJ, Viken RJ, Pulkkinen L, Kaprio J, Dick DM. Parental socialization and adolescents' alcohol use behaviors: predictive disparities in parents' versus adolescents' perceptions of the parenting environment. J Clin Child Adolesc Psychol. 2009;38(2):232–44.

Latza U, Hoffmann W, Terschüren C, Chang-Claude J, Kreuzer M, Schaffrath Rosario A, et al. Erhebung, Quantifizierung und Analyse der Rauchexposition in epidemiologischen Studien. Abschnitt 4.4.3: Variation des Fragebogens Aktivrauchen – Kurzversion (Erwachsene). Berlin: Robert Koch Institut; 2005.

Lissner L, Lanfer A, Gwozdz W, Olafsdottir S, Eiben G, Moreno LA, et al. Television habits in relation to overweight, diet and taste preferences in European children: the IDEFICS study. Eur J Epidemiol. 2012;27(9):705–15.

Marshall WA, Tanner JM. Variations in pattern of pubertal changes in girls. Arch Dis Child. 1969;44(235):291–303.

Marshall WA, Tanner JM. Variations in the pattern of pubertal changes in boys. Arch Dis Child. 1970;45(239):13–23.

Mazarello Paes V, Ong KK, Lakshman R. Factors influencing obesogenic dietary intake in young children (0–6 years): systematic review of qualitative evidence. BMJ Open. 2015;5(9): e007396.

Morris NM, Udry JR. Validation of a self-administered instrument to assess stage of adolescent development. J Youth Adolesc. 1980;9(3):271–80.

Pearson N, Atkin AJ, Biddle SJ, Gorely T, Edwardson C. Parenting styles, family structure and adolescent dietary behaviour. Public Health Nutr. 2010;13(8):1245–53.

Ravens-Sieberer U, Bullinger M. Assessing health-related quality of life in chronically ill children with the German KINDL: first psychometric and content analytical results. Qual Life Res. 1998;7(5):399–407.

Ravens-Sieberer U, Gosch A, Rajmil L, Erhart M, Bruil J, Duer W, et al. KIDSCREEN-52 quality-of-life measure for children and adolescents. Expert Rev Pharmacoecon Outcomes Res. 2005;5(3):353–64.

Reeske A, Spallek J, Bammann K, Eiben G, De Henauw S, Kourides Y, et al. Migrant background and weight gain in early infancy: results from the German study sample of the IDEFICS study. PLoS ONE. 2013;8(4):e60648.

Regber S, Novak M, Eiben G, Bammann K, De Henauw S, Fernandéz-Alvira JM, et al. Parental perceptions of and concerns about child's body weight in eight European countries—the IDEFICS study. Pediatr Obes. 2013;8(2):118–29.

Rideout VJ, Foehr UG, Roberts DF. Generation M^2: media in the lives of 8- to 18-year-olds. A Kaiser Family Foundation Study. Menlo Park, California: The Henry J. Kaiser Family Foundation; 2010.

Schneewind KA. Die Familienklimaskalen. In: Cierpka M, editor. Familiendiagnostik. Berlin: Springer; 1988. p. 232–55.

Slof-Op 't Landt MC, Dolan CV, Rebollo-Mesa I, Bartels M, van Furth EF, van Beijsterveldt CE, et al. Sex differences in sum scores may be hard to interpret: the importance of measurement invariance. Assessment. 2009;16(4):415–23.

Sprengeler O, Wirsik N, Hebestreit A, Herrmann D, Ahrens W. Domain-specific self-reported and objectively measured physical activity in children. Int J Environ Res Public Health. 2017;14 (3):E242.

Stice E, Telch CF, Rizvi SL. Development and validation of the eating disorder diagnostic scale: a brief self report measure of anorexia, bulimia, and binge eating disorder. Psychol Assess. 2000;12(2):123–31.

Suling M, Hebestreit A, Peplies J, Bammann K, Nappo A, Eiben G, et al. IDEFICS consortium. Design and results of the pretest of the IDEFICS study. Int J Obes (Lond). 2011;35(Suppl 1): S30–44.

United Nations Educational Scientific and Cultural Organization (UNESCO) Institute for Statistics. International Standard Classification of Education (ISCED) 1997. Montreal: UNESCO; 2006.

Vanaelst B, De Vriendt T, Ahrens W, Bammann K, Hadjigeorgiou C, Konstabel K, et al. Prevalence of psychosomatic and emotional symptoms in European school-aged children and its relationship with childhood adversities: results from the IDEFICS study. Eur Child Adolesc Psychiatry. 2012a;21(5):253–65.

Vanaelst B, Huybrechts I, De Bourdeaudhuij I, Bammann K, Hadjigeorgiou C, Eiben G, et al. IDEFICS consortium. Prevalence of negative life events and chronic adversities in European pre- and primary-school children: results from the IDEFICS study. Arch Public Health. 2012b;70(1):26.

Wallston KA. The validity of the multidimensional health locus of control scales. J Health Psychol. 2005;10(5):623–31.

Wallston KA, Wallston BS, DeVellis R. Development of the Multidimensional Health Locus of Control (MHLC) scales. Health Educ Monogr. 1978;6(2):160–70.

Whiteside SP, Lynam DR, Miller JD, Reynolds SK. Validation of the UPPS impulsive behaviour scale: a four-factor model of impulsivity. Eur J Pers. 2005;19:559–74.

WHO. International guide for monitoring alcohol consumption and related harm. Annex 8. Suggested questions for a 3 item and an 8 item set of questions about alcohol consumption. A. Module containing minimum required items (3 questions). Department of Mental Health and Substance Dependence, Noncommunicable Diseases and Mental Health Cluster. Geneva: World Health Organization; 2000.

Chapter 10
Instruments for Assessing the Role of Commercials on Children's Food Choices

Wencke Gwozdz and Lucia A. Reisch

Abstract Today's children are highly exposed to media and hence also to food advertising. Various strands of research suggest that exposure to advertising may contribute to childhood overweight. However, previous research has largely been deficient in identifying the causal impact of advertising on children's food choices. To address this, a toolbox of instruments related to the role of advertising in children's food choice has been developed. This study presents three research modules that are designed to shed new light on the question of whether food advertising affects children's dietary choices. The toolbox consists of three tools: (1) a children's questionnaire on advertising literacy, (2) an experimental design on children food knowledge and preferences and (3) an experimental design on active food choice with food advertisement stimuli.

10.1 Introduction

This chapter provides an overview of different instruments that were developed to assess the effects of advertising on children's food choices as a substudy of the IDEFICS study. Before the individual instruments are presented, we provide some background information and the overall rationale for the toolbox on the role of commercials on children's food choice.

On behalf of the IDEFICS and I.Family consortia.

W. Gwozdz · L. A. Reisch
Department of Management, Society and Communication,
Copenhagen Business School, Frederiksberg, Denmark

W. Gwozdz (✉)
Justus-Liebig-University Giessen, Giessen, Germany
e-mail: wencke.gwozdz@fb09.uni-giessen.de

© Springer Nature Switzerland AG 2019
K. Bammann et al. (eds.), *Instruments for Health Surveys in Children and Adolescents*, Springer Series on Epidemiology and Public Health,
https://doi.org/10.1007/978-3-319-98857-3_10

10.1.1   In Search of an Evidence Base for Policy-Makers

For years, public health organisations, consumer policy advocates and paediatricians have proposed stricter limitations or outright bans on food advertising aimed at children in order to reduce the prevalence of overweight children (e.g. IOM 2005; UK Department of Health 2008; WHO 2013). However, existing research provides only a weak scientific base for the justification of advertising restrictions on these grounds. In addition, the marketing to which children are exposed reaches beyond advertisements aired during children's television programmes. As the evidence remains mixed, policy-makers have called for research on whether advertising affects children's food patterns and, if it does, to what extent. This chapter describes an approach that could be taken in consumer research to help clarify the impact of commercial communication on children's diets and health. To this end, three interrelated instruments to measure advertising's effect on children's food choices were developed by the authors, critically assessed and validated with the support of the participating survey centres, and applied within the IDEFICS study to an international sample of European children aged six to ten years (Ahrens et al. 2011).

10.1.2   Focus of the Study

The marketing of food and beverages to children encompasses much more than explicit advertising messages in the mass media. Among the most important marketing techniques are food messages and product/brand placement embedded in television programming; programme-length commercials; school-based marketing; the tying of games, toys and other products with food products; viral and guerrilla marketing; and food messages embedded in children's books and play material (overview in Harris et al. 2009; Kelly et al. 2010; Mathios 2005). The research outlined in this chapter focuses on the traditional mass media commercial communication directed at children, which refers, for the most part, to television advertisements.

The main reason for this focus on TV is that the present study is about young children (six to ten years). Television is still the primary mass media through which this age group is exposed to commercial messages (Federal Trade Commission 2008; Livingstone 2005; Rideout 2017). Commercial messages on TV comprise overt advertisements as well as stealth marketing techniques, such as product and brand placement. While the latter are prohibited by law in TV programmes directed at children in the EU (EU 2007) and in the USA (Linn 2004), they are in fact commonplace in prime-time television programmes, where a large proportion of children's television viewing time occurs. This is why the term "prime-time diet" has been coined (e.g. Story and Faulkner 1990). Within the EU, the amended "Television without Frontiers" Directive on Audiovisual Media from 2007 (Audiovisual Media Services Directive 2007/65/EC; EU 2007) has created new possibilities for product placement and programme sponsorship for the food and beverage industry. Therefore, children within the EU are likely to be exposed to more "under the radar" persuasive food marketing in the near future.[1]

In addition to these commercial messages explicitly targeted at children, young consumers are incidentally exposed to all kinds of food and drink advertising (including advertising for products that are not age relevant) through mere exposure to a highly commercialised physical and medial environment. Through such effects as early brand imprinting, such incidental exposure to commercial messages has been shown to be nearly as effective as targeted exposure and this exposure can influence purchase decisions years later (Ferraro et al. 2009).

Increasingly, Internet and computer games play a role in commercial communication, particularly via product and brand placement and stealth marketing techniques such as "advergames"[2] (e.g. Montgomery and Chester 2007).[3]

10.1.3   Prior Research on the Influence of Television on Young Children's Diets

Many researchers propose that young children's television viewing habits shape their food knowledge, preferences and actual food choice and, hence, contribute to early onset obesity. Some researchers report that children's exposure to television advertising has been increasing in line with the rise in children's obesity (e.g. Cairns et al. 2013; IOM 2005; Hastings et al. 2003). The argument indicates that, first, television viewing lowers or replaces the time available for physical activity and reduces energy expenditure and, second, that young children are particularly susceptible to the persuasive content of advertising and programming and, therefore, to the "unhealthy" food that constitutes the bulk of the advertised food items on TV.

However, despite the plethora of studies on the influence of television on children's diets and health, a consensus on the "state of the research" has not been reached. While there is no scientific doubt about the fact that food marketing works (Hastings et al. 2003; Kunkel et al. 2004; McGinnies et al. 2006; Story and French 2004), there is a question about *how* it works—the causal effects and the relative strength of the influencing variables—and what can be done to "immunise" vulnerable groups, such as children and youth, from this influence (Harris et al. 2009).

Children's food behaviour cannot be disentangled from media use because young consumers are particularly susceptible to external influences. Within this age

---

[1]For instance, it is now legal for the sugar industry to sponsor a cooking show.

[2]Advergames are company-sponsored video or computer games in which brand images and messages are embedded in the content.

[3]The instruments reported in this chapter have been developed in the early 2010s; hence, we concentrated on television as major influencing media for this age group.

group, consumer competence (food literacy, media competence, etc.) is just being built up, family influences are gradually losing their predominance, and the material and symbolic consumption environments are gaining importance. Today, children experience purchasing and consumption situations more frequently and at an earlier stage because of an ubiquitous, highly commercialised media environment with new technological gadgets that offer an ever-increasing number of consumption opportunities (Ekström and Tufte 2007). Hence, the socialisation process of becoming a consumer is taking place earlier (Ekström and Tufte 2007). Whenever commercials are clearly separated from "normal" TV programmes, children are able to distinguish between them by the age of five (Mallalieu 2005). However, this understanding of the difference is mostly on a perceptual level—e.g. children understand that commercial spots are shorter—and it is not necessarily built on an understanding of the selling purpose of commercials (Kunkel et al. 2004; Roedder John 2008; Valkenburg and Cantor 2001; Young 2003). This latter level of understanding does not appear before children are seven to eight years old. From then on, children have a broader understanding of commercials even if they do not fully question the sent messages. They know that commercials do not always tell the truth and, therefore, they become more suspicious of advertising. Children aged seven to eleven become aware of the intention of advertising to sell products. Nevertheless, preferences for and familiarity with particular brands are developed at this stage (Jennings and Wartella 2007). Children typically enjoy watching advertising, while parents notice that commercials influence families' communication and shopping behaviour (Hastings et al. 2003). The media plays a major role in transmitting advertising messages to children, and it is, therefore, decisive for shaping consumption behaviour. Therefore, young children are particularly susceptible to commercial influences via media, which makes them ideal targets for preventive strategies.

Children are highly exposed to mass media. Children in the USA and Europe under the age of eight years watch, on average, more than two and a half hours of screen media per day with television still as the predominant channel (Rideout 2017). Basically, this exposure can have both negative and positive effects. On the one hand, public television and radio programmes present high-quality educative programmes and have been used as media partners in public campaigns for children's diets (e.g. Sesame Street). On the other hand, television viewing usually exposes children to advertising (Ofcom 2004), since ad-free children's channels are still an exception. While advertising aimed at children and included in children's television programmes is regulated in most European countries (see Hawkes 2007), children often watch other programmes in which food styles are portrayed, such as soap operas or cooking shows (Desrochers and Holt 2007). Moreover, while viewing television, energy intake rises through increased snacking, and fast food and pre-prepared meal consumption (Coon and Tucker 2002; Crespo et al. 2001; Temple et al. 2007). An estimated 20–25% of children's daily energy intake is consumed in front of the television (Matheson et al. 2004).

Television remains the most important marketing channel when it comes to children. However, computers, game systems and mobile phones are making significant inroads (Federal Trade Commission 2008; Livingstone 2005; Rideout 2017). Due to long hours in front of the TV, children from two to eleven years old are increasingly exposed to advertising—they are exposed to an estimated 25,000 commercials (food and non-food) per year in the USA (Coon and Tucker 2002; Desrochers and Holt 2007). About 20% of these ads are about food products (Desrochers and Holt 2007), and most of the advertised foodstuff is high in sugar, trans fats and/or salt, and poor in nutrients (Hawkes 2007). The "big five" group of food products—pre-sugared breakfast cereals, soft drinks, confectionary, savoury snacks and fast-food outlets—represents the majority of advertised foods (Cairns et al. 2009, 2013) and, therefore, tends to mould preferences for rather unhealthy food. Advertising aimed at children mainly concentrates on fun and taste, rather than on factors such as health and nutritional value (Hastings et al. 2003). Empirical evidence shows that such unhealthy advertising content often leads to unhealthier food choices (Borzekowski and Robinson 2001; Boyland et al. 2016; Lewis and Hill 1998; Taveras et al. 2006). Not only do overweight and obese children recognise advertised products significantly more often than normal weight children, but they also have a higher intake of advertised products (Coon and Tucker 2002; Halford et al. 2004). Moreover, a higher exposure to ads for unhealthy food leads to a lower intake of fruits and vegetables (Livingstone and Helsper 2004). On the other hand, some studies suggest a weak, positive relationship between exposure to healthy food commercials and the intake of fruits and vegetables (Klepp et al. 2007).

Overall, three lines of research suggest that exposure to advertising may contribute to childhood overweight:

1. Research on the correlation between television viewing habits and excess weight in childhood,
2. Research on the content of food advertising aimed at children (and, to a much lesser extent, on embedded product/brand placement in programming), and
3. Experimental studies of how food advertising affects children's consumption behaviour.

A large number of studies focus on the types of products that are advertised to children, or on the impact of these advertisements on nutritional knowledge, attitudes and behaviour. Policy-makers, in particular, are increasingly in need of "scientific evidence" that can inform public health policies. Therefore, in addition to purely academic studies, several encompassing and extensive literature reviews have been undertaken that also discuss policy implications (e.g. AAP 2001; Chambers et al. 2015; Coon and Tucker 2002; Harris et al. 2009; Hastings et al. 2003; Henry Kaiser Family Foundation 2004; Ippolito and Pappalardo 2002; Jenvey 2007; Kunkel et al. 2004; Livingstone and Helsper 2004; Ofcom 2004; Villani 2001; Young et al. 1996).

However, previous research has largely been deficient in identifying the causal impact of advertising on children's food choices. Furthermore, although there has been considerable research output in recent years (e.g. Adachi-Mejia et al. 2007;

Beales and Kulick 2013; Desrochers and Holt 2007; Ekström and Tufte 2007; Huang and Yang 2013; Ip et al. 2007; Kelly et al. 2007; Klepp et al. 2007; Robinson and Matheson 2007; Taveras et al. 2006; Temple et al. 2007), a sizeable portion of the empirical research in this area is relatively old (as noted by Ashton 2004). Today, children are in general much more "media literate" in general and at an earlier age than would have been the case when the older research was undertaken. At the same time, combined advertising pressure and exposure to multiple media sources have increased drastically over the past decade. Moreover, there are significant limitations to these studies, and there is ample room for improvement in the identification strategies used to assess whether, in fact, advertising "causes" poor nutritional outcomes and obesity or is simply an artefact of some other correlated behaviour.

This is the backdrop against which the toolbox of instruments related to the role of advertising in children's food choice has been developed. This study presents three research modules that are designed to shed new light on the question of whether food advertising affects children's dietary choices.

10.2   The Toolbox: A General Overview

Before describing each instrument in more detail, we provide a brief overview of the instruments and describe the development process.

10.2.1   Brief Overview of Instruments

Applying a mixed-method approach for the studies on the role of commercials in children's food choice allows for analyses of different aspects of this role. The instruments employed in this toolbox are:

- **Parent–child interviews**[4]

  Goal: To gain deeper insights into low socio-economic status families and their dietary behaviour as well as their physical activities with a special focus on barriers to health behaviour.
  Setting: Home
  Child's age: 6–8 years

---

[4]Developed by Jessica Dreas from the Bremen Institute for Prevention Research and Social Medicine (now: Leibniz Institute for Prevention Research and Epidemiology—BIPS), Germany, in collaboration with Eva Ossiansson and Barbro Johansson from the Gothenburg Research Institute at the University of Gothenburg, Sweden.

- **Ethnographic studies**[5]

  Goal: To obtain an understanding of what it means to be a child or a parent in today's consumer society, how everyday life is organised, and how problems and dilemmas that arise in relation to food and health are addressed.
  Setting: Home
  Child's age: 5–10 years

- **Questionnaire on children's knowledge about and attitudes towards food advertising**

  Goal: To analyse children's advertising literacy, i.e. their knowledge about and attitudes towards advertising
  Setting: School/classroom
  Child's age: 6–10 years

- **Experiments on children's food knowledge and preferences**

  Goal: To investigate children's knowledge about and preferences for food
  Setting: School/classroom
  Child's age: 6–10 years

- **Experiments on active food choices with food advertisements as stimuli**

  Goal: To assess the direct effect of TV advertising/branding on children's food choice
  Setting: School/classroom
  Child's age: 6–10 years

In the following sections, we present the three instruments that we developed for the school setting. The parent–child interviews focusing on families with low socio-economic status and the ethnographic studies were developed by other authors for the home setting and, therefore, will not be discussed further.

10.2.2   The Development Process

After a thorough review of existing empirical research, first drafts of the instruments were developed during 2008. Although all three tools were based on instruments already tested for objectivity, reliability and validity, the modifications and cross-cultural adaptations required that the instruments were tested again. Therefore, in December 2008 and January 2009, several pretests were carried out to check the cultural appropriateness of the children's questionnaire and the experiments. Content validity was assessed by a panel of academics working in applied

---

[5]Developed and carried out by Eva Ossiansson and Barbro Johansson from the Gothenburg Research Institute at the University of Gothenburg, Sweden.

nutrition research, who also conducted the pretesting in their home countries. These panel members provided comments on clarity and content in terms of cultural adequacy, cognitive complexity and nutritional appropriateness. In February 2009, all panel members met to discuss the appropriateness of the developed instruments given the experiences of the pretests. In addition, during that meeting, consensus was reached on how to maintain intercultural comparability while ensuring that the instruments were culturally adequate.

In order to ensure that the data collected was culturally comparable, the operating procedures had to be standardised. Accordingly, for the children's questionnaire and both choice experiments, the standard operating procedures (SOPs) (for access see Sect. 10.5) consisted of a brief summary of the respective tool together with field administration guidelines designed to standardise the field work. For instance, the guidelines explained what researchers should do before arriving at the school (e.g. ask teachers and parents for permission, brief teachers) and emphasised the need for advance clarification of the division of roles between teacher and researcher (i.e. the teacher as disciplinarian, the researcher as executor). These SOPs, cross-checked and improved with the help of the researchers in the field, also outlined environmental parameters like classroom setting and timing. For example, all tools had to be administered approximately two hours before lunch. Therefore, the entire procedure—from the introduction of the choice experiments or the children's questionnaire to the end of the activity—was predetermined and standardised in the SOPs.

The *children's questionnaire* is based on a questionnaire previously developed for teenagers on attitudes towards food advertising (Einstellung zur Lebensmittelwerbung—Kinderfragebogen, ELW-K; Diehl 2005). Given the younger age group, we reduced the number of questions and changed the answer format to a more children-friendly design. The selected questions were translated into the relevant languages and back-translated to ensure correct translation. The discriminant validity of the children's questionnaire was evaluated via factor analysis. Then, given the change in age group and the brevity of the questionnaire, the factor analysis was combined with Cronbach's alpha to measure instrument reliability and ensures that each dimension measured what was intended (see Gwozdz and Reisch 2011).

The food items used in the *choice experiments* were evaluated in terms of familiarity, availability and relevance for healthy/unhealthy nutrition. Likewise, face validity was established based on individual discussions with a convenience sample of children from the appropriate age group. For practical reasons, however, no test–retest reliability check was conducted on the whole instrument—not only was it necessary to minimise the amount of the children's time used by the field researchers, but the instruments had also already been tested for this age group in two different settings (Kopelman et al. 2007). For comparability reasons, the food items used in the *knowledge–preference experiment* were the same in all countries, which was possible after some minor changes (see Gwozdz and Reisch 2011).[6]

The *choice experiment* on the direct influence of advertising on children was based on Halford et al. (2004). The stimuli used for this experiment were cartoons and embedded food and toy advertisements. To ensure comparability, different cartoons and different advertisements were used in each country. The cartoon used was one of the most popular in the respective country with viewing rates serving as a decision base. Food advertisements were also chosen by popularity and awareness level. Here, market shares and pretests served as decision bases. Face validity was established based on individual discussions with a convenience sample of children from the appropriate age group as well as field researchers' assessments and discussions among panel members. No test–retest was undertaken because of the high workload of the field researchers and because this type of experiment had previously been validated and tested for reliability (e.g. Borzekowski and Robinson 2001; Halford et al. 2004, 2008).

Regarding ethical issues, no child took part in the survey or experiments without the consent of his or her parents. Moreover, we certify that this research followed all applicable institutional and governmental regulations on the ethical use of human volunteers. All methods used in this study have been approved by the ethics committees of the participating research institutions.

10.3   The Instruments

10.3.1   Children's Questionnaire on Advertising Literacy

The children's questionnaire on knowledge about and attitudes towards advertising is based on a questionnaire developed and validated by Diehl (Diehl 2005; Diehl and Hopf 2004). This instrument was originally developed for children aged eleven to sixteen. Pilot tests led to the assumption that a shortened version would be suitable for a younger target group (six to ten years), which was also suggested by the author himself (email dated April 25, 2008). The revised questionnaire included 9 items, rather than the original 17, as well as two items from the Children's Social Desirability for Food scale (C-SDF) (Baxter et al. 2004).

The questionnaire and the developed SOP were checked using pilot tests in Denmark and Germany and in pretests carried out in Germany, Italy, Spain and Sweden. Overall, about 110 children in five countries took part in the pilot tests and pretests. Given the results of these tests, the questionnaire presented in Fig. 10.1 and its corresponding SOP proved to be the most suitable.

---

[6]The procedures validating the children's questionnaire, and the experiment on children's knowledge and preferences has been documented in detail in Gwozdz and Reisch (2011).

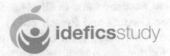

Setting ID: I_I_I_I_I_I_I

Child ID: I_I_I_I_I_I_I

What do you think about food commercials on TV?
Your view is important to us.

How old are you?   _____ years

Are you   □ 👤   □ 👤 ?

And now, please tick the smiley you think is most appropriate in your opinion.
Tick only one item per row!

	😊	🙂	🙁	☹️
1. TV food & drink advertisements offer things that taste well and are good for our body.	□	□	□	□
2. Without TV food & drink advertisement you would hardly know about existing yummy foods and sweets.	□	□	□	□
3. Advertisements give you the best tips what you should eat and drink.	□	□	□	□
4. Eating everything recommended by TV food & drink advertising will make you become chubby.	□	□	□	□
5. To eat healthy, you should not eat things offered by advertisements.	□	□	□	□
6. Advertisements convince people to buy food stuff that you should not eat or drink.	□	□	□	□
7. TV food & drink advertisements are fun and make you laugh.	□	□	□	□
8. Without food & drink advertisements, TV would be much more boring	□	□	□	□
9. After advertisements, you are mostly glad that it is over and you can keep on watching the movie.	□	□	□	□
10. Do you always eat everything on your plate even if you are not hungry?	□	□	□	□
11. Do you often watch TV or read while you eat a meal or a snack?	□	□	□	□

Well done!

Thanks for taking part!

Fig. 10.1 Children's questionnaire (based on Diehl 2005)

In place of the questionnaire's original response format, which was based on a scale of 1 = "disagree fully" to 4 = "agree fully", we use a child-friendly smiley scale to express the various nuances through different mouth shapes (see Fig. 10.2). As the questions investigating social desirability with regard to food preferences differ slightly in their phrasing, the response scale had to be adapted. Therefore, the smiley system employed ranges from 1 = "always" to 4 = "never". Overall, the smiley scale has been shown to be more appropriate for this age group than the use of numbers or words (Pecheux and Derbaix 1999). The questionnaire is self-administered—only the responsible researcher and the class teacher are in the classroom, and their role is only to introduce the instrument and to assist in case of questions. Completion of the questionnaire should not take more than 15 min, including the handing out and collection of the questionnaires. Further details on the procedure can be found in the detailed SOP.

The children's questionnaire comprises four dimensions; three are covered by Diehl's (2005) instrument, and one focuses on the social desirability of food preferences (Baxter et al. 2004). With the young age of the research group and the need to shorten the scale in mind, we picked three items for each of the three dimensions of the Diehl questionnaire, as well as two items on social desirability. Therefore, in its final version, the questionnaire includes eleven items.

The first dimension is about the *credibility and usefulness* of food commercials. If children perceive TV ads as a useful source of information about food and drink, they are more likely to believe the provided statements and it is likely that they will take information included in advertisements for granted. Another aim is to investigate whether children blend advertisement's suggestions with their own nutritional values (Diehl 2005), but pretests showed that the three questions on this issue could be difficult for children to understand. Therefore, guidelines for teachers and researchers on explaining these questions to children without influencing their choices were developed and provided in the SOP.

The second dimension is about *suspiciousness* towards food advertisements. The hypothesis underlying this dimension is that if children are suspicious of TV food commercials, they know that they cannot trust all of the information and, hence,

Fig. 10.2 "Smiley" system (response category)

Smiley	Meaning
☺	agree fully
😐	agree somewhat
🙁	disagree somewhat
☹	disagree fully

they question the advertising messages (Diehl and Hopf 2004). Pretests showed that the difficulties related to these three questions resemble those seen with the credibility dimension. Again, guidelines for how teachers and researchers can explain the questions to children without framing their answers are provided in the SOP.

The third dimension asks about the *entertainment factor* of TV commercials. It is hypothesised that children who are more suspicious and have less trust in the credibility of TV advertisements feel ads are less entertaining than children who are not as suspicious (Diehl 2005). This means that when children begin to understand the mechanisms behind advertisements, they will not enjoy commercials as much as they used to. Pretests did not show comprehension issues with the questions on this dimension.

While *credibility and usefulness* as well as the *entertainment factor* assess children's knowledge of food advertising, *suspiciousness* evaluates their attitudes towards TV advertising. Together, these dimensions provide a picture of children's advertising literacy.

The fourth dimension checks for the *social desirability* of the answers with regard to food preferences. The two items allow for judging whether the answers provided by the children are based on what they *think* they should have said or based on *conviction*. The items are taken from a social desirability scale that has been specifically developed for seven to fourteen-year-old children being surveyed on food issues (Baxter et al. 2004). The questions proved to be comprehensible in pretests, but it is important to introduce the altered meaning of the smiley answering category (see above).

In sum, the adapted children's questionnaire on knowledge about and the attitudes towards advertisements proved to be a suitable instrument in terms of validity and reliability in pilot tests, pretests and the field phase.

Three hundred and forty-eight children in six European countries (Belgium, Estonia, Germany, Hungary, Italy and Spain) answered the questionnaire. Knowledge about advertising was found, in general, to increase with age. One interesting finding was that the dimensions *credibility and usefulness* and *entertainment factor* go hand in hand; i.e., they were positively correlated. Furthermore, children were generally suspicious about advertising.[7]

10.3.2 Experiment on Children's Food Knowledge and Preferences

In the first choice experiment, children are presented with ten cards with photographs of pairs of food items, one showing a rather healthy food item and the

---

[7]The findings are partially presented in Reisch et al. (2013).

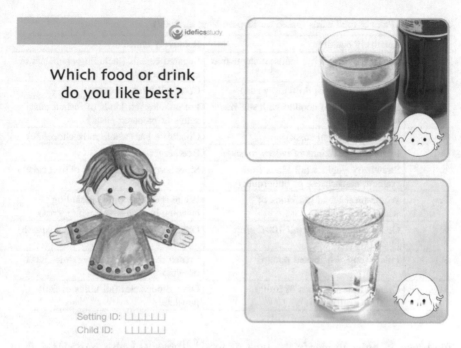

Fig. 10.3 Example from the experiment on children's food preferences [*Note* Food pictures printed with the permission of AID Infodienst Verbraucherschutz, Ernährung, Landwirtschaft e.V. and Klaus Arras (photographer)]

other one a rather unhealthy food item. This type of experiment was previously tested in the same context for test–retest reliability and validity (Calfas et al. 1991).

The food cards are printed in a (mother tongue) brochure in the style of a small magazine (see Fig. 10.3) in book format, with one food pair shown on each page. Table 10.1 shows the selected pairs, which are based on Kopelman et al. (2007) and adapted to available food cards[8] and cultural conditions, as shown by pretests. Pilot tests were carried out with ten children in Denmark, while pretests were undertaken in four survey centres (Germany, Italy, Spain and Sweden) with 39 children.

The pilot and pretests showed that the food examples (see Table 10.1) and the related procedures were most suitable for gathering information about children's preferences for and knowledge about food. Table 10.1 lists the food pairs that are presented in the magazine. The foods in each pair belong to similar food categories, such as "juice". In some cases, the original food containers are placed next to the

---

[8]The food cards are courtesy of the independent German governmental food expert service "AID Infodienst Verbraucherschutz, Ernährung, Landwirtschaft e.V.", which kindly allowed us to copy the cards for the experiments. The food cards are professionally photographed and are, therefore, suitable for our purpose.

Table 10.1 Pairs of food cards (based on Kopelman et al. 2007)

Number	Relatively healthy	Relatively unhealthy
1.	Sugar-free cereals (all kinds of sugar-free cereals)	Sugared cereals (including chocolate or crunchy cereals)
2.	Water (all kinds of drinking water)	Coke (all kinds of coke)
3.	Pasta (all kinds of noodles with self-made tomato sauce)	Pot noodles (all kinds of instant pasta soups or prepared pasta)
4.	Cereal bar (low in sugar)	Chocolate bar (whole milk chocolate)
5.	Roast beef (all kinds of fatless roasts)	Beefburger
6.	Strawberry yoghurt (all kinds fruit yoghurt, curd cheese or buttermilk)	Strawberry cake (all kinds of fruit cakes)
7.	Whole-meal bread (all kinds of whole-meal bread)	White bread all kinds, including ciabatta, baguettes and white toast)
8.	Orange juice (100%) (all 100% fruit juices)	Orange squash (all kinds of fruit squash)
9.	Potato (boiled or baked potato)	French fries (also fried potatoes, hash browns)
10.	Orange fruit (all kinds of fruits)	Orange popsicles (all kinds of fruit popsicles)

food item in order to clarify the type of food.[9] Table 10.1 also provides a short definition of each of the presented food and drink items. For instance, "water" is not generally understood as only sparkling water but encompasses all kinds of drinking water. By providing an explicit definition in the classroom, we assume that the experiment can take cultural differences into account while maintaining cross-national comparability by using the same food cards in every country.

The researcher introduces the setting and the topic to the class by highlighting that it is not a test situation but rather a gathering of opinions about food and drink (additional details are provided in the SOP). This is followed by an introduction to the magazine. Figure 10.3 provides an example of a page in such a magazine. A child's face is printed on each food picture, and the face is shown without a mouth. Children are instructed to draw a smile or a frown in each face, depending on their views. Pilot tests suggested that conducting the preference test first helps to reduce framing effects. Indeed, if children are asked to undertake the knowledge test first ("Which food or drink is the healthier one?"), the preferences that they indicate later would most likely be influenced in a socially desirable direction.

In the *preference test*, children are asked: "Which food or drink do you like best?" (see Fig. 10.3). In a "forced-preference choice" situation, children are asked to draw a smile and a frown on each page; i.e., they have to decide which one they prefer. This procedure has been shown to be most suitable in pilot tests. The underlying assumption is that children will generally prefer the rather unhealthy food.

---

[9]It is not possible to read the brand name, but if one knows the product, one is able to recognise the brand.

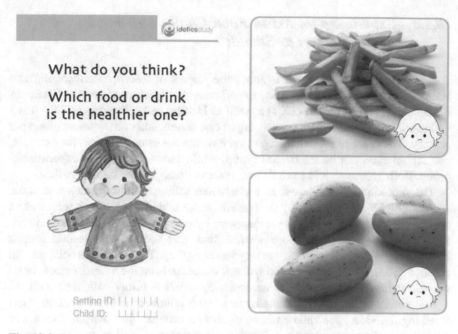

Fig. 10.4 Example from the experiment on children's food knowledge [*Note* Food pictures printed with permission of AID Infodienst Verbraucherschutz, Ernährung, Landwirtschaft e.V. and Klaus Arras (photographer)]

The *knowledge test* procedure is similar. However, before starting the experiment, the researcher provides an introduction to the concept of "health" ("Being healthy means that you can play outside, you don't get sick and you feel good"). Again, children have to draw in the missing mouths of the children in the pictures. The question used to prompt children's reaction is: "What do you think? Which food or drink is the healthier one?" (see Fig. 10.4). It is hypothesized that even if children prefer the unhealthy food, they are well aware of which choice is healthier.

More details about the procedure are available in the SOP. Overall, experiment 1 does not take more than 20 min. Pretests demonstrated that it is most suitable for children aged 8–10 (usually children that are in second or third grade).

We collected data from 335 children in six countries (Belgium, Estonia, Germany, Hungary, Italy and Spain). Like Kopelman and colleagues (2007), we found a discrepancy between food knowledge and preferences. While children showed good knowledge of what is relatively healthy and what is relatively unhealthy, they tend to prefer unhealthier foods. Therefore, knowledge did not seem to influence preferences (see also Reisch et al. 2013).

10.3.3 Experiment on Active Food Choice with Food Advertisements as Stimuli

The second choice experiment is about the impact of television advertising and branding on food choices. This experiment is developed on the basis of Borzekowski and Robinson (2001) as well as Halford and colleagues (2008). It is a within-subject, controlled trial consisting of one control and one treatment group per country. The order of presentation can vary within the sample so that, for example, one school class can be the control group, while another can be the experimental group. Both groups should have the same socio-demographic characteristics.

The procedure is as follows. In a classroom setting, children watch a cartoon, such as *The Flintstones*, *Scooby Doo* or *Vicky, the Little Viking*, which serves as an arbitrary reward. While the cartoon may vary by country, it has to meet two criteria. First, it must be aired on a national channel that shows advertising. Second, it must have the highest viewing rates in the targeted age group. The idea is that children will get involved in the programme and will not concentrate on the advertisements or on the researcher. In Germany, for example, *SpongeBob* fulfils both requirements. A commercial break with four advertisement spots is embedded in this cartoon. After watching the video, the children have to choose between four pairs of foods, one advertised and one not advertised. The latter must not be a well-known brand, but it should be very similar to the advertised item in terms of shape, colour and content. Both the treatment and control groups are presented with the same four food pairs and have to decide which food they prefer by drawing a smile and a frown.

The goal of this controlled trial is to measure the effect of advertisements on actual food choice. It is hypothesised that children who watch food commercials for certain branded products will prefer advertised brands significantly more often. If so, this could lead to a greater prevalence of overweight and obesity in children that are more exposed to commercials if those commercials promote unhealthy food.

In order to identify the advertisements' effect, we use a treatment group of about 25 children and a control group of about 25 children in each country. Children in the treatment groups are exposed to food advertisements for the four selected branded products. The control groups are exposed to a different stimulus—toy advertisements. To control for effects other than the change in stimulus, both groups receive the same introduction from the researcher, watch the same cartoon and have the same timeframe for the experiment. All factors that might influence children's food choice should be controlled and held constant to the greatest extent possible.[10]

---

[10]Obviously, we cannot control for previous experience and knowledge within the experiment. This can be partly compensated for at a later stage by connecting the collected experimental information to the rich IDEFICS study data. This even makes it possible to control for socio-demographic factors, media effects, and other lifestyle patterns or food habits, to mention just a few of the potentially influential factors.

We focus on healthy food as our advertising stimuli because little research has been conducted on the effects of healthy food advertising on children's food choices (Livingstone and Helsper 2004). Unhealthy food advertisements have been shown to affect children's food choices (Hastings et al. 2003). The question that arises here is whether healthy food advertisements increase the probability that a child will chose an advertised brand over a brand that is not advertised. If so, there would be a possibility to promote healthy foods and, therefore, increase positive diet behaviours, such as vegetable and fruit consumption.

It is not necessary to use exactly the same food commercials in every country. Nevertheless, the advertisements have to promote the same *type of products* (e.g. cereals, drinking water, cheese and fruit juice; see Table 10.2) in order to retain comparability across nations while taking cultural differences into account. The food commercials should cover the healthier versions of these food types. Table 10.2 reflects the brands that are easily accessible in each participating country and are well known and advertised on television. For some products, it is possible to use the same brand. This is particularly true for Kellogg's Special K in the cereals group and Babybel in the cheese group. Both meet the above-mentioned requirements and can, therefore, be used in every participating country. However, no mineral water or fruit juice brands are equally well known and advertised in most of the participating countries. Therefore, the most popular national brands are chosen. Table 10.2 presents the product types and brands that were selected by researchers in each participating country.

After showing the video, the researcher engages the children in a brief chat about the cartoon. The researcher might ask if the children liked the movie, what they liked best and what they did not like. After this "red herring" intervention, it is assumed that children have generally forgotten about the commercials. The researcher then pretends to play a "short quiz" game with the children in which they have to decide which food they *prefer*. The children are confronted with the four food pairs—one advertised, one not—and they have to choose one food. Matched pairs of foods are presented to the children in both groups. Here, the effects of advertisements can be analysed directly by comparing the food choice of the control group to the food choice of the treatment group.

About 250 children from four European countries (Belgium, Germany, Hungary and Spain) took part in the trial. There was a general preference among all of the children for branded food products over no-brand alternatives. Furthermore, those children exposed to food advertising chose the branded product significantly more often than did the children exposed to toy advertising. Therefore, modest effects of healthy food advertising on children's food preferences are indicated (see Hastings et al. 2003; Kunkel et al. 2004; McGinnies et al. 2006; Story and French 2004).

Table 10.2 Selected brands within the relevant product categories for experiment 2

Product category	Belgium	Germany	Hungary	Spain
Cereals	Kellogg's Special K	Kellogg's Special K	Jo reggelt	Kellogg's Special K
Water	Evian	Apollinaris	Naturaqua	Font Vella
Cheese	Babybel	Babybel	Tolle	Babybel
Fruit juice	Appelsientje	Hohes C	Happy Day	Zumosol

10.4 The Overall Benefit

The toolbox of instruments developed here can be used to assess the effects of advertising on children's food behaviour. In this respect, advertising does not only refer to the direct effect of television commercials on children's food choices. Instead, the overall aim is to assess the direct and indirect effects of advertising. Therefore, one instrument measures children's advertising literacy to obtain a picture of their understanding of advertising. Another instrument investigates children's food knowledge and preferences because classical consumer behaviour approaches, such as the theory of planned behaviour (TPB; see Ajzen 1991), predict that knowledge shapes preferences, which in turn creates intentions that consequently lead to an actual behaviour. Despite the focus of many intervention programmes on educational and informational approaches to steering food behaviour in a healthier direction, these approaches are usually not enough. While food knowledge is seen as a supporting factor, it does not directly lead to healthier food preferences, let alone to healthier food choices. Therefore, we also integrate the evaluation of knowledge and preferences in this toolbox. The last experiment (the cartoon) measures the direct effect of advertising and branding on children's food choices.

To get a broader picture of advertising's influence on children's food choices, the same children can be included in all three studies. This would make it possible to connect and compare the gathered data. In addition, to enhance the understanding of children's food choices, data on actual (observed) food choice is necessary. In this respect, the data collected from the above-described instruments can be merged with the overall IDEFICS study. The IDEFICS study not only includes information on the socio-demographic characteristics of the participating children and their families, but also a food diary (see Chap. 5 of this book) and other information about children's food behaviour (see Chap. 6 of this book).

10.5   Provision of Instruments and Standard Operating Procedures to Third Parties

All standard operating procedures (SOPs) described in this chapter can be accessed on the following website: www.leibniz-bips.de/ifhs after registration.

Each third partner using the SOPs provided in this chapter is kindly requested to cite this chapter as follows:

Gwozdz W, Reisch LA, on behalf of the IDEFICS consortium. Instruments for assessing the role of commercials on children's food choices. In: Bammann K, Lissner L, Pigeot I, Ahrens W, editors. Instruments for health surveys in children and adolescents. Cham: Springer Nature Switzerland; 2019. p. 209–230.

Acknowledgements   The development of instruments, the baseline data collection and the first follow-up work as part of the IDEFICS study (www.idefics.eu) were financially supported by the European Commission within the Sixth RTD Framework Programme Contract No. 016181 (FOOD).

We thank all families for participating in the extensive examinations of the IDEFICS study. We are also grateful for the support from school boards, headmasters and communities.

We are particularly thankful for the feedback received from the field teams in the participating IDEFICS countries, which helped us to develop and improve the instruments. We also thank the German AID Infodienst Verbraucherschutz, Ernährung, Landwirtschaft e.V. for permission to use their food cards. Finally, we wish to thank the children, parents and staff of the cooperating Danish–German school in Copenhagen, Denmark (St. Petri Dansk-Tysk Skole i København).

References

Adachi-Mejia AM, Longacre MR, Gibson JJ, Beach ML, Titus-Ernstoff L, Dalton MA. Children with a TV in their bedroom at higher risk for being overweight. Int J Obes (Lond). 2007;31 (4):644–51.

Ahrens W, Bammann K, Siani A, Buchecker K, De Henauw S, Iacoviello L, et al. IDEFICS consortium. The IDEFICS cohort: design, characteristics and participation in the baseline survey. Int J Obes (Lond). 2011;35(Suppl 1):S3–15.

Ajzen I. The theory of planned behavior. Organ Behav Hum Decis Process. 1991;50(2):179–211.

American Academy of Pediatrics (AAP), Committee on Public Education. Children, adolescents, and television. Pediatrics. 2001;107(2):423–6.

Ashton D. Food advertising and childhood obesity. J R Soc Med. 2004;97(2):51–2.

Baxter SD, Smith AF, Litaker MS, Baglio ML, Guinn CH, Shaffer NM. Children's social desirability and dietary reports. J Nutr Educ Behav. 2004;36(2):84–9.

Beales JH III, Kulick R. Does advertising on television cause childhood obesity? A longitudinal analysis. J Public Policy Mark. 2013;32(2):185–94.

Borzekowski DL, Robinson TN. The 30-second effect: an experiment revealing the impact of television commercials on food preferences of preschoolers. J Am Diet Assoc. 2001;101 (1):42–6.

Boyland EJ, Nolan S, Kelly B, Tudur-Smith C, Jones A, Halford JCG, et al. Advertising as a cue to consume: a systematic review and meta-analysis of the effects of acute exposure to unhealthy food and nonalcoholic beverage advertising on intake in children and adults. Am J Clin Nutr. 2016;103(2):519–33.

Cairns G, Angus K, Hastings G. The extent, nature and effects of food promotion to children: a review of the evidence to December 2008. Geneva: World Health Organization; 2009.

Cairns G, Angus K, Hastings G, Caraher M. Systematic reviews of the evidence on the nature, extent and effects of food marketing to children. A retrospective summary. Appetite. 2013;62:209–15.

Calfas KJ, Sallis JF, Nader PR. The development of scales to measure knowledge and preference for diet and physical behavior in 4- to 8-year-old children. J Dev Behav Pediatr. 1991;12 (3):185–90.

Chambers SA, Freeman R, Anderson AS, MacGillivray S. Reducing the volume, exposure and negative impacts of advertising for foods high in fat, sugar and salt to children: a systematic review of the evidence from statutory and self-regulatory actions and educational measures. Prev Med. 2015;75:32–43.

Coon KA, Tucker KL. Television and children's consumption patterns: a review of the literature. Minerva Pediatr. 2002;54(5):423–36.

Crespo CJ, Smit E, Troiano RP, Bartlett SJ, Macera CA, Andersen RE. Television watching, energy intake, and obesity in US children: results from the third national health and nutrition examination survey, 1988–1994. Arch Pediatr Adolesc Med. 2001;155(3):360–5.

Desrochers DM, Holt DJ. Children's exposure to television advertising: implications for childhood obesity. J Public Policy Mark. 2007;26(2):182–201.

Diehl JM. Macht Werbung dick? Einfluss der Lebensmittelwerbung auf Kinder und Jugendliche. Ernährungs-Umschau. 2005;52:40–6.

Diehl JM, Hopf A. Fernsehen, Süßwarenkonsum und Übergewicht bei Jugendlichen an Allgemein- und Berufsbildenden Schulen. Gießen: Fachbereich Psychologie, Justus-Liebig-Universität Gießen; 2004.

Ekström K, Tufte B, editors. Children, media and consumption. Gothenburg: Gothenburg University, Nordicom; 2007.

EU. Directive 2007/65/EC of the European Parliament and of the Council of 11 December 2007 amending Council Directive 89/552/EEC on the coordination of certain provisions laid down by law, regulation or administrative action in Member States concerning the pursuit of television broadcasting activities. Official Journal of the European Union, L332, Vol. 50: L 332/27-L 332/45; 2007.

Federal Trade Commission. Marketing food to children and adolescents: a review of industry expenditures, activities, and self-regulation: a federal trade commission report to congress. Washington, D.C.; 2008.

Ferraro R, Bettman JR, Chartrand TL. The power of strangers: the effect of incidental consumer brand encounters on brand choice. J Consum Res. 2009;35:729–41.

Gwozdz W, Reisch L. IDEFICS consortium. Instruments for analyzing the influence of commercials on children's food choices. Int J Obes (Lond). 2011;35(Suppl 1):S137–43.

Halford JCG, Gillespie J, Brown V, Pontin EE, Dovey TM. Effect of television advertisements for foods on food consumption in children. Appetite. 2004;42(2):221–5.

Halford JCG, Boyland EJ, Cooper GD, Dovey TM, Smith CJ, Williams N, et al. Children's food preferences: effects of weight status, food type, branding and television food advertisements (commercials). Int J Pediatr Obes. 2008;3(1):31–8.

Harris J, Brownell KD, Bargh JA. The food marketing defense model: Integrating psychological research to protect youth and inform public policy. Soc Issues Policy Rev. 2009;3(1):211–71.

Hastings G, Stead M, McDermott L, Forsyth A, MacKintosh A, Rayner M, et al. Review of the research on the effects of food promotion to children. Glasgow: Centre for Social Marketing, University of Glasgow; 2003.

Hawkes C. Regulating and litigating in the public interest: regulating food marketing to young people worldwide: trends and policy drivers. Am J Publ Health. 2007;97(11):1962–73.

Henry J. Kaiser Family Foundation. The role of media in childhood obesity—issue brief, February 2004. https://www.kff.org/other/issue-brief/the-role-of-media-in-childhood-obesity/. Accessed 29 Mar 2018.

Huang R, Yang M. Buy what is advertised on television? Evidence from bans on child-directed food advertising. J Public Policy Mark. 2013;32(2):207–22.

Institute of Medicine (IOM). Preventing childhood obesity: health in the balance. Washington, D. C.: National Academies Press; 2005.

Ip J, Mehta KP, Coveney J. Exploring parents' perception of television food advertising directed at children: a South Australian study. Nutr Diet. 2007;64:50–8.

Ippolito P, Pappalardo J. Advertising, nutrition, and health: evidence from food advertising 1977–1997. Washington, D.C.: Bureau of Economics Staff Report to the Federal Trade Commission; 2002.

Jennings NA, Wartella EA. Advertising and consumer development. In: Pecora N, Murray JP, Wartella EA, editors. Children and television—fifty years of research. Mahwah, NJ: Lawrence Erlbaum Associates; 2007. p. 149–82.

Jenvey VB. The relationship between television viewing and obesity in young children: a review of existing explanations. Early Child Dev Care. 2007;177(8):809–20.

Kelly B, Smith B, King L, Bauman A. Television food advertising to children: the extent and nature of exposure. Public Health Nutr. 2007;10(11):1234–40.

Kelly B, Halford JCG, Boyland EJ, Chapman K, Bautista-Castaño I, Berg C, et al. Television food advertising to children: a global perspective. Am J Publ Health. 2010;100(9):1730–6.

Klepp K-I, Wind M, de Bourdeaudhuij I, Rodrigo CP, Due P, Bjelland M, et al. Television viewing and exposure to food-related commercials among European school children, associations with fruit and vegetable intake: a cross sectional study. Int J Behav Nutr Phys Act 2007;4:46–54

Kopelman CA, Roberts LM, Adab P. Advertising of food to children: is brand logo recognition related to their food knowledge, eating behaviours and food preferences? J Publ Health. 2007;29(4):358–67.

Kunkel D, Wilcox B, Cantor J, Palmer E, Linn S, Dowrick P. Report of the APA task force on advertising and children: psychological issues in the increasing commercialization of childhood. Washington, D.C.: American Psychological Association; 2004.

Lewis MK, Hill AJ. Food advertising on British children's television: a content analysis and experimental study with nine-year olds. Int J Obes Relat Metab Disord. 1998;22(3):206–14.

Linn S. Food marketing to children in the context of a marketing maelstrom. J Public Health Policy. 2004;25(3/4):367–78.

Livingstone S. Assessing the research base for the policy debate over the effects of food advertising to children. Int J Advert. 2005;24(3):273–96.

Livingstone S, Helsper E. Advertising 'unhealthy' foods to children: understanding promotion in the context of children's daily lives. Report to Ofcom, London. 2004. http://eprints.lse.ac.uk/id/eprint/21757. Accessed 29 Mar 2018.

Mallalieu L, Palan K, Laczniak RN. Understanding children's knowledge and beliefs about advertising: a global issue that spans generations. J Curr Issues Res Advert. 2005;27:53–64.

Matheson DM, Killen JD, Wang Y, Varady A, Robinson TN. Children's food consumption during television viewing. Am J Clin Nutr. 2004;79(6):1088–94.

Mathios A. Research on the impact of food promotion and marketing on children's diets and strategies for improving this research. A Report to the Institute of Medicine, US, Working paper; 2005.

McGinnies JM, Gootman J, Kraak VI, editors. Food marketing to children and youth: threat or opportunity?. Washington, D.C.: Institute of Medicine of the National Academies; 2006.

Montgomery KC, Chester J. Food advertising to children in the New Digital Marketing Ecosystem. In: Ekström K, Tufte B, editors. Children, media and consumption. Gothenburg: Gothenburg University, Nordicum; 2007. p. 179–93.

Ofcom. Childhood obesity—food advertising in context. Children's food choices, parents' understanding and influence, and the role of food promotions. London: Ofcom; 2004.

Pecheux C, Derbaix C. Children and attitude toward the brand: a new measurement scale. J Advert Res. 1999;39(4):19–27.

Reisch L, Gwozdz W, Barba G, De Henauw S, Lascorz N, Konstabel K, Pigeot I. Experimental evidence on the impact of food advertising on children's knowledge about and preferences for healthful food. J Obes. 2013;Article ID 408582, 1–13.

Rideout V. The common sense census: media use by kids age zero to eight. San Francisco, CA: Common Sense Media. 2017. https://www.commonsensemedia.org/sites/default/files/uploads/research/csm_zerotoeight_fullreport_release_2.pdf. Accessed 29 Mar 2018.

Robinson TN, Matheson DM. Effects of fast food branding on young children's taste preferences. Arch Pediatr Adolesc Med. 2007;161(8):792–7.

Roedder John DR. Stages of consumer socialization: the development of consumer knowledge, skills, and values from childhood to adolescence. In: Haugvedt C, Herr P, Kardes F, editors. The handbook of consumer psychology. New York, NY: Lawrence Earlbaum Association; 2008. p. 1103–30.

Story M, Faulkner P. The prime time diet: a content analysis of eating behavior and food messages in television program content and commercials. Am J Publ Health. 1990;80(6):738–40.

Story M, French S. Food advertising and marketing directed at children and adolescents in the U.S. Int J Behav Nutr Phys Act. 2004;1:3.

Taveras EM, Sandora TJ, Shih M-C, Ross-Degnan D, Goldmann DA, Gillman MW. The association of television and video viewing with fast food intake by preschool-age children. Obesity. 2006;14(11):2034–41.

Temple JL, Giacomelli AM, Kent KM, Roemmich JN, Epstein LH. Television watching increases motivated responding for food and energy intake in children. Am J Clin Nutr. 2007;85(2):355–61.

UK Department of Health. Healthy weight, healthy lives: a cross government strategy for England. London: Department of Health; 2008.

Valkenburg PM, Cantor J. The development of the child into a consumer. J Appl Dev Psychol. 2001;22(1):61–72.

Villani S. Impact of media on children and adolescents: a 10-year review of the research. J Am Acad Child Adolesc. 2001;40(4):392–401.

World Health Organization. Marketing of foods high in fat, salt and sugar to children: update 2012–2013. Copenhagen: WHO Regional Office; 2013.

Young B. Does food advertising influence children's food choices? A critical review of some of the recent literature. Int J Advert. 2003;22:441–59.

Young B, Webley P, Hetherington M, Zeedyk S. The role of television advertising in children's food choice. Report commissioned by the UK Ministry of Agriculture, Fisheries & Food. 1996.

Chapter 11
Process Evaluation of the IDEFICS Intervention

Ilse De Bourdeaudhuij, Vera Verbestel, Lea Maes,
Annunziata Nappo, Charis Chadjigeorgiou, Dénes Molnár,
Éva Kovács, Gabriele Eiben, Holger Hassel, Katharina Gallois,
Kenn Konstabel, Luis A. Moreno, Michalis Tornaritis,
Natalia Lascorz Frauca, Toomas Veidebaum, Staffan Mårild
and Stefaan De Henauw

Abstract Process evaluation is an essential part of intervention evaluation that is often overlooked or reported limitedly. This chapter explains in detail how the process evaluation within the IDEFICS study was developed and how the different measures were built. For each intervention module, different measures were developed to integrate multiple perspectives on the implementation. All measures

On behalf of the IDEFICS consortium.

I. De Bourdeaudhuij (✉) · V. Verbestel · L. Maes · S. De Henauw
Ghent University, Ghent, Belgium
e-mail: Ilse.Debourdeaudhuij@UGent.be

A. Nappo
National Research Council, Avellino, Italy

C. Chadjigeorgiou · M. Tornaritis
Research and Education Institute of Child Health, Strovolos, Cyprus

D. Molnár · É. Kovács
University of Pécs, Pécs, Hungary

G. Eiben · S. Mårild
University of Gothenburg, Göteborg, Sweden

H. Hassel
Hochschule für Angewandte Wissenschaften Coburg, Coburg, Germany

K. Gallois
Leibniz Institute for Prevention Research and Epidemiology—BIPS, Bremen, Germany

K. Konstabel · T. Veidebaum
National Institute for Health Development, Tallinn, Estonia

L. A. Moreno · N. L. Frauca
University of Zaragoza, Zaragoza, Spain

© Springer Nature Switzerland AG 2019
K. Bammann et al. (eds.), *Instruments for Health Surveys in Children and Adolescents*, Springer Series on Epidemiology and Public Health,
https://doi.org/10.1007/978-3-319-98857-3_11

were based on the framework of Linnan and Steckler (2002) to ensure a theory- and evidence-based approach. As process measures used in research are seldom reported in manuscripts, most of the measures were newly developed with the IDEFICS study itself. The measures itself are added to the chapter to share these instruments with other researchers so that they can build on our measures to develop their own.

11.1   Why Process Evaluation?

Health promotion to induce behaviour change is best done as a well-planned process. This means that the development and evaluation of an intervention need to follow certain steps. The use of such a model of planned health education and behaviour change will considerably increase the chances in reaching effectiveness of the intervention (Bartholomew et al. 2006). The first step of this planned process is the analysis of the public health problems (e.g. obesity), and the second step is the analysis of the behaviours related with these health problems (e.g. nutrition and physical activity). The third step is the detection of the determinants that cause the behaviours (e.g. attitudes, knowledge, availability, parenting rules). Based on these previous steps, the intervention will be developed in the fourth step (e.g. the IDEFICS intervention) and implemented in the fifth step (e.g. one intervention community and one control community per IDEFICS country). The last and final step of the process of health promotion and behaviour change is the evaluation of the intervention. The most well-known form of evaluation is the effect evaluation: it measures whether the intervention yields the effects that were expected. A second form of intervention is less well known and is called the process evaluation. The process evaluation studies the level that the intervention was implemented as it was planned. In comprehensive multi-component interventions, the process evaluation can help disentangle the effects of each of the specific factors in the intervention. If the total intervention is not significant, the process evaluation can help us understand why this intervention did not yield the expected effects (Bartholomew et al. 2006; Linnan and Steckler 2002; Saunders et al. 2005).

11.2   The IDEFICS Intervention

The general aim of the IDEFICS intervention was the prevention of overweight and obesity in young children. The key messages selected to reach this aim are shown in Table 11.1.

Table 11.1 Overview of the IDEFICS key messages

Diet	Physical activity	Stress, coping and relaxation
Increase daily consumption of water	Reduce TV viewing	Strengthen parent–child relationships by spending more time together
Increase daily consumption of fruit and vegetables	Increase daily physical activity	Establish adequate sleep duration

Table 11.2 Overview of the IDEFICS intervention modules

	Community	School	Family	Individual
Diet	Module 1 Module 2 Module 3	Module 4 Module 8 Module 9	Module 10	Module 5
Physical activity	Module 1 Module 2 Module 3	Module 4 Module 6 Module 7	Module 10	Module 5
Stress, coping and relaxation	Module 1 Module 2 Module 3	Module 4	Module 10	Module 5

IDEFICS intervention modules
Module 1: Involvement of community partners
Module 2: Long-term media campaign and public relation strategy
Module 3: Lobbying for community environmental and policy interventions
Module 4: Building partnerships
Module 5: Education of children
Module 6: Environmental changes related to physical activity—the active playground
Module 7: Health-related physical education curricula
Module 8: Environmental changes and school policy related to water consumption
Module 9: Environmental changes and school policy related to fruit and vegetables
Module 10: Education of parents

These six key messages were the behavioural focus in the IDEFICS intervention. In each country, an intervention community and a control community were selected. The IDEFICS intervention was implemented in the whole intervention community on four levels: the community, the school, the family and the individual. Each of the key messages was addressed through each of these levels. The different levels of the IDEFICS intervention are reflected in Table 11.2. This table shows the overall structure of the IDEFICS intervention and is the framework in which the community-based intervention is elaborated. The intervention components were developed based on the intervention mapping protocol as described by Bartholomew et al. (2006). All intervention elements were summarised in ten modules which are briefly described below. A more detailed description about the development and content of these intervention modules can be found elsewhere (De Henauw et al. 2011; Verbestel et al. 2011, 2012). The results of the IDEFICS intervention are summarised in a supplement volume published in Obesity Reviews (Pigeot et al. 2015).

The first three modules are situated at the community level. Their aim is to develop a community platform (module 1), to develop and implement a public relations strategy (module 2) and to lobby at the policy and environmental level (module 3). The aim of the community platform is to lead and coordinate initiatives related to the IDEFICS key messages in the community.

Modules 4–9 are situated at the school level. In module 4, the school working groups are established. These working groups are responsible for the implementation of modules 5–9. Module 5 includes the classroom activities that are specifically focused on changing attitudes, knowledge, skills, self-efficacy and support of each individual child. In modules 6, 8 and 9, environmental interventions at the school level are encouraged (playground, water, fruit and vegetables). Module 7 focuses on the increase in activity in the physical education classes at school.

Module 10 focuses at parents and aims at increasing awareness, self-efficacy and skills using folders, children's homework, meetings with parents, etc.

In Table 11.3, the temporal pattern of the implementation of the IDEFICS intervention is shown. The effect evaluation of the intervention was conducted by comparing the main outcome parameter, namely body mass index, at two time points: a baseline measurement before the intervention (T_0) and a post-measurement after the intervention (T_1) (De Henauw et al. 2015). Further, outcome evaluations considered changes in behaviour (De Bourdeaudhuij et al. 2015a) and effects on markers of the metabolic syndrome (Mårild et al. 2015). In addition, more than 2 years after baseline (T_2) sustainability of behavioural change was assessed using a questionnaire mailed to all intervention participants (Nicholls et al. 2015). T_0 and T_1 are also referred to as the IDEFICS surveys, during which the participating children underwent a set of physical examinations (see Chap. 3 of this book) while their

Table 11.3 Timeline of the IDEFICS intervention activities in relation with the survey activities

	Year 1	Year 2	Year 3	Year 4	Year 5
	2006-2007	2007-2008	2008-2009	2009-2010	2010-2011
Sep					Intervention implementation
Oct					
Nov				Intervention implementation (only scientific supervision)	T_2
Dec					
Jan		T_0	Intervention adoption (support, scientific supervision)	T_1	
Feb					Intervention dissemination (no support, no scientific supervision)
Mar					
Apr					
May					
Jun		Intervention adoption (support, scientific supervision)			
Jul					
Aug					

parents reported—among others—behavioural aspects of their child (see Chap. 9 of this book).

The process evaluation of the IDEFICS intervention studied the implementation of the intervention during three time periods (De Bourdeaudhuij et al. 2015b; Verloigne et al. 2015). The first time period was the intervention **adoption phase**. This was the original implementation of the intervention situated between the baseline measurements T_0 and the post-measurements T_1 (June 2008 till August 2009). During this period, the intervention was implemented in the intervention communities with the support and supervision of the IDEFICS team in each participating country. Therefore, a member of the research staff was appointed in each participating country as the local "intervention programme manager" (IPM). The IPM worked closely together with the school working groups and the community platform to monitor and adjust the programme implementation throughout the whole intervention adoption period. An extensive intervention guide was developed, including the objectives for each module, a detailed description of their content and intervention materials to be used at the local level and to fulfil the intervention objectives. The adoption of the intervention was a process followed up closely between the countries in meetings and telephone conferences with the project partners.

The second time period was the intervention **implementation phase**. This phase is situated between the post-measurements at T_1 and the follow-up measurements at T_2 (September 2010 till December 2010). During this period, the schools and communities were encouraged to further implement the IDEFICS intervention with minimal support and supervision of the IDEFICS team. The aim was that the schools and communities implemented the IDEFICS key messages, strategies and methods in their everyday life and work. The idea was that the IDEFICS intervention became a sustainable intervention in this period.

Finally, the third time period was the **dissemination phase**. This phase was situated during and starting with the follow-up measurements at T_2 (from October 2010 on). This phase aimed at sustainability of the IDEFICS intervention in the intervention communities, and spontaneous initiatives have to be taken by the schools and local authorities to address the IDEFICS key messages.

11.3   A Model for Guiding Process Evaluation

Linnan and Steckler (2002) proposed a sequence of steps that guides programme developers and evaluators through the process of designing and implementing the process evaluation of public health interventions. One important step in the development of a process evaluation is the development of process evaluation questions. The aim of a process evaluation is to provide an answer to these questions. Linnan and Steckler (2002) described six components on which the development of the process evaluation questions can be based. These components are **fidelity**, **dose delivered**, **dose received**, **reach**, **recruitment** and **context**.

Fidelity refers to the quality of the implementation of the intervention. This means whether the intervention was delivered in accordance with how it was planned. As this component focuses specifically on quality, it means that it wants to evaluate whether the intervention was carried out both in the manner and the spirit that it was intended. An IDEFICS example might be whether primary school teachers exposed children to new fruits and vegetables and focused in this classroom activity on tasting fruits as it was intended by the intervention plan.

Dose delivered refers to the quantity of the components that were implemented. An IDEFICS example might be number of lessons that were delivered in one specific class on physical activity promotion and the proportion related to the intended dose.

Dose received is a construct related to the dose delivered and wants to detail how much of the dose delivered actually reached the participants. An IDEFICS example might be how many parents actually read the brochure on watching TV in their children.

Reach is the proportion of the intended audience to whom the programme is actually delivered. An IDEFICS example might be the proportion of the population in the intervention community that was actually reached by the initiatives of the stakeholders of the community.

Recruitment is a description of the strategy that was used to include participants in the programme. An IDEFICS example might be the strategy that was used to include the stakeholders of the intervention community in the community platform.

Context is a factor that refers to the aspects of the larger social environment that may affect implementation. An IDEFICS example might be whether the schools in the IDEFICS intervention participated in other interventions that also focused on nutrition and physical activity.

Implementation is an overall score that shows how the intervention was implemented. In fact, this is the final goal of the process evaluation measurement. It includes a combination of reach, fidelity, dose delivered and dose received. Different equations are used to compute this implementation score. Some authors used the product of those four components, and others argued for using an average score. When all four components are reported as a proportion, using a mean score will lead to higher implementation scores than using a multiplicative score. It might also be necessary to determine some optimal or minimal implementation score or to use some weighing factor across factors. Within the IDEFICS study, the implementation score was calculated adding up the four components. It might be useful to compare countries and explain possible differences in effects.

Table 11.4 reflects the key components of a process evaluation according to Saunders et al. (2005). In contrast with the components proposed by Linnan and

Table 11.4 Key components of a process evaluation according to Saunders et al. (2005)

Component	Explanation	Applications for formative use	Applications for summative use
Fidelity (quality)	Extent to which intervention was implemented as planned	Monitor and adjust programme implementation as needed to ensure theoretical integrity and programme quality	Describe and/or quantify fidelity of intervention implementation
Dose delivered (completeness)	Amount or number of intended units of each intervention or component delivered or provided by interventionists	Monitor and adjust programme implementation to ensure all components of intervention are delivered	Describe and/or quantify the dose of the intervention delivered
Dose received (exposure)	Extents to which participants actively engage with, interact with, are receptive to, and/or use materials or recommended resources; can include "initial use" and "continued use"	Monitor and take corrective action to ensure participants are receiving and/or using materials/resources	Describe and/or quantify how much of the intervention was received
Dose received (satisfaction)	Participant (primary and secondary audiences) satisfaction with programme, interactions with staff and/or investigators	Obtain regular feedback from primary and secondary targets, and use feedback as needed for corrective action	Describe and/or rate participant satisfaction and how feedback was used
Reach (participation proportion)	Proportion of the intended priority audience that participates in the intervention; often measured by attendance; includes documentation of barriers to participation	Monitor numbers and characteristics of participants; ensure sufficient numbers of target population are being reached	Quantify how much of the intended target audience participated in the intervention; describe those who participated and those who did not
Recruitment	Procedures used to approach and attract participants at individual or organisational levels; includes maintenance of participant involvement in intervention and measurement components of study	Monitor and document recruitment procedures to ensure protocol is followed; adjust as needed to ensure reach	Describe recruitment procedures

(continued)

Table 11.4 (continued)

Component	Explanation	Applications for formative use	Applications for summative use
Context	Aspects of the environment that may influence intervention implementation or study outcomes; includes contamination or the extent to which the control group was exposed to the programme	Monitor aspects of the physical, social, and political environment and how they impact implementation and needed corrective action	Describe and/or quantify aspects of the environment that affected programme implementation and/or programme impacts or outcomes

Steckler (2002), they differentiate dose received into exposure and satisfaction. For every component, an explanation is given together with its applications for formative and summative use. The formative use of process evaluation is important in the development of the programme and aims to adapt the implementation during the intervention process. The summative use of process evaluation mainly quantifies the level of implementation using each component. Its ultimate goal is to relate the dose of implementation with the effect of the intervention.

Within the IDEFICS intervention, summative use of the process evaluation components was monitored by the IDEFICS team within each country. The summative use of the process evaluation aimed to quantify the level of implementation. Therefore, numerous instruments were developed related to the different intervention modules within the IDEFICS intervention. These instruments will be discussed in the following paragraphs.

11.4   Process Evaluation Within the IDEFICS Modules

As mentioned before, a wide variety of process evaluation instruments were developed related to the intervention modules within the IDEFICS intervention. An overview of these instruments is shown in Table 11.5. Process evaluation instruments were developed for the community, school and family levels. Some of the process evaluation instruments were filled in each week during the whole intervention period (e.g., the classroom lessons in module 5), but most instruments were completed only once or twice in each of the three intervention periods.

Table 11.5 Overview of process evaluation instruments (numbers/letters refer to various instruments used to assess the process related to the modules 1 to 10)

		Sept 2008 (T_0)		Sept 2009 (T_1)		Oct 2010 (T_2)	
		IR[a]	CR[a]	IR[a]	CR[a]	IR[a]	CR[a]
Community	Reporting sheets for meetings of the community platform	1A		1A		1A	
	Questionnaire for IPM	1B		1B		1B	
	Local community actor		1C		1C		1C
	Reporting sheet for IDEFICS staff				2		2
	Questionnaire for local stakeholders	3A		3A	3B	3A	3B
School	Reporting sheets for meetings of the school working groups	4A		4A		4A	
	Interview with school working groups	4B		4B		4B	
	Questionnaire for headmasters		4C		4C		4C
	Questionnaire for kindergarten and primary school teachers	5A			5D	5C	5D
	Questionnaire for school working groups	5B					
	Environmental self-assessment (school working groups)	689A/B	689A	689A	689A	689A	689A
	Questionnaire for physical education teachers			7A	7B	7A	7B
	Questionnaire for kindergarten teachers			7C	7D	7C	7D
Parents	Questionnaire for parents			10A	10B	10A	10B
	Questionnaire for IPM			10C		10C	

[a]*IR* Intervention region, *CR* Control region

All process evaluation instruments were developed based on the theoretical model of Linnan and Steckler (2002) and Saunders et al. (2005) as outlined before. Below we will focus on each of the process evaluation instruments that were developed following the structure of the ten IDEFICS intervention modules.

For each module, the key questions will first be outlined in a table showing the theoretical base of the questionnaire. We will then refer to the questionnaires related

Table 11.6 Process evaluation questions for module 1

Component	Information needed for module 1
Fidelity (quality)	– Is a community platform established in the intervention region? Is one or more than one community platform established in the intervention region? – What is the composition and structure of the community platform? – Are stakeholders targeting low socioeconomic status (SES) and vulnerable groups included (e.g. migrants)? – Are all relevant stakeholders involved or are important stakeholders missing? – Who established the community platform? – Who coordinated the community platform after it was established? – Is the school platform integrated in the community platform? – Are schools integrated in the platform? – Has the community platform been stimulated to develop, organise and/or promote programmes and structural changes that encourage the health behaviours targeted by the IDEFICS intervention?
Dose delivered (completeness)	– How many meetings have been organised with the IPM, subcontractor or local coordinator? – How many meetings have been organised without the IPM, subcontractor or local coordinator?
Dose received (exposure)	– Did the community platform receive materials and/or education to support their operation? – Are the materials and/or educational opportunities used by the community platform? – To what extent was the community platform operating independently? – To what extent did the community platform receive support from the IPM, subcontractor or local coordinator?
Dose received (satisfaction)	– What is the attitude of the members of the community platform towards the information received about establishment, composition and expected operation of the community platform? – What is the attitude towards the concept of the community platform? – Do the members of the community platform think they get enough support from the IPM, subcontractor or local coordinator?
Reach (participation proportion)	– What is the number of participants in each meeting? – Does the composition of the community platform change? – How does the composition change and why? – What are barriers and facilitators to be part of the community platform?
Recruitment	– Is an existing community platform used, is an existing one extended or is a new one composed? – Which strategy has been used to compose the community platform? – Are new participants for the community platform recruited during the intervention period? How has this been done and why? – Which strategy has been used to recruit the stakeholders?

(continued)

Table 11.6   (continued)

Component	Information needed for module 1
Context	– Is the community platform also working on other health topics (e.g. in the scope of other projects)? – Are other community platforms in the community working on projects with the same and/or other health topics? – What are these topics about? – Are community platforms working on health topics in the control region? – About which health topics are these community platforms working?

to this module (for access see Sect. 11.7), and finally, we will give a short overview of the content of the questionnaire.

11.4.1   Process Evaluation Instruments Related to Module 1

Table 11.6 gives an overview of the process evaluation questions related to the process evaluation components of module 1.

For access to the questionnaires related to module 1 see Sect. 11.7.

Process evaluation 1A is a reporting sheet for the meetings of the community platform in the intervention regions. This sheet needs to be completed at every meeting of the community platform. It needs to be completed by a member of the community platform that is present at the meeting.

Process evaluation 1B is the first questionnaire for the person in charge of establishing the community platform in the intervention regions (logically the local IPM). It gives an idea of the establishment of the community platform, the stakeholders that are present within the platform, and the topics that these stakeholders are usually dealing with. A first measure needs to be filled in at the beginning of establishing the platform, right after T_0. A slightly adapted version needs to be filled in a second and third time at T_1 and T_2.

Process evaluation 1C is a short questionnaire asking for the existence of community platforms in the control region, possible stakeholders in these platforms and the topics they are usually working on. This questionnaire can be filled in by a person that has a central community position in the control region.

11.4.2   Process Evaluation Instruments Related to Module 2

Table 11.7 gives an overview of the process evaluation questions related to the process evaluation components of module 2.

For access to the questionnaire related to module 2 see Sect. 11.7.

Table 11.7 Process evaluation questions for module 2

Component	Information needed for module 2
Fidelity (quality)	– Was (part of) the campaign developed/financially supported/implemented by the community platform? – Did the community platform inform the community about the key messages, make the community aware about the key messages and promote the key messages as important components of long term health? – Were the window posters distributed/financed by the community platform or by the IDEFICS study (staff)?
Dose delivered (completeness)	– How many window posters were distributed for each key messages and how many times? – How many and which other IDEFICS-related public relation (PR) materials were provided to inform the community about the key messages, to make the community aware of them and to promote the key messages as important components of long term health?
Dose received (exposure)	– How many parents received the window posters (for each key message separately)? – How many parents received at least one version of all window posters? – How many parents received other IDEFICS-related PR materials?
Dose received (satisfaction)	– What was the opinion of the community/parents about the window posters and other IDEFICS-related PR materials?
Reach (participation proportion)	– What proportion of the parents received the window posters (for each key message separately)? – What proportion of the parents received at least one version of all window posters? – What proportion of the parents received other IDEFICS-related PR materials?
Recruitment	– Which strategies have been used to reach the parents? – Which strategies have been used to distribute the window posters and IDEFICS-related PR materials to the parents?
Context	– Did the parents in the control region receive materials about the IDEFICS key messages?

Process evaluation 2 is a reporting sheet that needs to be completed by the IDEFICS team. It details the distribution of the window posters and the relationship with the three objectives: information, awareness and promotion. This instrument also details the initiatives that were taken related to the public relations campaign. The reporting sheet has to be completed at T_1 and T_2.

Table 11.8 Process evaluation questions for module 3

Component	Information needed for module 3
Fidelity (quality)	– Did the stakeholder realise actions related to the prevention of obesity in the short/long term?[a] – Did the stakeholder make efforts to reach low SES and/or vulnerable groups?[a] – Did the stakeholders make efforts to reach both boys and girls through their initiatives?[a] – Did the stakeholder make a contribution to achieve the objective of the community platform to provide residents of the community to drink water at public places? – Did the stakeholder make a contribution to achieve the objective of the community platform to provide opportunities and possibilities for outdoor play to children in regions at risk in the community?
Dose delivered (completeness)	Which activities related to the prevention of obesity did the stakeholder already organise until now?[a] – Which additional activities related to the prevention of obesity did the stakeholder plan to organise, both at the short and the long term?[a] – Which activities related to the prevention of obesity did the stakeholder realise?[a] – Are new initiatives related to the four main parts of the module taken during the intervention adoption period (which were not described at the beginning)?[a] – What does the stakeholder plan in order to make a contribution to achieve the objective of the community platform to encourage residents of the community to drink water at public places? – Which contribution has been made by the stakeholder to achieve the objective of the community platform to encourage residents of the community to drink water at public places? – What does the stakeholder plan in order to make a contribution to achieve the objective of the community platform to provide opportunities and possibilities for outdoor play to children in regions at risk in the community? – Which contribution has been made by the stakeholder to achieve the objective of the community platform to provide opportunities and possibilities for outdoor play to children in regions at risk in the community?
Dose received (exposure)	– To what extent did inhabitants and/or the target population of the stakeholders engage with the intervention?
Dose received (satisfaction)	– What is the attitude of the stakeholder towards the information received about the operation within the community platform? – What is the attitude of the stakeholders towards the prevention of obesity at community level (concept of the community platform)? – What is the attitude of the stakeholder towards the prevention of obesity at inter and organisational level? – What is the attitude of the inhabitants/target population towards initiatives taken by the stakeholder? – Do the stakeholders think they receive enough support from the IDEFICS team[b] for the implementation of the interventions?

(continued)

244 I. De Bourdeaudhuij et al.

Table 11.8 (continued)

Component	Information needed for module 3
Reach (participation proportion)	– Which category of inhabitants/target population has been reached through the activities and how many have been reached? – What are barriers and/or facilitators for the inhabitants/target population to participate in the intervention(s)? – What are barriers and/or facilitators for stakeholders to implement the intervention(s)?
Recruitment	– How are the inhabitants/target population recruited for participation in the intervention(s)? – Did the stakeholder make additional efforts to recruit inhabitants/target population for participation in the intervention(s)?
Context	– Are other projects and/or initiatives, which target the same content as the IDEFICS project, running in both control region and intervention region? – Are stakeholders who are not part of the platform working about health-related topics and/or health topics which are part of the IDEFICS project?

[a]Question applies to both the organisational and inter-organisation levels
[b]IPM, subcontractor or local coordinator (not in pay of the IDEFICS study)

11.4.3   Process Evaluation Instruments Related to Module 3

Table 11.8 gives an overview of the process evaluation questions related to the process evaluation components of module 3.

For access to the questionnaires related to module 3 see Sect. 11.7.

Process evaluation 3A is a questionnaire that needs to be completed by each individual stakeholder that is a part of the community platform. The questionnaire gives a detailed view on the nature, tasks, goals, etc., that the stakeholders in the community platform have before they were involved within the IDEFICS project and during the further phases of the project. It has to be filled in at the beginning of the adoption period, immediately after T_0, and a slightly adapted version has to be filled in a second and a third time at T_1 and T_2. An adapted version of this questionnaire is also presented to the stakeholders in the intervention region that are not part of the community platform.

Process evaluation 3B is a questionnaire that needs to be completed by individual stakeholders in the control region. Comparable stakeholders need to be chosen in the control region compared to the intervention region. This questionnaire has to be completed at T_1 and T_2.

Table 11.9 Process evaluation questions for module 4

Component	Information needed for module 4
Fidelity (quality)	– Is a school working group been established in every school in the intervention region? – What is the composition of the school working groups? – Are persons targeting low SES included? – Are key individuals missing? – Has a continuous detection been done of what is going on in the school related to the key messages? – Did the school working group motivate the relevant teachers to implement modules 5 and 7?
Dose delivered (completeness)	– How many meetings have been organised with the IPM? – How many meetings have been organised without IPM?
Dose received (exposure)	Objectives to evaluate the use of the manuals about the different modules provided by the centre are formulated in the sections relevant for those modules.
Dose received (satisfaction)	– What is the attitude of the members of the school working groups towards the information received about establishment, composition and expected operation of the school working groups? – What is the attitude towards the concept of the school working groups? – Do the members of the school working groups think they get enough support from the IDEFICS team?
Reach (participation proportion)	– What is the number of participants in each meeting? – Does the composition of the school working groups change? – How does the composition change and why? – What are barriers and facilitators to be part of the school working groups?
Recruitment	– Is an existing school working groups used and/or extended? – Which strategy has been used to compose the school working groups? – Are new participants for the school working groups recruited during the intervention period? How has this been done and why?
Context	– Are the IDEFICS school working groups also working on other health topics (e.g. in the scope of other projects)? – Are other school working groups in the school working on projects with the same and/or other health topics? – What are these topics about and how are they implemented? – Are school working groups working on health topics in the control region? – About which health topics are these school working groups working and how are these implemented?

Table 11.10 Process evaluation questions for module 5

Component	Information needed for module 5
Fidelity (quality)	– Did teachers use the educational materials provided by the centre? – Did they receive the objectives from the matrices and did they use these to develop activities? – Did they receive nothing and developed activities related to the key messages on their own? – Have additional efforts been made by the teachers in order to involve parents? – Have additional efforts been made by the teachers in order to involve/ target low SES?
Dose delivered (completeness)	– What proportion of the intended intervention was actually delivered to the children (in terms of objectives)? – How many minutes/lessons of the classroom intervention were actually delivered to the children? – To what extent were all educational materials, designed for the intervention, used? – To what extent was all of the intended content covered? – To what extent were all of the activities used?
Dose received (exposure)	– What proportion of the educational materials did the children actually receive? – What proportion was read, viewed or otherwise used by the children? – To what extent did teachers make changes in their own curriculum to incorporate the IDEFICS classroom intervention?
Dose received (satisfaction)	– What was the attitude of the children towards the content of the classroom intervention? – What was the attitude of the teachers towards the intervention? – What were the reactions of the parents related to the content of the classroom intervention?
Reach (participation proportion)	– Did all the children between 2 and 9.9 year old receive the intervention? – How many did (not)? – Did some classes not participate?
Recruitment	– The reason for non-participation of children in the classroom intervention will be depending on the teachers. For this reason, this component of process evaluation is focussed at these actors: – What were the reasons and barriers for not delivering the intervention? – What were facilitators to implementing the healthy weeks in the classroom?
Context	– Are there factors that might influence programme implementation or intervention outcome? – Did other projects/actions trigger activities related to the topic of the IDEFICS intervention? – Are similar actions being performed in the control region? – Which activities have been organised at school level in the scope of the healthy week (did schools only deliver the classroom intervention or was the healthy week an opportunity to additionally highlight the key message at school level?) – Have teachers organised activities related to the other key messages during a healthy week? – Have teachers organised activities related to the key messages during the period between two healthy weeks?

11.4.4   Process Evaluation Instruments Related to Module 4

Table 11.9 gives an overview of the process evaluation questions related to the process evaluation components of module 4.

For access to the questionnaires related to module 4 see Sect. 11.7.

Process evaluation 4A is a reporting sheet for the meetings of the school working group. It has to be completed in the intervention community during each meeting of the school working group in each school.

Process evaluation 4B is the first interview with the members of the school working group in the intervention region. One interview has to be done with all the members of the school working group together, preferably related to a school working group meeting at the beginning of the intervention adoption period (after T_0). The members of the school working group do not have to be interviewed individually. This instrument gives an overview of the members, tasks, opinions, barriers, and history of each school working group. A slightly adapted version of the interview has to be completed at T_1 and T_2.

Process evaluation 4C is a questionnaire for the headmasters in the control region on the existence of school working groups independent of the IDEFICS intervention. One questionnaire has to be completed in every school that participated in the baseline survey in the control region. The aim of this questionnaire is to get an idea about the existence of school working groups in the control region and the topics that these school working groups are dealing with. The questionnaire has to be completed at T_0, T_1 and T_2.

11.4.5   Process Evaluation Instruments Related to Module 5

Table 11.10 gives an overview of the process evaluation questions related to the process evaluation components of module 5.

For access to the questionnaires related to module 5 see Sect. 11.7.

Ten versions of **process evaluation 5A** were developed. These instruments are related to module 5, which are the classroom teaching activities. Five questionnaires were developed for kindergarten, and five were developed for primary schools. Each of these five questionnaires addressed another key message (fruit and vegetables, water, physical activity, TV viewing, sleep duration). Each of these key messages was addressed two times during a "healthy week" in the classroom, apart from the key message about sleep duration which was undertaken only once. No separate process evaluation instruments were developed related to the sixth key message: strengthen parent–child relationships by spending more time together. This message was integrated in the nine healthy weeks about the other five key messages.

Table 11.11 Process evaluation questions for modules 6, 8 and 9

Component	Information needed for modules 6, 8, 9
Fidelity (quality)	– Are efforts made to involve parents in the implementation of these modules? – Are efforts made to target low SES children? – Did the school working groups stimulate other teachers to participate in the implementation of these intervention modules? – Did the school working groups promote the activities implemented for these modules at school?
Dose delivered (completeness)	– What is the initial stage of the school for these modules? – Which activities were planned to be implemented in the scope of these modules? – Which activities did the school working groups really implement for these modules?
Dose received (exposure)	– Did the school working groups use the manuals provided by the centre to select the activities that are planned to be implemented? – What is the opinion of the school working groups about the quality of the manuals provided by the centre, were they useful to elaborate these modules?
Dose received (satisfaction)	– What is the opinion of the school working groups related to the content of these modules? – What is the opinion of the school working groups towards activities implemented for these modules? – What is the attitude of children, other teachers and parents towards the content of these modules? – Do other teachers think they are enough involved in and informed about the implementation of these modules? – Are the activities for these modules implemented as intended at the beginning of the programme? – What are the reasons for not being able to implement the activities which were planned at the beginning of the programme?
Reach (participation proportion)	– Did children participate in the intervention activities related to these modules? – Did the activities reach the right target group (2–9.9 year old children)? – Are the activities related to these modules attractive for 2–9.9 year old children? – What can be a reason for non-participation of children in the activities implemented for these modules? – What are the reasons for not elaborating a certain module by the school working groups? – What are barriers/facilitators for elaborating or not elaborating certain modules?

Process evaluation 5B is a reporting sheet for the project leader of the school working group. The aim of this instrument is to make an inventory of the initiatives at the school level that were organised related to each of the healthy weeks. Healthy weeks typically include activities at the class level; however, it is encouraged to implement these classroom activities into a whole school approach.

Table 11.12 Process evaluation questions for module 7

Component	Information needed for module 7
Fidelity (quality)	– Are efforts made to involve parents in the implementation of this module? – Are efforts made to target low SES children? – Did the school working group stimulate physical education teachers to implement this module? – Did the school working group stimulate teachers in kindergarten to implement this module?
Dose delivered (completeness)	– Which guidelines do physical education teachers implement at the beginning and at the end of the programme? – How many opportunities are provided to the children in kindergarten to be physically active during the day (apart from the official breaks at the playground)? – How are these opportunities provided?
Dose received (exposure)	– Did the physical education teachers and teachers in kindergartens use the materials received from the centre or are other resources used? – What is the opinion of the physical education teacher about the quality of the guidelines provided by the centre? – What is the opinion of teachers in kindergarten about the information received from the centre? Were they useful to implement this module? – Did the school working group stimulate physical education teachers to implement this module during the year? – Did the school working group stimulate teachers in kindergarten to implement this module during the year?
Dose received (satisfaction)	– What is the opinion of the physical education and kindergarten teacher about the content of this module? – What is the attitude of the children and parents towards the content of this module? – What are reasons for not being able to implement this module?
Reach (participation proportion)	– Did all the children between 2 and 9.9 year old receive the intervention? – How many did (not)? – Did some classes not participate? – What are reasons for not implementing this module? – What or are barriers/facilitators for (not) implementing this module?
Recruitment	– How did the school working group stimulate physical education and kindergarten teachers to implement this module?
Context	– To what extent do physical education teachers apply the health-related physical education guidelines at the beginning and at the end of the programme, in both the control region and intervention region? – How many opportunities do teachers in kindergarten provide to the children to be physically active during the day (apart from the official breaks at the playground) in the control region? – Are other projects and/or initiatives, which focus on health-related physical education and increasing time spent in kindergarten, running at school: in both the control region and intervention region?

Process evaluation 5C is a reduced version of process evaluation 5A. It has to be completed by kindergarten and primary school teachers in the intervention region at T_2. Its aim is to assess the extent to which teachers still integrated the key messages into their classroom activities during the second phase of the intervention. A slightly adapted version of this questionnaire, process evaluation 5D, has to be completed by kindergarten and primary school teachers in the control region at T_1 and T_2.

11.4.6 Process Evaluation Instruments Related to Modules 6, 8 and 9

Table 11.11 gives an overview of the process evaluation questions related to the process evaluation components of modules 6, 8 and 9.

For access to the questionnaires related to modules 6, 8 and 9 see Sect. 11.7.

Process evaluation 689A is a self-assessment instrument that needs to be completed before the intervention and at T_1 and at T_2 to make an inventory of the environmental initiatives that were taken by the schools related to modules 6, 8 and 9. This instrument needs to be completed in the control region and the intervention region. In the intervention region, one member of every school working group is the best choice to complete this questionnaire. In the control region, this questionnaire can be completed by one member of each participating school; this can be the headmaster or another member of the school staff who has enough information about these topics.

Process evaluation 689B is a reporting sheet for the project leaders of the school working groups in the intervention region. It is a sheet in which the schools of the intervention region write down their objectives for the coming years related to modules 6, 8 and 9. The sheet already contains the specific possible targets related to the three modules to give the schools an overview of all possible strategies that can be taken.

11.4.7 Process Evaluation Instruments Related to Module 7

Table 11.12 gives an overview of the process evaluation questions related to the process evaluation components of module 7.

For access to the questionnaires related to module 7 see Sect. 11.7.

Process evaluation 7A is an instrument for physical education (PE) teachers in primary schools. Its aim is to get an idea of the initiatives that the PE teachers took to include the health-related PE in their lessons, to make the lessons more active and to stress the transfer of activities outside the PE context. It has to be completed by the PE teachers of the intervention schools at T_1 and T_2. A comparable instrument was developed, process evaluation 7B, for the PE teachers of the control regions, to get insight into the health-related PE principles in the PE courses of all control region schools.

Process evaluation 7C is an instrument for the kindergarten teachers/pedagogues in the intervention region. It aims to get an idea of the initiatives that these teachers take to make the kindergarten time as active as possible. The questionnaire has to be completed by the kindergarten teachers/pedagogues in the participating kindergartens at T_1 and T_2. A comparable instrument, process evaluation 7D, was also developed for the kindergarten teachers/pedagogues in the control region.

Table 11.13 Process evaluation questions for module 10

Component	Information needed for module 10
Fidelity (quality)	– Were the folders financially supported/distributed by the community platform? – Did the community platform or IDEFICS staff organise additional initiatives to educate parents? – Were special efforts made to reach low SES parents?
Dose delivered (completeness)	– How many folders were distributed for each key messages and how many times? – How many and which other initiatives were organised to educate parents?
Dose received (exposure)	– How many parents received the folders (for each key message separately)? – How many parents received at least one version of all folders? – How many parents were involved in IDEFICS activities for parents (through the school and/or community)? – How many parents were aware of IDEFICS activities for parents (through the school and/or community)?
Dose received (satisfaction)	– What was the opinion of the parents about the folders and IDEFICS activities for parents?
Reach (participation proportion)	– What proportion of the parents received the folders (for each key message separately)? – What proportion of the parents received at least one version of all folders? – What proportion of the parents was aware of IDEFICS activities for parents (through the school and/or community)? – What proportion of the parents was involved in IDEFICS activities for parents (through the school and/or community)?
Recruitment	– Which strategies have been used to reach and to educate the parents? – Which strategies have been used to distribute the folders?
Context	– Did the parents in the control region receive folders/materials about the IDEFICS key messages? – Were the parents in the control region involved in activities for parents (through the school and/or community)? – Were the parents aware of activities for parents (through the school and/or community)

11.4.8   Process Evaluation Instruments Related to Module 10

Table 11.13 gives an overview of the process evaluation questions related to the process evaluation components of module 10.

For access to the questionnaire related to module 10 see Sect. 11.7.

Process evaluation 10A is an instrument that was added to the parental questionnaire distributed during the surveys at T_1 and at T_2, and it reports the initiatives that parents have seen or participated in, in the schools of their child or in the community related to the IDEFICS intervention. A comparable instrument, process evaluation 10B, was also developed for the parents of the control region.

Process evaluation 10C is a reporting sheet to be completed by the IDEFICS team. It details the distribution of the folders and the initiatives taken to educate parents. The reporting sheet has to be completed at T_1 and T_2.

11.5   A Combination of Methods and Analyses

It is clear from what is reported before that a wide variety of instruments was developed for the process evaluation. This is a typical situation as process evaluation uses often a wide range of methods, combining quantitative data collection methods such as surveys, checklists, number of members attending meetings, and qualitative data collection methods such as structured interviews, observations, content analysis.

Typical for the use of a wide range of methods is also a wide range of possible analyses in using the data. Most process evaluation analyses use descriptive methods (Steckler and Linnan 2014). The process instruments will be used to describe the level of implementation across the theoretical constructs (fidelity, dose delivered, dose received, etc., see above), for the different settings, for the different schools within one country and for the different countries and communities in the whole project.

However, it is clear that descriptive analyses are not the only objective of the IDEFICS process evaluation. A major objective will be to compose different composite instruments of implementation and to use these implementation scores as mediators of the effectiveness of the intervention within and between countries.

11.6   Experiences with the IDEFICS Process Evaluation

It is clear that the more detailed a process evaluation is, the more information will be derived from it, and the more insight we can get into the mechanisms through which an intervention may work. In Belgium, more detailed analyses on the process evaluation were performed. Here, it became clear that the IDEFICS intervention was able to prevent unfavourable changes in sedentary time and light physical activity in Belgium schools which showed medium or high intervention process scores (Verloigne et al. 2015). However, to get such detailed information is also the biggest challenge in process evaluation: to be able to let the stakeholders in the field complete the process evaluation instruments or participate in the interviews.

We especially experienced a lot of problems motivating teachers during the whole process to fill in the questionnaires. As we wanted a detailed idea of the exposure time of the children and the content of the classroom lessons, we asked teachers to fill in a process evaluation measure after every "healthy week" which was nine times during the first year of the IDEFICS intervention. This was perceived to be a large burden for teachers which resulted in a very large variation in response proportions across countries, across schools and even across teachers within schools. Furthermore, problems occurred to retrieve completed questionnaires from the control region at the level of the community and the schools. This may be due to the fact that the direct contact was more elaborate in the intervention region.

Triangulation is considered desirable in process evaluations, but limited resources may force researchers to restrict data collections and analyses. Linnan and Steckler (2002) indicated that it is recommended to get an answer on all possible process evaluation questions; however, if not possible, the questions about reach, dose and fidelity should be prioritised. Although data collection for the process evaluation of the IDEFICS intervention was limited, it is in principle possible to report on these minimal requirements. The obtained information led to the conclusion that parental exposure and involvement in the IDEFICS intervention in all countries were much less than aimed for where higher levels of parental exposure were not shown to be related to more favourable changes in body mass index (BMI) z-scores (De Bourdeaudhuij et al. 2015b). However, we were not able to assess the reasons for the low parental exposure which might be due to the diverse focus, high intensity or duration of the IDEFICS intervention.

11.7   Provision of Instruments and Standard Operating Procedures to Third Parties

All instruments described in this chapter including the General Survey Manual that provides among other all standard operating procedures can be accessed on the following website: www.leibniz-bips.de/ifhs after registration.

Each third partner using the instruments provided in this chapter is kindly requested to cite this chapter as follows:

De Bourdeaudhuij I, Verbestel V, Maes L, Nappo A, Chadjigeorgiou C, Molnár D, Kovács E, Eiben G, Barba G, Hassel H, Gallois K, Konstabel K, Moreno LA, Tornaritis M, Frauca NL, Veidebaum T, Mårild S, De Henauw S, on behalf of the IDEFICS consortium. Process evaluation of the IDEFICS intervention. In:

Bammann K, Lissner L, Pigeot I, Ahrens W, editors. Instruments for health surveys in children and adolescents. Cham: Springer Nature Switzerland; 2019. p. 231–255.

Acknowledgements The development of instruments, the baseline data collection and the first follow-up work as part of the IDEFICS study (www.idefics.eu) were financially supported by the European Commission within the Sixth RTD Framework Programme Contract No. 016181 (FOOD). The most recent follow-up including the development of new instruments and the adaptation of previously used instruments was conducted in the framework of the I.Family study (www.ifamilystudy.eu) which was funded by the European Commission within the Seventh RTD Framework Programme Contract No. 266044 (KBBE 2010–14).

We thank all families for participating in the extensive examinations of the IDEFICS and I. Family studies. We are also grateful for the support from school boards, headmasters and communities.

We also thank Gianvincenzo Barba from the Institute of Food Sciences, National Research Council (Avellino, Italy) who unexpectedly passed away before this book was completed for his valuable contributions to the IDEFICS/I.Family studies.

References

Bartholomew LK, Parcel GS, Kok G, Gottlieb NH. Planning health promotion programs: an intervention mapping approach. 1st ed. San Fransisco: Jossey-Bass; 2006.

De Bourdeaudhuij I, Verbestel V, De Henauw S, Maes L, Huybrechts I, Mårild S, IDEFICS consortium, et al. Behavioural effects of a community-oriented setting-based intervention for prevention of childhood obesity in eight European countries. Main results from the IDEFICS study. Obes Rev. 2015a;16(Suppl 2):30–40.

De Bourdeaudhuij I, Verbestel V, De Henauw S, Maes L, Mårild S, Moreno LA, IDEFICS consortium, et al. Implementation of the IDEFICS intervention across European countries: perceptions of parents and relationship with BMI. Obes Rev. 2015b;16(Suppl 2):78–88.

De Henauw S, Verbestel V, Mårild S, Barba G, Bammann K, Eiben G, IDEFICS consortium, et al. The IDEFICS community oriented intervention program. A new model for childhood obesity prevention in Europe. Int J Obes (Lond). 2011;35(Suppl 1):S16–23.

De Henauw S, Huybrechts I, De Bourdeaudhuij I, Bammann K, Barba G, Lissner L, IDEFICS consortium, et al. Effects of a community-oriented obesity prevention programme on indicators of body fatness in pre-school and primary school children. Main results from the IDEFICS study. Obes Rev. 2015;16(Suppl 2):16–29.

Linnan L, Steckler A. Process evaluation for public health interventions and research. An overview. In: Linnan L, Steckler A, editors. Process evaluation for public health interventions and research. San Fransisco: Jossey-Bass; 2002. p. 1–23.

Mårild S, Russo P, Veidebaum T, Tornaritis M, De Henauw S, De Bourdeaudhuij I, IDEFICS consortium, et al. Impact of a community based health-promotion programme in 2- to 9-year-old children in Europe on markers of the metabolic syndrome, the IDEFICS study. Obes Rev. 2015;16(Suppl 2):41–56.

Nicholls SG, Pohlabeln H, De Bourdeaudhuij I, Chadjigeorgiou C, Gwozdz W, Hebestreit A, IDEFICS consortium, et al. Parents' evaluation of the IDEFICS intervention: an analysis focussing on socio-economic factors, child's weight status and intervention exposure. Obes Rev. 2015;16(Suppl 2):103–18.

Pigeot I, De Henauw S, Baranowski T, editors. The IDEFICS (Identification and prevention of Dietary- and lifestyle-induced health EFfects In Children and infantS) trial outcomes and process evaluations. Obes Rev. 2015;16 Suppl 2:2–3.

Saunders RP, Evans MH, Joshi P. Developing a process-evaluation plan for assessing health promotion program implementation: a how-to guide. Health Promot Pract. 2005;6:134–47.

Steckler A, Linnan L, editors. Process evaluation for public health interventions and research. San Francisco: Jossey-Bass; 2014.

Verbestel V, De Henauw S, Maes L, Haerens L, Mårild S, Eiben G, et al. Using the intervention mapping protocol to develop a community-based intervention for the prevention of childhood obesity in a multi-centre European project: the IDEFICS intervention. Int J Behav Nutr Phys Act. 2011;8:82.

Verbestel V, De Henauw S, Mårild S, Storcksdieck S, Celemín LF, Gallois K, et al. The IDEFICS Intervention Toolbox—a guide to successful obesity prevention at community level. In: Maddock J, editor. Public health—social and behavioral health. InTech: Rijeka; 2012. http://www.intechopen.com/books/public-health-social-and-behavioral-health/the-idefics-inter vention-toolbox-a-guide-to-successful-obesity-prevention-at-community-level. Accessed 29 Mar 2018.

Verloigne M, Ahrens W, De Henauw S, Verbestel V, Mårild S, Pigeot I, IDEFICS consortium, et al. Process evaluation of the IDEFICS school intervention: putting the evaluation of the effect on children's objectively measured physical activity and sedentary time in context. Obes Rev. 2015;16(Suppl 2):89–102.

Chapter 12
Assessment of Sensory Taste Perception in Children

Hannah Jilani, Jenny Peplies and Kirsten Buchecker

Abstract In health research, sensory taste perception and preference have rarely been examined. Especially in children, it is challenging to conduct sensory taste perception and preference tests due to their still-developing cognitive and physiological abilities. In the IDEFICS and I.Family studies, four different instruments were developed to assess sensory taste perception and preference in children, adolescents and their parents across Europe. A taste threshold test and a taste preference test were adapted to be used in children from the age of 6 years onwards in the IDEFICS study. A food and beverage preference questionnaire and a taste intensity test were adapted to be used in I.Family. The taste preference test and the taste intensity test were conducted with standardised real foods to obtain results that are relevant for real-life conditions. The taste threshold test was conducted with standardised solutions. All test procedures were standardised across the participating countries, and all materials were supplied centrally and tested for suitability. Experiences in the surveys showed that these four instruments were suitable to be used in children and adolescents. The game-like character of the sensory test module enhanced the acceptance of this survey module and made it quite popular among the participating children. Furthermore, the sensory tests were reported to be the participants' favourite procedure during the surveys. In conclusion, these tests were feasible to be conducted in large-scale studies across Europe.

On behalf of the IDEFICS and I.Family consortia

H. Jilani (✉)
Leibniz Institute for Prevention Research and Epidemiology—BIPS, Bremen, Germany
e-mail: jilani@leibniz-bips.de

J. Peplies
Institute for Public Health and Nursing Research (IPP), Working Group Epidemiology of Demographic Change, University of Bremen, Bremen, Germany

K. Buchecker
Department of Food Science, Technologie-Transfer-Zentrum (TTZ Bremerhaven), Bremerhaven, Germany

K. Buchecker
University of Applied Sciences Bremerhaven, Bremerhaven, Germany

© Springer Nature Switzerland AG 2019
K. Bammann et al. (eds.), *Instruments for Health Surveys in Children and Adolescents*, Springer Series on Epidemiology and Public Health, https://doi.org/10.1007/978-3-319-98857-3_12

257

12.1 Assessment of Sensory Taste Perception

Sensory taste perception differs substantially between subjects. But it is evident that how people perceive the taste of foods influences their food choice and how much they eat (Sorensen et al. 2003). Therefore, the global aims of the assessment of sensory perception in the IDEFICS and I.Family studies (Ahrens et al. 2011, 2017) were to investigate the variation of sensory taste perception in European children and adolescents and its association with overweight, obesity, metabolic syndrome and food choice. Relating sensory taste perception with health outcomes presented an innovative research field resulting in novel insights in this area.

Previously, the majority of methods commonly applied to assess sensory perception, e.g. during the evaluation of newly developed foods by industry, were designed to work with adults. Studies on sensory testing in children are still rare. Some studies, however, provided an insight into requirements for sensory work with children. Guinard, for instance, published in 2001 a review on sensory and consumer testing with children (Guinard 2001), and Popper and Kroll reviewed the current state of knowledge in 2004 (Popper and Kroll 2005). These reviews, including their recommendations, are summarised in the international standard guidelines on sensory evaluation by children and minors, and some very general examples are given (ASTM 2013). Nevertheless, before the start of the IDEFICS and I.Family studies, there was a lack of validated methods for sensory testing with children, especially for the assessment of taste thresholds. Consequently, specific test procedures, tailor-made for the application in young children, had to be developed. During the course of the IDEFICS and I.Family studies, four methods to assess sensory taste perception and preference were adapted for the use in children and adolescents.

Previous publications using sensory data from the IDEFICS and I.Family studies have investigated associations between taste sensitivity/preferences and food intake as well as weight status or have assessed correlates of taste preferences and have described the development of the methods (Knof et al. 2011; Lanfer et al. 2012, 2013; Lissner et al. 2012). A special challenge was to design the test for application in different European countries. Since gold standards were missing, the newly developed tests needed to be validated in terms of reliability and repeatability.

12.2 Implications for Sensory Testing with Children

During childhood, the physical and cognitive abilities are still less developed than those of adults (Doty and Shah 2008), and thus, different approaches are needed when planning sensory testing with children. Tests have to be easy for the investigator to conduct and for the children to understand. Additionally, children have a short attention span, implying that the whole test procedure must not take too long. The way of explaining the test to the children has to be motivating to get the consent of the children and keep them attending until they completed the whole test (Knof et al. 2011).

Furthermore, the decision-making process of children is strongly influenced by adult approval and reaction. Commonly, children tend to respond affirmatively to positively phrased questions or change their opinion on enquiry by an adult immediately (Guinard 2001). A simple question like "are you sure?" can easily turn a "yes" into a "no".

Besides the psychological development, there are also differences in the physiological development: children have about five times more taste buds, and their foliate papillae are larger and more abundant compared to those of adults. Nevertheless, this does not consequently lead to higher taste sensitivity, due to the fact that children's innervation of taste papillae is not fully developed. The development of the taste apparatus carries on through childhood (Plattig 1984). A small number of studies reported thresholds for children to be similar to those of adults (Anliker et al. 1991). Most publications, however, found young children's sensitivity to be about a magnitude lower than the one reported for adults (Glanville et al. 1964; James et al. 1997).

It can be summarised that for sensory testing with children, there are four main challenges.

1. To attract and motivate children to participate in the test procedure and to keep the motivation up throughout the whole test duration. Therefore, it works best to arrange the test procedure as a (board) game and introduce it to the children with a small story. This offers the possibility for direct interaction and involvement. Due to the game-like character of the procedure, children hardly notice taking part in a test, which prevents them from pretending or cheating in order to achieve better results.
2. To cope with the cognitive abilities of children, most notably reflected in a short attention span, distractibility, as well as difficulties in task comprehension. Thus, the procedure needs to be easily understandable and attractive for the participating children. The test should therefore last no longer than 15 min. This is crucial in order to receive good results. If children get bored, their answers will be influenced by their impatience to finish the game as soon as possible.
3. To eliminate any influence of the performing experimenter as children of this age are easily led by adults. The experimenter's relationship with the child is of great importance. In particular, special attention of the performing experimenter has to be paid on the language and phrasing of questions. This should be done in a way that avoids influencing the child's decisions. Furthermore, appropriate tone and body language is of high importance to help the children to make them feel comfortable. To exclude distraction from parents, guardians or caregivers, they should ideally wait in another room.
4. To account for the limited physiological development of children, i.e. the less-developed taste apparatus and the smaller hands compared to those of

adults. Children are accustomed to kid-sized furniture and materials at home as well as their school environments. Suitable equipment, for instance small cups, will arouse the children's interest and thus increase willingness to participate. To account for the children's underdeveloped taste apparatus, the range of concentrations of applied test solutions needs to be adapted.

Test environments are most suitable when they are familiar to the children. Ideally, the tests are performed in pre-school or school setting. In addition, the test environment should be bright and decorated in a child-friendly manner which, however, should not be too colourful in order to avoid distraction.

12.3 Performance on European Level—The Need for Standard Operating Procedures (SOPs) and Standardisation

Procedures for application within the framework of a multi-centre study have to provide comparable results on a cross-national level. In the IDEFICS and I.Family studies, all survey teams were trained at a central training session previous to the survey to assure standardised test performance and preparation of test solutions in each survey centre (for access see Sect. 12.8). This central training was conducted by experts and included lessons on behaviour, the used vocabulary and the phrasing of questions, as well as lessons on handling the equipment for preparation of test solutions and setting up the test environment. Detailed SOPs were provided to each survey centre.

The test substances, even if they appear simple such as sucrose or sodium chloride, were also standardised. A central supply was established for all test material: food samples, test substances and equipment for preparation of test solutions, as well as equipment such as drinking cups were purchased centrally and shipped to the survey centres. As an example, to avoid anti-caking and flow-regulating agents which are commonly applied by industry, food samples were purchased centrally without additives and provided to the survey centres pre-packaged and "ready-to-use" for the preparation of the test solutions. Taking into consideration that tap water quality differs substantially among the European countries, demineralised water was used for all test samples and procedures.

Accordingly, the selection of appropriate food samples is also very challenging on a cross-national level. For example, a juice which is well accepted in one country can be broadly rejected in other countries and recipes may differ by country.

12.4   General Considerations

For children, as minors, parental or guardian consent is required in addition to an oral consent given by the children to participate in the test procedures. Food intolerances in terms of food allergies and food sensitivities are highly prevalent in Europe. Especially, the sensitivity for monosodium glutamate and gluten (coeliac disease) is widely spread in Europe. Therefore, parents needed to be asked for particular food allergies of their children before the tests.

Performing experimenters were not allowed to use fragrance or perfumed hand cream and to consume cigarettes, coffee or bubblegum prior to the tests. It was assured that participating children were neither hungry nor saturated. Ideally, they had had their last meal one hour previous to the test sessions. Peppermint chewing gums or sweets with a strong taste were not allowed one hour prior to the tests.

Test environments were instructed to be bright, friendly decorated and colourful rooms, where children feel comfortable. It was pointed out that there should be no undesired odours like strong smell from kitchens or disinfectants.

12.5   Test Designs of Sensory Taste Perception Tests

After taking into consideration the aforementioned challenges, four different test procedures were developed to be implemented in the different surveys of the IDEFICS and I.Family studies.

1. As the taste qualities, sweet, salty, bitter and umami (the taste for monosodium glutamate) appeared to be most important in the context of overweight and obesity, and these qualities were selected for the *taste sensitivity tests*. In the literature, salty and umami tastes have been shown to be associated with increased appetite (He et al. 2008; Bellisle 1999; Rogers and Blundell 1990) and the sweet taste characterises many calorically dense foods. The bitter taste, however, is characteristic for a variety of vegetables, such as broccoli or Brussels sprouts, which are low in calories and often rejected by young children.
2. Besides taste sensitivity for basic taste qualities, *taste preferences* for sweet, salty, umami, aroma and fat were assessed. Aromas have recently been discussed in literature to be linked to increased appetite and thus to contribute to overweight and obesity (Azadbakht and Esmaillzadeh 2008). The role of fat appears to be even clearer: fat is the macronutrient with the highest energy density.
3. Furthermore, a food and beverage preference questionnaire was recommended for the use in epidemiological studies as a proxy for sensory taste perception (Duffy et al. 2009). For this purpose, a *food and beverage preference questionnaire* that assesses preferences for sweet, bitter, salty and fatty was developed for I.Family.

4. In a subsample of the I.Family children, a *taste intensity test* for sweet and fatty was conducted to assess the perceived taste intensity, taste preference and taste sensitivity. The use of suprathreshold intensities was recommended due to its impact on everyday life's decisions regarding food choice (Snyder and Bartoshuk 2009).

Generally, for all four test procedures, children from the age of 6 years and older were invited to participate. Pre-testing showed that children under the age of 6 years often did not comply with the test procedure and that it was not possible to obtain reliable answers from them (Suling et al. 2011).

12.5.1 Threshold Testing

As a measure of taste sensitivity, the detection threshold was assessed as the lowest concentration of a stimulus that must be exceeded, in order to have any taste effect (Pfaffmann et al. 1971). Reliance on cognitive resources is minimised for this methodology. In addition, to deal with response bias in terms of experience and expectation, the paired comparison forced-choice technique was used (Linschoten et al. 2001).

12.5.1.1 Test Procedure

The basic test design for the sensory threshold tests was based on the Deutsche Industrie Norm (DIN, German Industry Standard) 10,959 for adults which works with ten aqueous solutions with increasing concentrations of the corresponding test substance. For our purpose, the test design had to be adapted to the physical and psychological development of children. First, the number of test solutions was reduced to five. Furthermore, an additional cup of demineralised water was provided and the children were instructed to compare each test solution with this cup to identify a deviant taste.

The threshold tests were arranged as a board game (Fig. 12.1) to attract and motivate the children to take part in the test procedure. For each basic taste, a row of five test solutions with increasing concentrations of stimuli was presented in small cups, with a volume of 20 ml to the children at the lower end of the board.

The experimenter introduced the board game with a small background story: the children were told to be "taste detectives". They learned that some cups on the board may contain pure water, whereas some other may taste different and they would have to find the deviant cups. The children were advised to compare the test solutions with an extra cup of demineralised water. In case that the test solution from the board tasted like the water in the cup, they had to place it on a water icon on the upper left side of the board. If the child tasted a difference, they had to place the test solution on the crossed water icon on the upper right of the board. Between

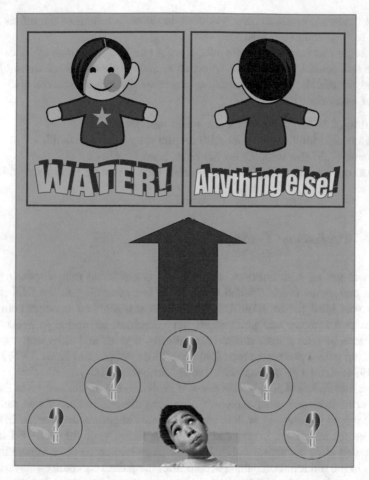

Fig. 12.1 Game board for taste threshold testing. The board was printed in A3 and laminated. *Source* Ahrens and IDEFICS consortium (2015)

the different solutions, the children neutralised the taste in their mouth with demineralised water. The whole test procedure did not exceed 15 min.

12.5.1.2 Test Samples

The test solutions were prepared by the survey centres on-site. Therefore, for each basic taste quality a concentrated stock solution had to be prepared from the corresponding test substance. Using this stock solution, the survey centres had to prepare the five test solutions by dilution in demineralised water. The survey centres received small packages with the test substances in the correct amounts needed to prepare the stock solution. This was done in order to minimise the efforts for the survey centres and avoid mistakes.

To assure that the stimuli were adequate for children, the range of concentration of each test substance was about an order of magnitude above the threshold level reported for adults. The concentration ranges of the test substances were (in the order of assessment):

1. sucrose (8.8–46.7 mmol/l) for the sweet taste threshold,
2. sodium chloride (3.4–27.4 mmol/l) for the salty taste threshold,
3. caffeine (0.26–1.3 mmol/l) for the bitter taste threshold,
4. monosodium glutamate (0.6–9.5 mmol/l) for the umami taste threshold.

12.5.2 Preference Testing

Preference testing with children is by far less complicated than threshold testing. For the preference tests, a paired comparison test according to the DIN standard 10,959 was used in the IDEFICS study. This test allowed a direct comparison between two samples and is a simple, very common technique to evaluate taste preferences. Several studies showed that children 6 years and older were capable of performing paired preference tests (Guinard 2001; Popper and Kroll 2005; Kimmel et al. 1994; Kroll 1990; Léon et al. 1999; Liem et al. 2004).

A preference test is an affective test and evaluates the higher degree of liking for one over at least one other sample. Comparing the preference of two samples is called a paired preference test. It is one of the most important approaches in sensory testing, as the test design is easy and thus allows focusing on the presented samples. It goes well with the sensory abilities of young children to discriminate the preferences in the offered food pairs. Furthermore, the paired comparison forced-choice technique was used: the children had to make a preference decision between the two samples. If children could or would not make a choice, no result was reported to avoid additional stress on the children.

12.5.2.1 Test Procedure

To create a very easy, child-friendly test design, a simple game board was developed for the preference test (Fig. 12.2). During the test, it was placed on a table in front of the children. In each test sequence, the children had to compare the sensory pleasure of a basic sample and a modification of it. Each pair was presented inside the two circles at the bottom of the board. The children were asked to place their preferred sample on the happy smiley at the top of the board. Between each test sequence, the children rinsed their mouth with demineralised water to avoid adaptation.

Fig. 12.2 Game board used for preference testing. The board was printed in A4 format and laminated. *Source* Ahrens and IDEFICS consortium (2015)

12.5.2.2   Food Samples

The food samples were selected according to two main criteria: the sensory acceptance by school children aged 6 years and above in all participating countries and the representativeness of the food samples for the evaluated taste quality. Crackers were used to test salty, fatty and umami taste preferences, and apple juice was used to assess the preference for sweet taste and aroma.

Food Samples for Sweet and Aroma

As reference for the sweet and aroma taste preferences, a clear natural apple juice was selected, with an addition of 0.53% sucrose to ensure proper acceptance of the juice. To evaluate the taste preference for sweetness, the amount of sucrose in the reference juice was increased to 3.11%. To evaluate the taste preferences for aroma, 0.05% apple aroma (nature identical, SENSIENT®) was added to the basic apple juice (Table 12.1).

All juices were presented on the board (Fig. 12.2) in 20 ml cups. The small sample quantities were chosen in order to prevent the children from becoming saturated. All survey centres were instructed to serve the juices at 18 ± 2 °C. The order of assessment was sweet followed by aroma.

Food Samples for Salty, Fatty and Umami

To evaluate the preferences for salt, fat and umami, a cracker was developed. To increase the attractiveness for young children, the crackers were heart-shaped (Fig. 12.3).

Table 12.1 Overview on recipes for apple juices applied to assess preferences for the sweet taste and aroma

	Apple juice (%)	Sucrose (%)	Aroma (%)
Reference	99.47	0.53	–
Sweet taste	96.89	3.11	–
Aroma taste	99.42	0.53	0.05

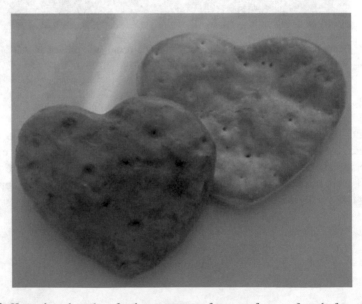

Fig. 12.3 Heart-shaped crackers for the assessment of taste preferences for salt, fat and umami

Table 12.2 Overview on recipes for crackers applied to assess preferences for the salty, fatty and umami taste

	Flour/water (%)	Salt (%)	Fat (%)	MSG (%)	DAWE (%)
Reference	91.3	0.7	8	0	0
Salt	89.4	**1.6**	8	0	1
Fat	81.3	0.7	**18**	0	0
Umami	89.3	0.7	8	1	1

Source Knof et al. (2011)
DAWE diacetyl tartaric ester, MSG monosodium glutamate

The reference crackers for all tests were produced according to a basic recipe containing wheat flour, water, 0.7% salt and 8% fat, finished with soda lye (0.5% aqueous solution, purchased from Carl Roth Chemicals). To evaluate the taste preference for fat, the amount of fat included in the basic recipe was increased from 8 to 18%. To evaluate the taste preference for salt, the amount of salt was increased from 0.7 to 1.6%. Additionally, 1% of an emulsifying agent (DAWE, diacetyl tartaric ester) was added. To evaluate the taste preference for umami, 1% of monosodium glutamate and 1% emulsifier were added to the basic recipe (Table 12.2).

The order of test assessment was first fat then salt and umami last. This order was selected due to the fact that the umami taste remains on the taste buds for a long time and would thus affect subsequent taste experiments.

12.5.3   Food and Beverage Preference Questionnaire

In I.Family, a food and beverage preference questionnaire was developed to assess preferences for sweet, bitter, salty and fatty that could be applied in children/adolescents as well as in adults. This questionnaire did not require high cognitive abilities from the participants. The food and beverage preference questionnaire was compiled based on existing tools (Deglaire et al. 2012; Vereecken et al. 2013). Additionally, bitter food items were compiled from studies that investigated the bitter taste perception by reviewing the literature. Thus, the questionnaire assessed preferences for the sweet, fatty, bitter and salty taste. It contains pictures of relevant food and drink items to be used in all age groups (Fig. 12.4). In total, the questionnaire consisted of 63 items including single foods (e.g. banana, spinach), mixed foods (e.g. hot dog, kebab), condiments (e.g. jam, mayonnaise) and drinks (e.g. coke, lemonade).

12.5.3.1   Test Procedure

Participants were asked to indicate how much they liked the taste of the food presented on the pictures using a five-point smiley face Likert scale, ranging from

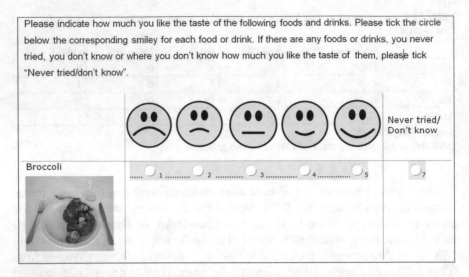

Fig. 12.4 Example (screenshot) from the food and beverage preference questionnaire. *Source* Jilani et al. (2017)

disliking to liking. Thus, the variable of liking for each food and drink item ranged from 1 to 5, with 1 meaning "do not like at all" and 5 meaning "like very much". Additionally, participants could indicate that they do not know or have never tasted the specific food item. A pre-test was conducted in every country to ensure the feasibility of all food items across countries.

12.5.3.2 Taste Preference Scores

Foods that were ranked by at least 75% of the participants (e.g. less than 25% of the participants never tried or did not know the food) were used for further analyses. Participants were excluded when they had more than 20 items missing or "Never tried/Don't know" answers. Furthermore, a sex- and age-specific factor analysis was conducted to gain more accurate information about the factorial structure of food preference. The strata were younger boys (<12 years), younger girls (<12 years), older boys (≥ 12 years), older girls (≥ 12 years) and their mothers and fathers. A food or drink item was considered to belong to a particular factor if the factor loading was greater than 0.30 on that factor. The factor analysis explained between 32 and 41% of the overall variance of the variables (fathers 41%, mothers 39%, older girls 36%, older boys 38%, younger boys 37% and younger girls 32%). The obtained factors were used to conduct a content analysis in order to assign the factors to the taste modalities sweet, salty, fatty and bitter. Food and drink items with no load on one of the factors were not included in further analyses.

Scores for liking of the specific taste quality were computed by calculating the mean liking of the foods and drinks included in each of the four categories. Scores were calculated individually for younger boys, younger girls, older boys, older girls as well as their mothers and fathers. The sum of the ratings for the foods and drinks was calculated and divided by the number of foods and drinks that were included in the specific taste modality group.

12.5.4   Taste Intensity Test

For the last survey of I.Family, a new sensory taste perception test was applied. Perceived taste intensity for different concentrations of sugar and fat was assessed in a smaller subsample in every participating country. At that time, a more advanced technique could be implemented because all participating children were at least 8 years old. Cold whipped vanilla pudding was chosen as matrix to measure perceived taste intensity (Mennella et al. 2012). Children are in most cases familiar with pudding, which increased the acceptance and adherence to the test procedures. It can be varied easily in sugar and fat concentrations, and due to its fluidity, the sweet and fatty taste can diffuse easily in the oral cavity. Children with at least one parent present participated in this test.

12.5.4.1   Test Procedure

The test was organised in two different blocks (fatty/sweet). It started with either sweet or fat in a randomised order. Participants had to rate three cups of pudding with different sugar concentrations and three cups of pudding with different fat concentrations on a nine-point-scale (Fig. 12.5) and on a "generalised Labelled Magnitude Scale" (gLMS) developed by Green et al. (1996) and modified by Bartoshuk et al. (2004). Finally, they were asked to indicate their favourite pudding of the fat and the sweet block placing it on a happy smiley (Fig. 12.5). The three samples were presented in counterbalanced order in 20 ml plastic cups to level out potential confounding effects (Zandstra and de Graaf 1998). To test fatty taste perception, the term "creamy" was used to avoid negative associations to fat.

Between each test sequence, the participants rinsed their mouth with demineralised water to avoid adaptation and took a 2–3 min break. The test continued with the second block following the same procedure. The pudding samples were presented under a red light in order to mask colour differences.

12.5.4.2   Test Samples

Cold whipped vanilla pudding (RUF Schlemmer Crème, vanilla flavour) was chosen as flavour carrier with different concentrations of sugar and fat. The first concentration step was the same for both test blocks (sweet/fatty) and contained 14.5% sugar and 3.1% fat. For testing sweet taste perception, the proportion of fat

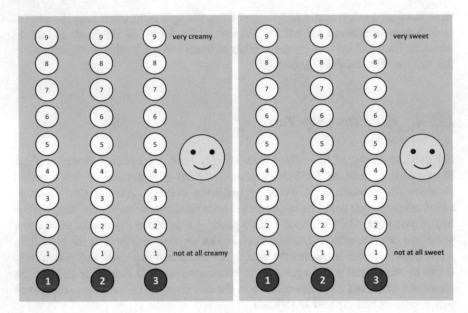

Fig. 12.5 Game board used for intensity testing. The board was printed in A3 format and laminated

Table 12.3 Overview of recipes for vanilla pudding applied to assess preferences for the sweet and fatty taste

	Sucrose[a] (%)	Fat[b] (%)
Reference	14.5	3.1
Second concentration step	24.1	6.8
Third concentration step	36.2	14.1

[a]Fat concentration was kept stable at 3.1%
[b]Sugar concentration was kept stable at 14.5%

was kept stable and the amount of sugar was modified to 24.1% in a second concentration step and to 36.2% in a third concentration step (Table 12.3). Sucrose was used to modify the sugar concentration. For testing fatty taste perception, the proportion of sugar was kept stable and the amount of fat was modified to 6.8% in a second concentration step and to 14.1% in a third concentration step (Table 12.3). Cream was centrally purchased and shipped to the survey centres and used to modify the fat concentration.

12.6 Test–Retest Reliability

To assess the test–retest reliability, the preference and threshold tests were performed over two consecutive mornings under identical conditions, partially with different experimenters. For threshold testing, it was assessed if the threshold levels,

Table 12.4 Test–retest correlation for the threshold test procedure ($N = 40$)

Taste quality	Cohen's κ
Sucrose	0.81
Sodium chloride	0.75
Caffeine	0.68
Monosodium glutamate	0.77

Source Excerpt from Table 3 in Knof et al. (2011)

Table 12.5 Test–retest correlation for the taste preference test procedure ($N = 40$)

Preference for	Cohen's κ
Sweet taste	0.77
Aroma taste	0.78
Fatty taste	0.77
Salty taste	0.86
Umami taste	0.80

Source Excerpt from Table 4 in Knof et al. (2011)

measured on the second day, were lower, higher or matched exactly to the threshold values measured on the previous day.

For the preference tests, it was assessed if the children's choice from the consecutive session matched their choice from the previous session. In total, 40 children (aged 6–10 years) participated in the retest session for threshold testing and 20 (aged 6–10 years) for preference testing. These groups were homogenous in terms of age and sex.

Test–retest reliability was determined by comparing the two scores of the consecutive sessions. To assess intra-rater reliability of the developed methods, weighted Cohen's Kappa (κ) coefficients were calculated.

Analysis of test–retest results for threshold testing shows a strength of agreement that is rated to be "almost perfect" for the detection of sucrose, according to Landis and Koch (1977). For the detection of sodium chloride, caffeine and MSG, the strength of agreement is rated to be "substantial" (Table 12.4). For preference testing, the degree of stability between the sessions is rated to be "substantial", for the sweet, aroma, fatty and umami taste. For the salty taste preference, the strength of agreement again is "almost perfect" (Table 12.5).

This shows that sensory testing with children is reliable, provided that the applied methods are adapted to the special requirements.

12.7 Experiences from the Surveys

A subsample of 20% of the school children who participated in the IDEFICS study was selected to perform the battery of sensory tests (threshold and preference tests) in the baseline survey. Sensory testing was restricted to children 6 years of age and older because experiences in the pre-test showed that pre-school children often did not comply with the test procedure and that it was not possible to obtain reliable answers from them (Suling et al. 2011). Altogether, 1861 children from eight countries participated in the taste threshold tests and 1718 in the taste preference tests in the IDEFICS study (Ahrens et al. 2011). In I.Family, 7841 children and 5938 parents filled in the food and beverage preference questionnaire as well as 985 children and 788 parents participated in the taste intensity test. In addition, 1046 children and 58 parents participated in the taste preference test.

As reported by the survey centres or discovered during the site visits performed by the central quality control unit of the project, several problems occurred during the examinations. The survey centres could not always guarantee for the best possible test conditions. It was, for example, sometimes difficult to find bright, colourful and friendly decorated rooms in the schools and to guarantee the absence of undesired odours and sources of distraction, as the survey personnel depended on the schools to offer them appropriate rooms for the examination.

Since sensory tests were largely unknown to the experimenters, the detailed description of test procedures in the general survey manual, the central training, the provision of SOPs and the site visits of the coordinating centre to all survey centres turned out to be very important. Otherwise, non-compliance to the SOPs would have occurred, e.g. terminating the test sequence of the threshold test once the child detected the first test solution deviant from water or conducting the preference tests in the wrong order (first crackers, second juice).

The survey centres complained about the time-consuming preparation of test solutions for the threshold and intensity tests (despite the pre-packaged portions of chemicals that were supplied). The workload attributed to the preference tests was much smaller since all test materials were delivered "ready-to-use" by the coordinating centre. In general, the experiences from the survey underline the beneficial effect of a central supply of consumables. Especially multi-centre studies depend on careful standardisation of test materials to obtain comparable results from different settings and countries.

Finally, all centres reported that the game-like character of the sensory test module enhanced the acceptance of this survey module and made it quite popular among the participating children. Furthermore, the sensory tests were reported to be the participants' favourite procedure during the surveys. In general, all four test procedures were age-appropriate according to the study populations of the IDEFICS and I.Family studies as they never turned out to require too high cognitive abilities.

12.8   Provision of Instruments and Standard Operating Procedures to Third Parties

All instruments described in this chapter including the general survey manuals that provide among other all standard operating procedures can be accessed on the following website: www.leibniz-bips.de/ifhs after registration.

Each third partner using the instruments provided in this chapter is kindly requested to cite this chapter as follows:

Jilani H, Peplies J, Buchecker K, on behalf of the IDEFICS and I.Family consortia. Assessment of sensory taste perception in children. In: Bammann K, Lissner L, Pigeot I, Ahrens W, editors. Instruments for health surveys in children and adolescents. Cham: Springer Nature Switzerland; 2019. pp. 257–275.

Acknowledgements The development of instruments, the baseline data collection and the first follow-up work as part of the IDEFICS study (www.idefics.eu) were financially supported by the European Commission within the Sixth RTD Framework Programme Contract No. 016181 (FOOD). The most recent follow-up including the development of new instruments and the adaptation of previously used instruments was conducted in the framework of the I.Family study (www.ifamilystudy.eu) which was funded by the European Commission within the Seventh RTD Framework Programme Contract No. 266044 (KBBE 2010–14).

We thank all families for participating in the extensive examinations of the IDEFICS and I.Family studies. We are also grateful for the support from school boards, headmasters and communities.

References

Ahrens W, IDEFICS consortium. Sensory taste preferences and taste sensitivity and the association of unhealthy food patterns with overweight and obesity in primary school children in Europe—a synthesis of data from the IDEFICS study. Flavour. 2015;4:8.

Ahrens W, Bammann K, Siani A, Buchecker K, De Henauw S, Iacoviello L, et al. IDEFICS consortium. The IDEFICS cohort: design, characteristics and participation in the baseline survey. Int J Obes (Lond). 2011;35(Suppl 1):S3–15.

Ahrens W, Siani A, Adan R, De Henauw S, Eiben G, Gwozdz W, I.Family consortium, et al. Cohort profile: the transition from childhood to adolescence in European children – how I. Family extends the IDEFICS cohort. Int J Epidemiol. 2017;46(5):1394–5j.

Anliker JA, Bartoshuk L, Ferris AM, Hooks LD. Children's food preferences and genetic sensitivity to the bitter taste of 6-n-propylthiouracil (PROP). Am J Clin Nutr. 1991;54(2):316–20.

ASTM. Standard guide for sensory evaluation of products by children and minors. Designation: E2299 – 13. West Conshohocken, PA: ASTM; 2013.

Azadbakht L, Esmaillzadeh A. Fast foods and risk of chronic diseases. JRMS. 2008;13(1):1–2.

Bartoshuk LM, Duffy VB, Green BG, Hoffman HJ, Ko CW, Lucchina LA, et al. Valid across-group comparisons with labeled scales: the gLMS versus magnitude matching. Physiol Behav. 2004;82(1):109–14.

Bellisle F. Glutamate and the UMAMI taste: sensory, metabolic, nutritional and behavioural considerations. A review of the literature published in the last 10 years. Neurosci Biobehav Rev. 1999;23(3):423–38.

Deglaire A, Méjean C, Castetbon K, Kesse-Guyot E, Urbano C, Hercberg S, et al. Development of a questionnaire to assay recalled liking for salt, sweet and fat. Food Qual Prefer. 2012;23 (2):110–24.

Doty RL, Shah M. Taste and smell. In: Marshall MH, Janette BB, editors. Encyclopedia of infant and early childhood development. San Diego: Academic Press; 2008. p. 299–308.

Duffy VB, Hayes JE, Sullivan BS, Faghri P. Surveying food and beverage liking: a tool for epidemiological studies to connect chemosensation with health outcomes. Ann N Y Acad Sci. 2009;1170:558–68.

Glanville EV, Kaplan AR, Fischer R. Age, sex, and taste sensitivity. J Gerontol. 1964;19(4):474–8.

Green BG, Dalton P, Cowart B, Shaffer G, Rankin K, Higgins J. Evaluating the 'Labeled Magnitude Scale' for measuring sensations of taste and smell. Chem Senses. 1996;21(3): 323–34.

Guinard JX. Sensory and consumer testing with children. Trends Food Sci Technol. 2001;11: 273–83.

He K, Zhao LC, Daviglus ML, Dyer AR, Van Horn L, Garside D, et al. Association of monosodium glutamate intake with overweight in Chinese adults: the INTERMAP study. Obesity. 2008;16(8):1875–80.

James CE, Laing DG, Oram N. A comparison of the ability of 8-9-year-old children and adults to detect taste stimuli. Physiol Behav. 1997;62(1):193–7.

Jilani HS, Intemann T, Bogl LH, Eiben G, Molnar D, Moreno LA, I.Family consortium, et al. Familial aggregation and socio-demographic correlates of taste preferences in European children. BMC Nutrition. 2017;3:87.

Kimmel S, Sigman-Grant MJ, Guinard JX. Sensory testing with young children. Food Technol. 1994;48:92–9.

Knof K, Lanfer A, Bildstein MO, Buchecker K, Hilz H, IDEFICS consortium. Development of a method to measure sensory perception in children at the European level. Int J Obes (Lond). 2011;35(Suppl 1):S131–6.

Kroll BJ. Evaluating rating scales for sensory testing with children. Food Technol. 1990;44:78–86.

Landis JR, Koch GG. The measurement of observer agreement for categorial data. Biometrics. 1977;33(1):159–74.

Lanfer A, Knof K, Barba G, Veidebaum T, Papoutsou S, De Henauw S, IDEFICS consortium, et al. Taste preferences in association with dietary habits and weight status in European children: results from the IDEFICS study. Int J Obes (Lond). 2012;36(1):27–34.

Lanfer A, Bammann K, Knof K, Buchecker K, Russo P, Veidebaum T, et al. Predictors and correlates of taste preferences in European children: the IDEFICS study. Food Qual Prefer. 2013;27(2):128–36.

Léon F, Couronne T, Marcuz MC, Köster EP. Measuring food liking in children: a comparison of non verbal methods. Food Qual Prefer. 1999;10(2):93–100.

Liem DG, Mars M, de Graaf C. Consistency of sensory testing with 4- and 5-year-old children. Food Qual Prefer. 2004;15(6):541–8.

Linschoten MR, Harvey LO, Eller PM, Jafek BW. Fast and accurate measurement of taste and smell thresholds using a maximum-likelihood adaptive staircase procedure. Percept Psychophys. 2001;63(8):1330–47.

Lissner L, Lanfer A, Gwozdz W, Olafsdottir S, Eiben G, Moreno LA, et al. Television habits in relation to overweight, diet and taste preferences in European children: the IDEFICS study. Eur J Epidemiol. 2012;27(9):705–15.

Mennella JA, Finkbeiner S, Reed DR. The proof is in the pudding: children prefer lower fat but higher sugar than do mothers. Int J Obes (Lond). 2012;36(10):1285–91.

Popper R, Kroll JJ. Conducting sensory research with children. J Sens Stud. 2005;20(1):75–87.

Plattig KH. The sense of taste. In: Piggot JR, editor. Sensory analysis of foods. New York: Elsevier; 1984. p. 1–22.

Pfaffmann C, Bartoshuk LM, McBurney DH. Taste psychophysics. In: Beidler LM, editor. Handbook of sensory physiology. New York: Springer; 1971. p. 75–101.

Rogers PJ, Blundell JE. Umami and appetite: effects of monosodium glutamate on hunger and food intake in human subjects. Physiol Behav. 1990;48(6):801–4.

Snyder DJ, Bartoshuk LM. Epidemiological studies of taste function: discussion and perspectives. Ann N Y Acad Sci. 2009;1170:574–80.

Sorensen LB, Moller P, Flint A, Martens M, Raben A. Effect of sensory perception of foods on appetite and food intake: a review of studies on humans. Int J Obes Relat Metab Disord. 2003;27(10):1152–66.

Suling M, Hebestreit A, Peplies J, Bammann K, Nappo A, Eiben G, IDEFICS consortium, et al. Design and results of the pretest of the IDEFICS study. Int J Obes (Lond). 2011;35(Suppl 1): S30–44.

Vereecken C, Covents M, Parmentier J, Maes L. Test-retest reliability and agreement between children's and parents' reports of a computerized food preferences tool. Public Health Nutr. 2013;16(1):8–14.

Zandstra EH, de Graaf C. Sensory perception and pleasantness of orange beverages from childhood to old age. Food Qual Prefer. 1998;9(1–2):5–12.

Chapter 13
Physical Fitness

Mirko Brandes, Germán Vicente-Rodríguez, Marc Suling,
Yannis Pitsiladis and Karin Bammann

Abstract Previous research indicates growing evidence that physical fitness is a powerful marker for individual health perspectives. Therefore, the IDEFICS and I. Family studies included measures of physical fitness and aimed to explore the relationship of physical fitness to youth health. However, given the complex structure of individuals' physical fitness, relevant test items had to be chosen wisely. In this chapter, we will introduce the complex construct of human physical fitness and its components, and briefly describe selected test batteries available for the assessment of physical fitness in youth. Afterwards, we will describe the test battery applied in the IDEFICS and I.Family studies in detail, which is a combined test battery of EUROFIT items, the backsaver sit and reach test, and the 20-m shuttle run. The protocol was well accepted by the children in the IDEFICS study and fitted to the small amount of time provided for the assessment of physical fitness. In I.Family, only handgrip strength was measured as a strong predictor for general health. The fitness measures of both studies contributed to the valuable database that is now available for analysis.

On behalf of the IDEFICS and I.Family consortia

M. Brandes (✉) · M. Suling · K. Bammann
Leibniz Institute for Prevention Research and Epidemiology—BIPS,
Bremen, Germany
e-mail: brandes@leibniz-bips.de

G. Vicente-Rodríguez
GENUD (Growth, Exercise, Nutrition and Development) Research Group,
University of Zaragoza, Zaragoza, Spain

G. Vicente-Rodríguez
Department of Public Health, Ghent University, Ghent, Belgium

Y. Pitsiladis
University of Brighton, Eastbourne, UK

K. Bammann
Working Group Epidemiology of Demographic Change,
Institute for Public Health and Nursing Research (IPP),
University of Bremen, Bremen, Germany

© Springer Nature Switzerland AG 2019
K. Bammann et al. (eds.), *Instruments for Health Surveys in Children
and Adolescents*, Springer Series on Epidemiology and Public Health,
https://doi.org/10.1007/978-3-319-98857-3_13

277

13.1 Physical Fitness

13.1.1 Rationale and Definition

There exists no unique and clear definition of physical fitness although efforts have been undertaken for long to find one. Already Caspersen et al. (1985) saw the need of a standardised terminology to obtain comparable results and to gain a better understanding of the relation between physical fitness, physical activity, exercise and health. In contrast to physical activity (see Chap. 7, of this book) that seeks to survey the type, duration, frequency and intensity of an activity carried out as a process, physical fitness measures a status that is rather stable over a certain period of time. Physical activity and physical fitness are weakly associated (Martínez Vizcaíno et al. 2008). This weak association may be explained by the fact that the validity and reliability of the measurements vary strongly between physical activity and physical fitness (see Martínez Vizcaíno et al. 2008). Moreover, physical fitness is supposed to be primarily determined by physical activity, but is also influenced by non-modifiable factors such as age, sex and genotype, as well as by modifiable factors such as smoking, obesity and medication (Lee et al. 2010). Consequently, physical fitness and physical activity were measured independently in the IDEFICS (Ahrens et al. 2011) and I.Family (Ahrens et al. 2017) studies.

One well-accepted definition of physical fitness is given in the glossary of the Report of the Surgeon General on Physical Activity and Health (US Department of Health and Human Services 1996), which goes back to Caspersen et al. (1985). It defines physical fitness as "a set of attributes that people have or achieve that relates to the ability to perform physical activity." The Report of the Surgeon General explicates physical fitness as the "ability to carry out daily tasks with vigour and alertness, without undue fatigue, and with ample energy to enjoy leisure-time pursuits and to meet unforeseen emergencies," which follows the idea of Clarke (1971) as presented in the first issue of the Physical Fitness Research Digest. This annotation uses an undetermined wording, e.g. the measurement of undue fatigue, and therefore it is not very stringent.

In the 1990s, two consensus conferences have been held with the intent to find a standardised terminology and understanding of physical fitness, activity and health (Bouchard et al. 1990, 1994). In the latter reference, physical fitness is understood as a composition of morphological fitness, bone strength, muscular fitness, flexibility, motor fitness, cardiovascular fitness and metabolic fitness.

Recent efforts to standardise the terminology refrain from claiming to give the one and only definition but rather give one "definition that is consistent with experts" (Corbin et al. 2000). Corbin et al. (2000) thus present the following Table 13.1 describing the aspects of physical fitness and its multi-dimensional hierarchical nature which will be discussed in more detail in the following section.

Skill- or performance-related fitness is typically associated with those fitness aspects that vary with a sport activity (e.g. distance running vs. weightlifting), i.e. that are necessary for a good sports performance, whereas health-related fitness comprises the components that are closely related to health (Howley 2001). Performance-related fitness is sometimes termed motor fitness. Obviously, health- and skill-related fitness aspects interact strongly and a general motor ability is required (Vedul-Kjelsås et al. 2012). Physiological fitness components are related to biological systems that are influenced by one's level of habitual physical activity and do not measure performance (Bouchard et al. 1990; Corbin et al. 2000).

The classification of body composition as a health-related fitness component is debatable. Bouchard et al. (1994) classify body composition as a morphological fitness aspect as this covers body composition factors such as body circumferences, body fat content and regional body fat distribution whereas, e.g. Howley (2001) or Caspersen et al. (1985) categorise it as a health-related fitness component which is more common today.

However, the most recent position stand of the American College of Sports Medicine (ACSM) still follows the approach to find an expert consent and describes physical fitness as a "physiological state of well-being and that reduces the risk of hypokinetic disease, a basis for participation in sports and good health, which enables one to complete task of daily living. Components include cardiorespiratory endurance, muscle strength endurance, flexibility and body composition" (Donnelly et al. 2016). These rather broad definitions implicate a careful decision on what measures of physical fitness are included in study protocols, in particular, when children and adolescents are studied which is the case in the IDEFICS and I.Family studies. Consequently, the assessment of physical fitness in both studies is based on reference standards following the complex construct of physical fitness (De Miguel-Etayo et al. 2014).

Table 13.1 Components describing physical fitness. Adapted from Corbin et al. (2000)

Physical fitness components		
Health-related	Skill-related	Physiological
Body composition	Agility	Metabolic fitness
Cardiovascular fitness	Balance	Morphological fitness
Flexibility	Coordination	Bone integrity
Muscular endurance	Power	Other
Muscular strength	Speed	
	Reaction time	
	Other	

13.1.2 Physical Fitness Components

This section describes briefly the components used above to assess the term of physical fitness. It is based on the glossary from the Report of the Surgeon General (US Department of Health and Human Services 1996) and the review by Corbin et al. (2000).

Health-related fitness components:

- *Body composition* describes the relative amounts of the body components. These include muscle, fat, bone and other vital body parts (see also Chap. 3 of this book).
- *Cardiovascular fitness, cardiorespiratory fitness and cardiorespiratory endurance* are often used synonymously in the literature. They describe the ability of the circulatory and respiratory systems to supply oxygen when being sustainably physical active.
- *Flexibility* describes the range of motion available at a joint.
- *Muscular endurance* covers the ability of the muscle to continue to perform without fatigue.
- *Muscular strength* describes the ability of the muscle to exert force.

Skill-related fitness components:

- *Agility* describes the ability to rapidly change the position of the entire body in space with speed and accuracy.
- *Balance* describes the ability to maintain equilibrium while stationary or moving.
- *Coordination* describes the ability to use the senses, such as sight and hearing, together with body parts in performing motor tasks smoothly and accurately.
- *Power* is the rate at which one can perform work.
- *Speed* is the ability to perform a movement within a short period of time.
- *Reaction time* covers the time elapsed between stimulation and the beginning of the reaction to it.

Physiological fitness components:

- *Metabolic fitness* describes the state of metabolic systems and variables that can be altered by an increased physical activity or regular endurance exercise without the requirement of a training-related increase of maximal oxygen uptake (VO_2 max). This includes blood sugar levels, blood lipid levels and blood hormone levels (Corbin et al. 2000).
- *Morphological fitness* describes fitness that is related to body composition, e.g. body fat content and distribution, waist-to-hip ratio.
- *Bone integrity or bone strength* is described by the area of bone, bone mineral content or density and bone structural properties.

13.2 Importance of Physical Fitness

The most important purpose of physical fitness assessment in children and adolescents is its use as a predictor for later health outcomes. Ortega et al. (2008) give a
detailed review on the association of physical fitness with obesity, cardiovascular
disease, skeletal health, cancer and mental health. They focus on cardiorespiratory
fitness, muscular fitness and speed/agility as physical fitness components. Ortega
et al. (2008) report strong association of obesity and cardiorespiratory fitness levels,
association of cardiovascular risk factors and cardiorespiratory and muscular fitness
and association of skeletal health and muscular fitness and speed/agility.
Cardiorespiratory fitness and muscular fitness support among other compensation
of chemotherapy-induced neuropathy and muscular atrophies of cancer patients. In
addition, association of cardiorespiratory fitness with depression, anxiety mood
status and self-esteem is reported. Ruiz et al. (2009) published a systematic review
that takes additionally into account quality of life and lower back pain. For lower
back pain, no relationship with body composition can be established from the
literature search and inconclusive evidence is available on the relationship of lower
back pain and flexibility.

There is evidence that cardiovascular diseases are determined during childhood,
i.e. risk factors track into adulthood (Raitakari et al. 2003; Andersen et al. 2004;
Högström et al. 2014). As cardiovascular diseases are the most frequent causes of
mortality in the European Union (EU) (Eurostat 2017), the assessment of
health-related fitness components which are risk factors for cardiovascular diseases
is most important (e.g. Ortega et al. 2008; Kvaavik et al. 2009).

However, it should not be forgotten that 3.5 million osteoporotic fractures occur in
Europe every year, representing a substantial and increasing burden on healthcare
systems in many countries (Kanis et al. 2017). Strength and speed are directly related
to bone quality (Vicente-Rodriguez 2006). These fitness components can be enhanced
by intervention, e.g. training, and prevention (e.g. Ruiz et al. 2009) and the promotion
of a healthy lifestyle beginning during childhood is crucial (Terre 2008).

At the same time, it must be recognised that the genetic background and social
factors largely determine physical fitness in children. Therefore, the modification of
individual and social determinants of physical activity must be in the focus, even if this
will not affect the level of physical fitness directly (Martínez Vizcaíno et al. 2008).

Moreover, surveying physical fitness of children offers the opportunity to
monitor children's health and the efficacy of prevention programmes (Ortega et al.
2008; Finger et al. 2014).

13.3 Measurement of Physical Fitness Components

The following section discusses the measurement of physical fitness components.
We will focus on components that were included in the IDEFICS and I.Family
studies (see Sect. 13.4). The measurement of health-related fitness aspects is highly

developed as physiological dimensions are studied where these measurements can be obtained most exactly in a laboratory setting. However, laboratory methods typically require expensive equipment and are personnel intensive. They are therefore not feasible in large-scale population-based studies where appropriate surrogate measures have to be used instead. In contrast to physiological dimensions, laboratory methods to measure skills like balance or agility are rare. Hence, valid field methods have to be used and strict protocols for studies, General Survey Manuals (for access see Sect. 13.6) were worked out that provide detailed protocols for all examinations to be followed by trained field staff.

Cardiovascular endurance describes an individual's aerobic capacity, e.g. the ability to supply oxygen to the working muscles during an activity (Morrow et al. 2000). It is captured best by the maximal oxygen consumption (VO_2 max) that is measured during an exhaustive exercise. In a laboratory setting, an exercise is conducted, e.g. on a treadmill, cycloergometer or a step-bench and the expired gases are monitored, i.e. by a gas analysis system, to determine the maximum exhaustion reached. When laboratory testing is not feasible, e.g. in large epidemiological studies, field methods have to be applied. These methods aim to estimate the maximal oxygen consumption from other parameters as Morrow et al. (2000) report: From a step test, for example, VO_2 max can be estimated by assessing the heart rate after exercise and the one-minute recovery heart rate, and exploiting the linear relationship between workload, heart rate and VO_2 max. The Rockport one-mile walk test accounts for sex, weight, age and ending heart rate to obtain a valid VO_2 max estimate. The 20 m shuttle run test (also known as the beep test) measures how often running between two lines 20 m apart in time to recorded beeps (in an increasing frequency) is accomplished. It can be performed by children and has a longstanding history (e.g. Tomkinson et al. 2003). The recorded shuttles are transformed to VO_2 max values (e.g. Leger and Lambert 1982) or used as a score without transformation. Lang and colleagues demonstrate that the 20-m shuttle run test is a very useful and powerful indicator for population health in children and youth (Lang et al. 2018).

The gold standard to assess flexibility in a laboratory setting is radiography, although feasibility is limited due to radiation (Miller 1985). A flexometer allows direct assessment of the possible range of motion. Alternatively, the sit and reach test which specifically measures the flexibility of the hip back (mainly lower back) and hamstring muscles, by measuring how far forward an individual is able to bend, can be applied. The backsaver sit and reach test, a modified version, measures the flexibility of the right and left leg separately (Chillon et al. 2010). It can be easily accomplished by children. When analysing results, it should be borne in mind that a limitation of this procedure is that people with long arms and/or short legs would get a better result.

Muscular strength and endurance can be measured in a laboratory setting with the help of computerised dynamometers, which track force, work, torque and power generated throughout a range of motion. Controlling the speed of the movement can be realised by isokinetic dynamometers. Strength is defined as the peak force measurement whereas endurance is captured by fatigue rates in force production during a set of repetitions (Morrow et al. 2000). Field methods focus on particular muscle groups, e.g. the upper or lower body. Muscular endurance is typically assessed by counting the number of pull-up, push-ups or sit-ups an individual can accomplish which is not feasible for small children. Therefore, muscular strength instead of muscular endurance is measured to describe the muscular fitness of a child. The force that is generated by a contracting muscle can be measured with a cable tensiometer in a laboratory setting. A field method that provides equivalent information is a one-repetition maximum test. For example, weights for weightlifting or the bench press are increased such that the individual is able to perform one repetition only. Muscular isometric strength of children can be easily assessed using dynamometers; i.e. handgrip. The dynamic strength of the lower extremities can be measured withstanding broad jump or vertical jump tests. In both cases, the leg power can be calculated by the distance that was overcome, which can be transformed into Watts (e.g. Sayers et al. 1999).

Balance as one important skill-related fitness aspect can be measured either static or dynamic; that is the ability to maintain equilibrium when stationary, respectively, when moving. A laboratory method to assess balance is computerised dynamic posturography. Force plates or similar devices are used to measure ground reaction forces. From these ground reaction forces, among others, centre of pressure, dis placements, sway of the centre of mass, equilibrium score, postural stability index (PSI) can be computed (for a review of methods see Chaudhry et al. 2011). The measurement obtained by performing a Flamingo or other balance tests is the time an individual can maintain static equilibrium on one leg. Protocols describe when equilibrium is lost, e.g. the supporting foot moves in any direction or the non-supporting foot touches the ground. It can easily be accomplished by children.

Agility is the ability to move quickly and to change directions while maintaining control and balance. It therefore has an important speed component. There exists no laboratory method to assess agility. A common field method that can be accomplished by children is a modified shuttle run (e.g. Ortega et al. 2008). The time elapsed while running as quickly as the individual can between two markers covers the speed aspect, the pick-up and dropping off an item cover the control and balance aspect. This method can be performed in groups. Protocols describe the exact distance between markers and the numbers of shuttles to be completed.

Table 13.2, an adaption and extension of the table presented in Caspersen et al. (1985), summarises the measurements that have been discussed in detail. Wood (2008) provides online an extensive list of fitness tests.

According to Castro-Piñero et al. (2010), the following conclusions on the validity of the field methods can be drawn:

1. The 20m shuttle run test is most appropriate to assess cardiorespiratory fitness. Equations by Barnett (1993, equation (b)) and Ruiz et al. (2008) yield best VO_2 max estimates.
2. The backsaver sit and reach test has moderate validity to assess hamstring and low back flexibility.

Table 13.2 Field and laboratory methods to assess aspects of physical fitness (Morrow et al. 2000)

Fitness aspect	Outcome	Laboratory method	Examples of field methods
Cardiovascular fitness	Maximum oxygen uptake	Monitoring of expired gas during treadmill, etc. exercise	Distance run, step test, 20-m shuttle run
Flexibility	Range of motion of a joint or group of joints	Radiography	Flexometer, sit and reach test
Muscular endurance	Amount of performed work, either relative or absolute (i.e. repetitive performance at a fixed resistance)	Computerised dynamometer	Pull-ups, push-ups, sit-ups
Muscular strength, power	Maximal force generated by the contracting musculature	Computerised dynamometer	1-repetition maximum test, handgrip strength test, standing broad jump, vertical jump test
Balance	Centre of pressure, displacements	Computerised dynamic posturography	Flamingo balance test, stork balance stand test
Speed, agility	Time		Sprint, shuttle run

3. The handgrip strength test with an extended elbow and adapted grip span is a valid test to assess upper body maximal strength. Due to the small number of studies available in the literature, there is limited evidence that the standing broad jump can assess explosive leg power validly.

Field methods for fitness testing often lack validity and reliability and further research is needed here (e.g. Ortega et al. 2008 and above).

13.4 Assessment of Physical Fitness in the IDEFICS and I.Family Studies

A number of physical fitness test batteries have been developed over the last four decades where the most popular test batteries that are applicable to children and/or adolescents are compared in the following. Table 13.3 covers the FitnessGram (Plowman and Meredith 2013), EUROFIT (Adam et al. 1988), the International Physical Fitness Test (Rosandich 2008) and the Movement Assessment Battery for Children (M-ABC, Henderson et al. 2007). Castro-Piñero et al. (2010) provide a systematic review on the criterion-related validity of existing field-based fitness tests used in children and adolescents, including components of FitnessGram, EUROFIT and the IPTF.

Table 13.3 Comparison of selected fitness test batteries for children and adolescents

Test	Age group	Aim	Items
FitnessGram (Plowman and Meredith 2013)	Kindergarten to college age (5–21 years)	Promotion of regular physical activity among all youth, particularly activity patterns that lead to reduced health risk and improved health-related physical fitness	Six tasks Aerobic capacity Body composition Muscular strength, endurance Flexibility
EUROFIT (Adam et al. 1988)	School age (6+ years)	Tracking of physical fitness	Ten tasks Anthropometry Balance Speed, agility Flexibility Muscular strength, endurance Cardiorespiratory endurance
International Physical Fitness Test (Rosandich 2008)	9–19 years	Tracking of physical fitness, based on norms collected on Arab youth	Six tasks Anthropometry Muscular strength, endurance Cardiorespiratory endurance Speed, agility
Movement Assessment Battery for Children-2 (M-ABC) (Henderson et al. 2007)	3–16 years	Assessment of children's motor skills dis-abilities and determination of intervention strategies	Eight tasks Manual dexterity Ball skills Static/dynamic balance

Obviously, all tests differ in the age groups they address and the exercises to be conducted. Only the M-ABC is suitable for the whole age range surveyed in the IDEFICS study but has a strong focus on motor abilities. It was therefore decided to use a modified EUROFIT test because the EUROFIT test offers a sound assessment of most physical fitness aspects. Furthermore, single to all items of the EUROFIT tests are widely used in other European studies investigating aspects of physical fitness and health, for example, in Spain (Fonseca Del Pozo et al. 2017) and Greece (Arnaoutis et al. 2018) which allows comparability of results. The following tests were included in the IDEFICS protocol:

1. Flamingo balance test
2. Backsaver sit and reach

3. Handgrip strength
4. Standing broad jump
5. 40-m sprint
6. 20-m shuttle run test

The reasons for using a shortened EUROFIT version were the limited time that was available for single measurements to not further increase the burden for the participating children, in particular, since the assessment of physical fitness was not the major focus of the IDEFICS study. Furthermore, only children 6 years and older were asked to participate in the physical fitness assessment. At a younger age, children are not able to understand and conduct some of the requested exercises correctly. The pre-test showed that children at kindergarten age were not able to complete the requested exercises in reasonable time (Suling et al. 2011). Only the handgrip item was continued in I.Family because it required the least amount of time and effort. Moreover, muscular strength has shown to be a valid and feasible predictor of all-cause mortality (Garcia-Hermoso et al. 2018) and is positively associated with blood pressure in youth (Zhang et al. 2018).

13.5 Practical Aspects When Assessing Children's Fitness

Several recommendations can be given based on the experiences the field staff gained from the fitness tests, by this expanding the findings of the pre-tests published previously (Suling et al. 2011). In general, the children who participated in the IDEFICS study enjoyed the fitness tests, in particular, the 20-m shuttle run test. Some test items, such as the Flamingo balance test, were easy and quick to apply, whereas sufficient space was crucial to conduct the 20-m shuttle run test and the 40-m sprint test. It would be therefore highly recommendable to use a whole gym, if available, such that clearly defined stations are available for each test item.

Especially for the 20-m shuttle run test, ensuring maximal exhaustion is mandatory. From our practical experiences, we cannot recommend to have each child run the test individually. Instead, we highly recommend (a) to let the children run in groups of 5–10 children, each child on a separate track, and (b) to have an experienced pacemaker from the study team, running on a separate track alongside. Thus, it is possible to measure many children simultaneously, ensure a sound implementation of the test protocol and ensure maximum exhaustion of the children.

13.6 Provision of Instruments and Standard Operating Procedures to Third Parties

All standard operating procedures (SOPs) described in this chapter are provided by the General Survey Manuals that can be accessed on the following website: www.leibniz-bips.de/ifhs after registration.

Each third partner using the SOPs provided in this chapter is kindly requested to cite this chapter as follows:

Brandes M, Vicente-Rodríguez G, Suling M, Pitsiladis Y, Bammann K, on behalf of the IDEFICS and I.Family consortia. Physical fitness. In: Bammann K, Lissner L, Pigeot I, Ahrens W, editors. Instruments for health surveys in children and adolescents. Cham: Springer Nature Switzerland; 2019. p. 277–289.

Acknowledgements The development of instruments, the baseline data collection and the first follow-up work as part of the IDEFICS study (www.idefics.eu) were financially supported by the European Commission within the Sixth RTD Framework Programme Contract No. 016181 (FOOD). The most recent follow-up including the development of new instruments and the adaptation of previously used instruments was conducted in the framework of the I.Family study (www.ifamilystudy.eu) which was funded by the European Commission within the Seventh RTD Framework Programme Contract No. 266044 (KBBE 2010-14).

We thank all families for participating in the extensive examinations of the IDEFICS and I. Family studies. We are also grateful for the support from school boards, headmasters and communities.

References

Adam C, Klissouras V, Ravazzolo M, Renson R, Tuxworth W. EUROFIT: European test of physical fitness. Rome, Italy: Council of Europe, Committee for Development of Sport; 1988.

Ahrens W, Bammann K, Siani A, Buchecker K, De Henauw S, Iacoviello L, et al. IDEFICS consortium. The IDEFICS cohort: design, characteristics and participation in the baseline survey. Int J Obes (Lond). 2011;35(Suppl 1):S3–15.

Ahrens W, Siani A, Adan R, De Henauw S, Eiben G, Gwozdz W, et al. I.Family consortium. Cohort profile: the transition from childhood to adolescence in European children—how I. Family extends the IDEFICS cohort. Int J Epidemiol. 2017;46(5):1394–1395j.

Andersen LB, Hasselstrøm H, Grønfeldt V, Hansen SE, Karsten F. The relationship between physical fitness and clustered risk, and tracking of clustered risk from adolescence to young adulthood: eight years follow-up in the Danish Youth and Sport Study. Int J Behav Nutr Phys Act. 2004;1(1):6.

Arnaoutis G, Georgoulis M, Psarra G, Milkonidou A, Panagiotakos DB, Kyriakou D, et al. Association of anthropometric and lifestyle parameters with fitness levels in Greek schoolchildren: results from the EYZHN program. Front Nutr. 2018;5:10.

Barnett A, Chan L, Bruce I. A preliminary study of the 20-m multistage shuttle run as a predictor of peak VO2 in Hong Kong Chinese students. Pediatr Exerc Sci. 1993;5(1):42–50.

Bouchard C, Shephard RJ, Stephens T, editors. Exercise, fitness, and health: a consensus of current knowledge. Champaign, IL: Human Kinetics Books; 1990.

Bouchard C, Shephard RJ, Stephens T, editors. Physical activity, fitness, and health: international proceedings and consensus statement. Champaign, IL: Human Kinetics Books; 1994.

Caspersen CJ, Powell KE, Christenson GM. Physical activity, exercise, and physical fitness: definitions and distinctions for health-related research. Public Health Rep. 1985;100(2):126–31.

Castro-Piñero J, Artero EG, España-Romero V, Ortega FB, Sjöström M, Suni J, et al. Criterion-related validity of field-based fitness tests in youth: a systematic review. Br J Sports Med. 2010;44(13):934–43.

Chaudhry H, Bukiet B, Ji Z, Findley T. Measurement of balance in computer posture-graphy: comparison of methods. A brief review. J Bodyw Mov Ther. 2011;15(1):82–91.

Chillon P, Castro-Piñero J, Ruiz JR, Soto VM, Carbonell-Baeza A, Dafos J. Hip flexibility is the main determinant of the back-saver sit-and-reach test in adolescents. J Sports Sci. 2010;28(6): 641–8.

Clarke H. Basic understanding of physical fitness. President's Counc Phys Fitness Sports: Phys Fitness Res Digest. 1971;1:1.

Corbin CB, Pangrazi RP, Franks BD. Definitions: health, fitness and physical activity. President's Counc Phys Fitness Sports Res Digest. 2000;3:9.

De Miguel-Etayo P, Gracia-Marco L, Ortega FB, Intemann T, Foraita R, Lissner L, et al. IDEFICS consortium. Physical fitness reference standards in European children: the IDEFICS study. Int J Obes (Lond). 2014;38(Suppl 2):S57–66.

Donnelly JE, Hillman CH, Castelli D, Etnier JL, Lee S, Tomporowski P, et al. Physical activity, fitness, cognitive function, and academic achievement in children: a systematic review. Med Sci Sports Exerc. 2016;46(6):1197–222.

Eurostat (European Commission), editor. Eurostat regional yearbook 2017. Louxembourg: Publications Office of the European Union; 2017. https://doi.org/10.2785/257716.

Finger JD, Mensink GBM, Banzer W, Lampert T, Tylleskär T. Physical activity, aerobic fitness and parental socio-economic position among adolescents: the German Health Interview and Examination Survey for Children and Adolescents 2003–2006 (KiGGS). Int J Behav Nutr Phys Act. 2014;11:43.

Fonseca Del Pozo FJ, Alsono JV, Alvarez MV, Orr S, Cantarero FJL. Physical fitness as an indicator of health status and its relationship to academic performance during the prepubertal period. Health Promot Perspect. 2017;4:196–204.

Garcia-Hermoso A, Cavero-Redondo I, Ramírez-Vélez R, Ruiz J, Ortega FB Lee DC, et al. Muscular strength as a predictor of all-cause mortality in apparently healthy population: a systematic review and meta-analysis of data from approximately 2 million men and women. Arch Phys Med Rehabil. 2018. [Epub ahead of print]. https://doi.org/10.1016/j.apmr.2018.01. 008.

Henderson SE, Sugden DA, Barnett AL. Movement assessment battery for children—2 Examiner's manual. London: Harcourt Assessment; 2007.

Högström G, Nordström A, Nordström P. High aerobic fitness in late adolescence is associated with a reduced risk of myocardial infarction later in life: a nationwide cohort study in men. Eur Heart J. 2014;35(44):3133–40.

Howley ET. Type of activity: resistance, aerobic and leisure versus occupational physical activity. Med Sci Sports Exerc. 2001;33(6 Suppl):S364–9.

Kanis JA, Cooper C, Rizzoli R, Abrahamsen B, al-Daghri NM, Brandi ML, ESCEO, et al. Identification and management of patients at increased risk of osteoporotic fracture: outcomes of an ESCEO expert consensus meeting. Osteoporos Int. 2017;28(7):2023–34.

Kvaavik E, Klepp K-I, Tell GS, Meyer HE, Batty GD. Physical fitness and physical activity at age 13 years as predictors of cardiovascular disease risk factors at ages 15, 25, 33, and 40 years: extended follow-up of the Oslo Youth Study. Pediatrics. 2009;123(1):80–6.

Lang JJ, Belanger K, Poitras V, Janssen I, Tomkinson GR, Tremblay MS. Systematic review of the relationship between 20 m shuttle run performance and health indicators among children and youth. J Sci Med Sport. 2018;21(4):383–97.

Lee DC, Artero EG, Sui X, Blair SN. Mortality trends in the general population: the importance of cardiorespiratory fitness. J Psychopharmacol. 2010;24(4 Suppl):27–35.

Leger LA, Lambert J. A maximal multistage 20-m shuttle run test to predict VO2 max. Eur J Appl Physiol Occup Physiol. 1982;49(1):1–12.

Martínez Vizcaíno V, Salcedo Aguilar F, Franquelo Gutiérrez R, Solera Martínez M, Sánchez López M, Serrano Martínez S, et al. Assessment of an after-school physical activity program to prevent obesity among 9- to 10-year-old children: a cluster randomized trial. Int J Obes (Lond). 2008;32(1):12–22.

Miller P. Assessment of joint motion. In: Rothstein J, editor. Measurement in physical therapy. New York: Churchill Livingstone; 1985.

Morrow JR, Jackson AW, Disch JG, Mood DP. Measurement and evaluation in human performance. 2nd ed. Champaign, IL: Human Kinetics Books; 2000.

Ortega FB, Ruiz JR, Castillo MJ, Sjöström M. Physical fitness in childhood and adolescence: a powerful marker of health. Int J Obes (Lond). 2008;32:1–11.

Plowman SA, Meredith MD, editors. Fitnessgram/Activitygram reference guide. 4th ed. Dallas, TX: The Cooper Institute; 2013.

Raitakari OT, Juonala M, Kähönen M, Taittonen L, Laitinen T, Mäki-Torkko N, et al. Cardiovascular risk factors in childhood and carotid artery intima-media thickness in adulthood: the Cardiovascular Risk in Young Finns study. J Am Med Assoc. 2003;290(17): 2320–2.

Rosandich TP. An international physical fitness test for the Arab world. Sports J. 2008;19.

Ruiz JR, Castro-Piñero J, Artero EG, Ortega FB, Sjöström M, Suni J, et al. Predictive validity of health-related fitness in youth: a systematic review. Br J Sports Med. 2009;43(12):909–23.

Ruiz JR, Ramirez-Lechuga J, Ortega FB, Castro-Piñero J, Benitez JM, Arauzo-Azofra A, et al. Artificial neural network-based equation for estimating VO2max from the 20 m shuttle run test in adolescents. Artif Intell Med. 2008;44(3):233–45.

Sayers SP, Harackiewicz DV, Harman EA, Frykman PN, Rosenstein MT. Cross-validation of three jump power equations. Med Sci Sports Exerc. 1999;31(4):572–7.

Suling M, Hebestreit A, Peplies J, Bammann K, Nappo A, Eiben G, et al. IDEFICS consortium. Design and results of the pretest of the IDEFICS study. Int J Obes (Lond). 2011;35(Suppl 1): S30–44.

Terre L. Behavioral medicine review: promoting healthy lifestyles in pediatric popula-tions. Am J Lifestyle Med. 2008;2(1):37–9.

Tomkinson GR, Léger LA, Olds TS, Cazorla G. Secular trends in the performance of children and adolescents (1980–2000): an analysis of 55 studies of the 20 m shuttle run in 11 countries. Sports Med. 2003;33:285–300.

U.S. Department of Health and Human Services. Physical activity and health: a Report of the Surgeon General. Atlanta, GA: U.S. Department of Health and Human Services, Centers for Disease Control and Prevention, National Center for Chronic Disease Prevention and Health Promotion; 1996.

Vedul-Kjelsås V, Sigmundsson H, Stensdotter AK, Haga M. The relationship between motor competence, physical fitness and self-perception in children. Child Care Health Dev. 2012;38 (3):394–402.

Vicente-Rodríguez G. How does exercise affect bone development during growth? Sports Med. 2006;36(7):561–9.

Wood RJ. Complete guide to fitness testing. 2008. https://www.topendsports.com/testing/. Accessed 04 Apr 2018.

Zhang R, Li C, Liu T, Zheng L, Li S. Handgrip strength and blood pressure in children and adolescents: Evidence from NHANES 2011 to 2014. Am J Hypertens. 2018. [Epub ehead of print]. https://doi.org/10.1093/ajh/hpy032.

Chapter 14
Interview on Kinship and Household

Leonie-Helen Bogl, Jaakko Kaprio, Claudia Brünings-Kuppe,
Lauren Lissner and Wolfgang Ahrens

Abstract As parents transmit their genes to their children and also provide the rearing environment, the family profoundly shapes the development and behaviour of a growing child. In the European I.Family study, we aimed to quantify the degree of familial resemblance in anthropometric measures and indices of obesity, cardio-metabolic risk factors, diet quality, taste preference and indicators of sleep using a pedigree file. Familial resemblance can arise from shared genes and shared environments and in the case of spousal correlations, assortative mating or social homogamy. This chapter explains the instrument used in I.Family to assess household composition and size and to identify biological and non-biological relationships in the household. We describe the design of the kinship interview and the challenges encountered in its implementation.

On behalf of the I.Family consortium

L.-H. Bogl (✉) · C. Brünings-Kuppe · W. Ahrens
Leibniz Institute for Prevention Research and Epidemiology—BIPS,
Bremen, Germany
e-mail: bogl@leibniz-bips.de

L.-H. Bogl · J. Kaprio
Institute for Molecular Medicine (FIMM), University of Helsinki,
Helsinki, Finland

L. Lissner
Section for Epidemiology and Social Medicine (EPSO), Department of Public
Health and Community Medicine, Sahlgrenska Academy,
University of Gothenburg, Gothenburg, Sweden

W. Ahrens
Faculty of Mathematics and Computer Science, University of Bremen,
Bremen, Germany

© Springer Nature Switzerland AG 2019
K. Bammann et al. (eds.), *Instruments for Health Surveys in Children
and Adolescents*, Springer Series on Epidemiology and Public Health,
https://doi.org/10.1007/978-3-319-98857-3_14

14.1 The Role of the Family in Children's Development

The family is important in the development of children and adolescents. Parents, siblings and other relatives provide the closest personal, social and psychological support to foster the physical and mental development of a young human. Thus, familial influences are seen not only on normal traits, such as growth, eating behaviours and physical activity, but also when these are disturbed as in obesity or sedentary behaviour. Parents influence the development of their children directly through multiple mechanisms such as genetic makeup, parental norms and modelling of parental behaviours and indirectly through choosing neighbourhoods. The role of parents is a major one during infancy and early childhood. Their influence decreases as the child grows up and becomes exposed to other environments like day care, school and peer groups. In adolescence, peer influences play a much greater role, as the child becomes more independent of his or her family.

Family members share social, psychological and economic environments, but only biological relatives are also genetically related. Parents and siblings are considered first-degree relatives, sharing on average 50% of segregating genes (Thomas 2004), while grandparents, aunts and uncles are defined as genetically more distant second-degree relatives. In a pedigree (family tree), various biological and social relationships can be identified. Family members generally resemble each other more on most characteristics including obesity and food intake compared to two unrelated individuals from the same community (Bogl et al. 2017; Chaput et al. 2014). Familial resemblance can be attributed both to material and psycho-social factors in the family and to genetic relatedness of family members. The relative roles of genetic and non-genetic influences for siblings are readily documented using twin studies (Polderman et al. 2015). In order to study the causes and consequences of familial resemblance, information of the family and its constituents needs to be collected and documented. For this purpose, an instrument was created in I.Family based on experiences of the research group and prior literature.

14.2 The Interview

The design of the interview was a challenging task. We had to assess not only the social and the biological relationships within a family but also the composition of the household and—in case that parents were separated—the household(s) to which the child belonged. In addition, the interview had to allow for more than one participating child and for all possible combinations of biological and non-biological relationships between family members living in different households as is often the case in so-called blended families. All these requirements resulted in a complex instrument not suitable for self-completion (for access see Sect. 14.7).

The interview was mainly conducted with one parent or legal guardian using a computer-assisted telephone interviewing (CATI) or computer-assisted personal interviewing (CAPI). In case of technical problems, a paper version was used as a backup for both, face-to-face or telephone interview. A flowchart depicting the branching structure of the instrument to assess family relationships and household composition is shown in Fig. 14.1.

The kinship interview was conducted by contacting the households of the children who already participated in the IDEFICS study. The child who already participated in the IDEFICS study was set as the so-called index child. If a family had multiple children who already participated in the IDEFICS study, the older/oldest child was chosen as the main index child. At the beginning of the interview, a set of questions was asked to inquire information about the relationship of the interviewee to the chosen index child and to ensure that the interview was taking place at the main household, where the child lived 50% or more of the time. If a child lived 50% or more in another household, the phone number of the parent living with that index child in the other household was asked so that this second household could be contacted later as well. If there was another index child living 50% or more in the current (first) household, the interview was restarted for that other index child. If there was no other index child living 50% or more in the household, the interview was continued with the current index child despite the fact that this child lived 50% or less in that household. This was done because it was not certain that the second household where the child lived 50% or more of the time could always be reached. The second household was also contacted, if possible, after completing the interview with the first household.

After the information on the household was inquired, the interviewer asked about the number of children and adults above the age of 18 in the household. The following information was inquired for adults: name, sex, age and the relationship to the chosen index child. This was repeated for as many adults as there were in the household. The interview inquired the following information for children: IDEFICS ID number (for all children who already had participated in the IDEFICS study), the child's birth date, the child's sex, the name of his/her school and the relationship of that child to the chosen index child. The questions were repeated for all children in the household. A final question inquired information on the presence and number of other biological sibling(s) or half-siblings living outside this household. The interviewer assigned one of the following family relationship codes for each individual in the household presented in Table 14.1. Each person was assigned a kinship ID number.

Table 14.2 gives an overview of the household types and the average number of household members in I.Family by the eight countries as assessed by the kinship interview. The most common household type was a child or siblings living with both biological parents (74%). Households in which a child or full siblings lived with only one biological parent comprised 11% of all households, of which 90% were single-mother households. Finally, 14% of the households were blended families, which included various combinations of step-parents, single-parents, half-siblings or other household members. Overall, half- or step-siblings were present in 6% of the households, of which most included half-siblings (5% half-siblings, 1% step-siblings).

Fig. 14.1 Flow chart illustrating the branching structure of the instrument to assess family relationships and household composition

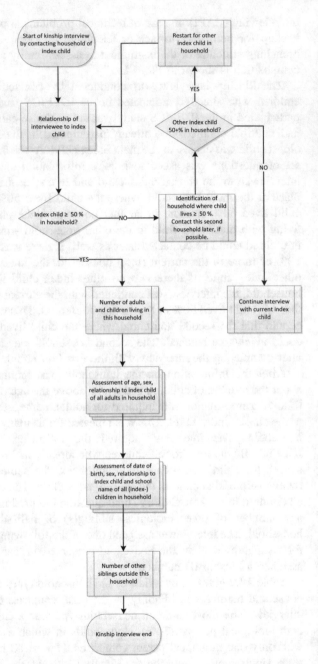

Table 14.1 Assignment of codes to family members with i1 denoting the chosen index child in the household

Code	Person in household
i1	*Chosen index child in household*
01	Biological mother of i1
02	Biological father of i1
03	Biologically unrelated female adult who can be step-mother/adoptive mother/foster mother/new partner of biological mother or father of i1
04	Biologically unrelated male adult who can be step-father/adoptive father/foster father/new partner of biological mother or father of i1
05	Other adult (any relationship, biologically related or unrelated)
11	Biological sibling of i1 (this code has also to be used for siblings who already had participated in the IDEFICS study, i.e. for non-chosen index children)
12	Half-sibling of i1 (same biological mother or same biological father)
13	Non-biological sibling of i1 (e.g. adopted sibling, foster sibling, child of step-father/step-mother unrelated to i1)

Table 14.2 Household types in I.Family by country

Household types		Italy	Estonia	Cyprus	Belgium	Sweden	Germany	Hungary	Spain	All
Households where child(ren) lived with both biological parents[a]	n	844	313	1027	65	427	506	470	254	3906
	%	85.2	60.3	82.1	72.2	77.4	66.9	61.5	75.8	74.3
Households where child(ren) lived with one biological parent[b]	n	51	72	108	11	79	116	116	45	598
	%	5.1	13.9	8.6	12.2	14.3	15.4	15.2	13.4	11.4
All other households[c]	n	96	134	116	14	46	134	178	36	754
	%	9.7	25.8	9.3	15.6	8.3	17.7	23.3	10.8	14.3
Number of household members (mean)	n	4.2	3.9	4.4	4.3	4.1	4.0	3.9	4.0	4.1

Note [a]A two-parent household, where a child lived with both biological parents, either as a single child or with full siblings
[b]A single-parent household, where a child lived with one biological parent, either as a single child or with full siblings
[c]A so-called blended family where a child lived with non-biological parents such as step-parents and/or step- or half-siblings and/or other adults in the household (various combinations possible, and first-degree relatives may also be present)

The interview collected information on all household members; thus, it also included relationship information of non-participants. I.Family aimed to recruit at least one parent and in the case of siblings, at least one sibling of the index children who already had participated in the IDEFICS study. On average, 2.9 out of 4.1

family members living in a household were recruited in I.Family. Although 14.3% of the index children lived in household where non-biologically related relatives or non-first-degree relatives such as step-parents, step- or half siblings or other adults (e.g. aunt/uncle or grandparents) were present, the index children were more likely to participate in I.Family with their first-degree relatives (biological parents and their biological siblings). Thus, out of the participating family members for whom we have data, 97% were first-degree relatives.

Because at the time of the interview, it was not clear yet which household members would participate in the I.Family study, the kinship file included a kinship ID (identification) number for all persons living in the household but not the individual ID number which has been used for all other data in the study. Thus, we had to use three different approaches to merge the individual ID numbers to the kinship data:

1. For the IDEFICS children, the linkage was possible via the IDEFICS ID number.
2. For newly participating children, the family ID number, the sex and the birthdate were used.
3. The age of adult family members was partly reported by other family members. Because this information was considered as less valid than self-reported age, data were merged via the family ID number, the sex and the age allowing for an error range of ±2.5 years.

14.3 Creation of a Pedigree File

A pedigree file that describes the biological and non-biological relationships between individuals in the dataset is typically required by most statistical genetic analysis programs for family data. Siblings can be identified by having common parents. Full siblings will have the same mother and father ID numbers, while half-siblings will only share either the mother or father ID. Although pedigrees can become complex, most commonly only the five following variables are needed to create the pedigree file: a family identifier (family ID number), an identifier for the individual (individual ID number), two parent identifiers (father ID and mother ID numbers) and an indicator of each individual's sex.

A blank parental ID number is commonly used for individuals whose parents are not in the pedigree and this indicates that the individual is a founder. Founders are assumed to be biologically unrelated. Some software requires that either both parents are unknown or both parents are known where knowledge refers to identity and not knowledge about phenotypes or genotypes. In order to correctly identify biological and non-biological relationships in the sample, this may require the creation of fictitious parental ID numbers for individuals who did not participate in the study. As an example of how family relationships may be labelled in a pedigree

Table 14.3 Extract of a pedigree file used in the analysis of biological and non-biological relationships in a family

Family ID number	Individual ID number	Father ID number	Mother ID number	Sex	Phenotype data
FAM001	ID004F			Male	Not available
FAM001	ID005			Female	Available
FAM001	ID006	ID004F	ID005	Male	Available
FAM001	ID007	ID004F	ID005	Female	Available

Note The fictitious ID number (ID004F) was created for the non-participating father

file, Table 14.3 shows a small pedigree consisting of two siblings and their parents, where a fictitious father ID number has been created to indicate that the siblings are full siblings.

14.4 Analysis of Family Data

Family studies are useful to assess whether a trait of interest runs in families. Family resemblance can arise from shared genes and shared environments and in the case of spousal correlations from assortative mating or social homogamy (Thomas 2004). Often the first question to address is whether a specific trait is influenced by genetic differences at all. If a trait is only weakly genetically determined, this may have important implications for gene-finding efforts, and for efforts to influence the trait value through interventions. For quantitative traits, familial correlations can be estimated for pairs of relatives using a covariance-based measure. The degree of resemblance between two family members of the same classes of individuals (e.g. sibling pairs) can be estimated by the intraclass correlation coefficient (ICC) and the degree of resemblance between two family members from different classes of individuals (e.g. parent–offspring) by the interclass correlation coefficient. Higher correlation coefficients imply a stronger familial resemblance.

In I.Family, we calculated intra- and interclass correlations by using the FCOR programme of the Statistical Analysis for Genetic Epidemiology software package (SAGE, version 6.3) (Elston and Gray-McGuire 2004). FCOR calculates multivariate familial correlations with their asymptotic standard errors without assuming multivariate normality of the traits across family members (Keen and Elston 2003). It calculates familial correlations for all relative pair types available in the pedigree file (see Sect. 14.3).

If a trait aggregates in families, the next step is to quantify the contributions of genetic and environmental factors to phenotypic variation. Family and twin studies are widely used to quantify the proportion of phenotypic variance attributable to genetic effects. Twin studies as a unique case of family studies are analysed with complex modelling and variance decomposition methods that are described in detail elsewhere (Neale and Maes 2004). Family studies can include nuclear families (parents and their offspring) or extended pedigrees (grandparents, parents, offspring, cousins, etc.). Heritability from twin or extended family studies refers to the proportion of the total variance in a particular trait that is explained by genetic factors only. It is important to remember that phenotypic data on nuclear families alone do not enable the estimation of the relative contribution of genetic and shared environmental components on phenotypic variation. Family studies that have mainly data only on first-degree relatives can be used to assess only overall "familiality", i.e., the proportion of phenotypic variance attributable to the combined effects of all familial influences (Kendler and Neale 2009). Other common terms for familiality previously used as synonyms in the literature are maximal heritability and transmissibility.

In I.Family, we estimated "familiality" using a maximum-likelihood variance component method implemented in Sequential Oligogenic Linkage Analysis Routines (SOLAR) (Southwest Foundation for Biomedical Research). The variance decomposition method is based on the fact that biologically related relatives share a certain amount of genes identical by descent (IBD) and relatives living in the same household share environmental factors. Thus, the correlations between any pair of relatives depend on their degree of genetic and shared environmental relationships. For example, biological siblings and parents and their offspring share 50% of their segregating genes IBD, while spouse pairs are assumed not to share any genes. All types of relative pairs living in the same household are matched for shared environmental factors, and differences among biologically related family members are attributable to their unique environmental factors. Greater familial resemblance for biological than non-biological siblings or for monozygotic (100% of genetic variation IBD) than dizygotic twins (50% of genetic variation IBD) would thus suggest a genetic contribution to the phenotype.

14.5 Parenting Style in I.Family

In addition to kinship and household structure, the family questionnaire (FQ) (see Chap. 9 of this book) assessed several aspects of parenting style to study influences on diet and other health-related factors. Questions about the family, not specific to one child, were answered by the father or mother. Topics here included description of the family atmosphere, joint activities and rules about media use (Latendresse et al. 2009; Rideout et al. 2010).

In the parental questionnaire (PQ) (see Chap. 9 of this book), mothers and fathers gave their views on parental versus school responsibilities about healthy lifestyles, parental engagement in their children's activities, and authoritarian versus permissive parenting styles were described (questions taken from the respective IDEFICS questionnaires).

In the teen questionnaire (TQ), children 12 years and older reported rules about being out at night (Pearson et al. 2010), and in addition answered "mirror image" questions describing their own perceptions of the family atmosphere, which correspond to those answered by their parents (Latendresse et al. 2009).

14.6 Challenges

Modern family structures can be quite complex as well as dynamic over time. Thus, the design and implementation of the kinship interview was a challenging task. Our experience showed that some aspects of the interview can be further improved, and that the training of the interviewer is very important. We have noticed that some of the interviewers mistakenly assigned the relationship code "i1" for more than one child in a household (despite the instruction to assign the code "i1" only for the oldest index child in case there was more than one index child in the household). This led to the fact that for sibling pairs for which both children were assigned the relationship code "i1", it is not possible to tell whether they are full siblings, half-sibling or non-biological siblings. Furthermore, the relationship code "05" which stands for "Other adult (any relationship, biologically related or unrelated)" was intended for other adults that did not fit into categories "01–04". However, the formulation obviously has led to some confusion among the interviewers and the code "05" was also assigned to some of the step-parents (for which the relationship codes 03 or 04 were intended). Therefore, if the instrument is used in the future, we recommend reformulating the category "05" to "Other adult (any other relationship, for example aunt/uncle or grandparents)". All of the three categories (03–05) comprise adults that are non-first-degree relatives. In I.Family, such family members were excluded from the analysis of familial resemblance since this analysis was restricted to biological parents and full siblings. In other settings, characterisation of second-degree relatives may also be desirable and so the coding would needed to be appropriately modified.

In I.Family, the examination of family members was restricted to those living in the same household as the index child. This limits the possibility of the analyses to distinguish between genetic and non-genetic familial effects. Although a substantial proportion of children did live in blended families, their proportion in the study sample was much smaller because the recruitment of such family members was not a central aim of I.Family. In fact, in case the response proportion was so good that the survey centres needed to decide which children should be included in the study, biological siblings were prioritized over non-biologically related siblings. Studies of first-degree relatives can tell us whether a trait is familial or not, but they cannot disentangle genetic from familial environmental sources of resemblance. It is also important to remember that familial correlations and the relative importance of familial vs. non-familial factors can vary among populations depending on genetic and environmental circumstances. With the advent of molecular genetic techniques and large-scale genotyping, genetic relationships can be confirmed and polygenic risk scores can be used to provide additional information about the actual strength of the relationship for any relative pair with respect to the study trait.

14.7   Provision of Instruments and Standard Operating Procedures to Third Parties

All instruments described in this chapter including the General Survey Manual that provides among other all standard operating procedures can be accessed on the following website: www.leibniz-bips.de/ifhs after registration.

Each third partner using the instruments provided in this chapter is kindly requested to cite this chapter as follows:

Bogl L-H, Kaprio J, Brünings-Kuppe C, Lissner L, Ahrens W, on behalf of the I. Family consortium. Interview on kinship and household. In: Bammann K, Lissner L, Pigeot I, Ahrens W, editors. Instruments for health surveys in children and adolescents. Cham: Springer Nature Switzerland; 2019. p. 291–301.

Acknowledgements The development of instruments, the baseline data collection and the first follow-up work as part of the IDEFICS study (www.idefics.eu) were financially supported by the European Commission within the Sixth RTD Framework Programme Contract No. 016181 (FOOD). The most recent follow-up including the development of new instruments and the adaptation of previously used instruments was conducted in the framework of the I.Family study (www.ifamilystudy.eu) which was funded by the European Commission within the Seventh RTD Framework Programme Contract No. 266044 (KBBE 2010–14).

We thank all families for participating in the extensive examinations of the IDEFICS and I. Family studies. We are also grateful for the support from school boards, headmasters and communities. We greatly appreciate the input provided by Marcus Zaja, Leibniz Institute for Prevention Research and Epidemiology—BIPS, Bremen, Germany.

References

Bogl LH, Silventoinen K, Hebestreit A, Intemann T, Williams G, Michels N, et al. Familial resemblance in dietary intakes of children, adolescents, and parents: Does dietary quality play a role? Nutrients. 2017;9(8).

Chaput JP, Perusse L, Despres JP, Tremblay A, Bouchard C. Findings from the Quebec Family Study on the etiology of obesity: genetics and environmental highlights. Curr Obes Rep. 2014;3:54–66.

Elston RC, Gray-McGuire C. A review of the 'Statistical Analysis for Genetic Epidemiology' (S. A.G.E.) software package. Hum Genomics. 2004;1(6):456–9.

Keen KJ, Elston RC. Robust asymptotic sampling theory for correlations in pedigrees. Stat Med. 2003;22(20):3229–47.

Kendler KS, Neale MC. "Familiality" or heritability. Arch Gen Psychiatry. 2009;66(4):452–3.

Latendresse SJ, Rose RJ, Viken RJ, Pulkkinen L, Kaprio J, Dick DM. Parental socialization and adolescents' alcohol use behaviors: predictive disparities in parents' versus adolescents' perceptions of the parenting environment. J Clin Child Adolesc Psychol. 2009;38(2):232–44.

Neale MC, Maes HHM. Methodology for genetic studies of twins and families. Dordrecht: Kluwer Academic Publisher; 2004.

Pearson N, Atkin AJ, Biddle SJ, Gorely T, Edwardson C. Parenting styles, family structure and adolescent dietary behaviour. Public Health Nutr. 2010;13(8):1245–53.

Polderman TJ, Benyamin B, de Leeuw CA, Sullivan PF, van Bochoven A, Visscher PM, et al. Meta-analysis of the heritability of human traits based on fifty years of twin studies. Nat Genet. 2015;47(7):702–9.

Rideout VJ, Foehr UG, Roberts DF. Generation M2: media in the lives of 8–18 year-olds. In: Kaiser family foundation. 2010. http://www.kff.org/entmedia/upload/8010.pdf. Accessed 29 Mar 2018.

Thomas DC. Statistical methods in genetic epidemiology. New York: Oxford University Press; 2004.

Printed in the United States
By Bookmasters